P9-DUP-350

Handbook of Experimental Pharmacology

Volume 185/I

Wolfhard Semmler • Markus Schwaiger
Editors

Molecular Imaging I

Contributors

S. Aime, G. Antoni, C. Burtea, H. Dahnke, W. Dastrù, L. Vander Elst, S. Foster,
R. Gobetto, P. Hauff, G. Henry, M.S. Judenhofer, M. Kachelrieß, B. Långström,
S. Laurent, K. Licha, M. Lindner, R.N. Muller, C. Pfannenberg, B.J. Pichler,
M. Reinhardt, D. Santelia, T. Schaeffter, R.B. Schulz, W. Semmler, V.C. Spanoudaki,
U. Speck, A. Viale, S.I. Ziegler

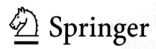 Springer

Prof. Dr. rer. nat. Dr. med. Wolfhard Semmler
Leiter der Abteilung für Medizinische Physik
in der Radiologie (E 020)
Forschungsschwerpunkt Innovative
Krebsdiagnostik und -therapie (E)
Deutsches Krebsforschungszentrum
Im Neuenheimer Feld 280
69120 Heidelberg
Germany
wolfhard.semmler@dkfz.de

Prof. Dr. med. Markus Schwaiger
Nuklearmedizinische Klinik und
Poliklinik
Klinikum rechts des Isar des
Technischen Universität München
Ismaninger Str. 22
81675 München
Germany
markus.schwaiger@tum.de

ISBN 978-3-540-72717-0   e-ISBN 978-3-540-72718-7

Handbook of Experimental Pharmacology ISSN 0171-2004

Library of Congress Control Number: 2007943479

Cover Design: WMXDesign GmbH, Heidelberg

Printed on acid-free paper

9 8 7 6 5 4 3 2 1

springer.com

Foreword

Bayer Schering Pharma welcomes Springer Verlag's endeavor to open its well-known Handbook of Pharmacology to the exciting field of molecular imaging and we are pleased to contribute to the printing costs of this volume.

In principle, noninvasive diagnostic imaging can be divided into morphological/anatomical imaging on the one hand, with CT/MRI the most important imaging technologies, and molecular imaging on the other. In CT/MRI procedures, contrast agents are injected at millimolar blood concentrations, while today's molecular imaging technologies such as PET/SPECT use tracers at nanomolar blood concentrations. Morphological imaging technologies such as X-ray/CT/MRI achieve very high spatial resolution. However, they share the limitation of not being able to detect lesions until the structural changes in the tissue (e.g., caused by cancer growth) are large enough to be seen by the imaging technology. Molecular imaging offers the potential of detecting the molecular and cellular changes caused by the disease process before the lesion (e.g., a tumor) is large enough to cause the kind of structural changes that can be detected by other imaging modalities. On the other hand, molecular imaging methods suffer from a rather poor level of spatial resolution, although current PET machines are better than SPECT devices.

The current diagnostic imaging revolution of fusing conventional diagnostic imaging (CT, MRT) with molecular imaging technologies (PET, SPECT) combines the strength of molecular imaging — i.e., detecting pathophysiological changes at the onset of the disease — with the strength of morphological imaging — i.e., high structural resolution. Today, already more than 95% of new PET scanners installed are PET/CT scanners. PET/CT fusion imaging is currently the fastest-growing imaging technology. And PET/MRI fusion scanners are also on the horizon. The trend toward specialized imaging centers, where all the required equipment is available in one facility, is expected to continue. The former technology-driven focus in diagnostic imaging research looks set to change into a more disease-oriented one.

Fusion imaging will make it possible to detect the occurrence of a disease earlier than is possible today. This is significant, because the likelihood of successful therapeutic interventions increases the earlier diseases are diagnosed. Furthermore, because a disease can be characterized at the molecular level, patients can be stratified for a given therapy and therapeutic responses monitored early on and in a quantitative manner. The growing pressure for selection, early therapy monitoring and justification (outcome) of a specific treatment will have a significant impact on molecular imaging procedures. Hence, molecular imaging technologies are now an integral part of both research and development (early clinical prediction of drug distribution and efficiency) at most pharmaceutical companies.

Bayer Schering Pharma (BSP) has always been a pioneer in the research and development of new imaging agents for "classic" modalities like CT and MRI. In line with this history and BSP's focus on innovation, we are now fully committed to breaking new ground in molecular imaging, especially in research and development of radio-tracers like PET imaging agents.

A strong and active partnership with academia is essential in order to be successful in the exciting new field of molecular imaging. We want to help make innovative imaging solutions invented in university research labs available to the patients. Furthermore, the low doses of "tracers" injected make it possible to perform clinical research studies under the microdosing/exploratory IND regulations. This will help molecular imaging move into the hospital and, hopefully, also generate early and fruitful collaborations between academia, clinic, regulatory authorities and the pharmaceutical industry.

Bayer Schering Pharma, Berlin   *Matthias Bräutigam and Ludger Dinkelborg*

Preface

"Molecular imaging (MI) is the in vivo characterization and measurement of biologic processes on the cellular and molecular level. In contradistinction to 'classical' diagnostic imaging, it sets forth to probe such molecular abnormalities that are the basis of disease rather than to image the end results of these molecular alterations" (Weissleder and Mahmood 2001).[a]

Imaging has witnessed a rapid growth in recent decades. This successful development was primarily driven by impressive technical advances in structural imaging; i.e., fast computer tomography (CT) and magnetic resonance imaging (MRI). In parallel, functional imaging emerged as an important step in the diagnostic and prognostic assessment of patients addressing physiological functions such as organ blood flow, cardiac pump function and neuronal activity using nuclear, magnetic resonance and ultrasonic techniques. More recently the importance of molecular targets for diagnosis and therapy has been recognized and imaging procedures introduced to visualize and quantify these target structures. Based on the hypothesis that molecular imaging provides both a research tool in the laboratory and a translational technology in the clinical arena, considerable funding efforts in the US and Europe were directed to accelerate the development of this imaging technology. In addition, the industry responded to the new demand with the introduction of dedicated imaging equipment for animal research as well as multimodality imaging (PET/CT), used to combine high-resolution imaging with the high sensitivity of tracer techniques.

Molecular imaging has been applied academically in neuroscience with emphasis on cognition, neurotransmission and neurodegeneration. Besides this established area, cardiology and oncology are currently the fastest growing applications. Vascular biology provides new targets to visualize atherosclerotic plaques, which may lead to earlier diagnosis as well as better monitoring of preventive therapies. Labeling of cells allows localization of inflammation or tumors and labeled stem-cell tracking of these cells in vivo. The noninvasive biologic characterization of tumor tissue in animals and humans opens not only exciting new research strategies but also appears

---

[a] Weissleder R, Mahmood U (2001) Molecular imaging. Radiology 219:316–333

promising for personalized management of cancer patients, which may alter the diagnostic and therapeutic processes.

Detection and characterization of lesions, especially tumors, remains challenging, and can be only achieved by using specific tracers and/or contrast media. The past decade has seen the development of specific approaches that use labeled antibodies and fragments thereof. However, in general only a relatively low target-to-background ratio has been attained due to the slow clearance of unbound antibody. Other target-specific approaches include labeled proteins, peptides, oligonucleotides, etc. Due to the low concentration of proteins, such as receptors in the target (e.g., tumors, cells), imaging requires highly sensitive probes addressing these structures. Whereas this challenge does not affect the use of positron emission tomography (PET) nor single photon emission tomography (SPECT) because of their high physical sensitivity, optical imaging methods (OT) as well as magnetic resonance imaging (MRI) have limitations: low penetration depth (OT) and inherent low physical sensitivity (MRI prevents straightforward imaging strategies for both latter modalities). PET and SPECT have been successfully used in the past for molecular imaging, employing imaging probes such as monoclonal antibodies, labeled peptides [i.e., somatostatine analogues (Octreotide)], and labeled proteins such as ^{99m}Tc-AnnexinV, etc. Specific imaging probes for OT and MR are under development. However, OT is likely to remain an experimental tool for investigations in small animals, and will be used in humans only for special indications, where close access to targets can be achieved by special imaging devices such as endoscopy or intraoperative probes. In recent years, molecular imaging with ultrasound devices has developed quickly and the visualization of targeted microbubbles offers not only identification of specific binding but also the regional delivery of therapeutics after local destruction of the bubbles by ultrasound.

Achieving disease-specific imaging requires passive, or better yet, active accumulation of specific molecules to increase the concentration of the imaging agent in the region of interest. Marker substrates as well as reporter agents can be used to visualize enzyme activity, receptor or transporter expression. The introduction of new imaging agents requires a multistep approach, involving the target selection, synthetic chemistry and preclinical testing, before clinical translation can be considered. Target identification is supported by molecular tissue analysis or by screening methods, such as phage display. Subsequently, further development requires methods to synthesize macromolecules, minibodies, nanoparticles, peptide conjugates and other conjugates, employing innovative biotechnology tools for specific imaging with high accumulation in the target area. This process involves optimization of the target affinity and pharmacokinetics before in-vivo application can be considered. Amplification of the imaging signal can be enhanced by targeted processes which involve internalization of receptors, transport mechanisms or enzymatic interaction with build-up of labeled products. (i.e., phosphorylated deoxyglucose). Reporter gene imaging provides not only high biological contrast if a protein, which does not occur naturally, is expressed after gene transfer but also leads to signal amplification if tissue-specific promoters in combination with enzymatic or transporter activity are used.

The development process usually produces numerous candidates, of which only a few pass preclinical evaluation with the promise of clinical utility. The most suitable substances have to undergo in-depth toxicological evaluation before the regulatory process for clinical use can be started. Currently, this is the major rate-limiting step in the process and requires not only the biological qualification of the compound but also the necessary financial support for the clinical testing required by the regulatory agencies.

With the increasing interest in the experimental and clinical application of molecular imaging, many institutions have created research groups or interdisciplinary centers focusing on the complex development processes of this new methodology. The aim for this textbook of molecular imaging is to provide an up-to-date review of this rapidly growing field and to discuss basic methodological aspects necessary for the interpretation of experimental and clinical results. Emphasis is placed on the interplay of imaging technology and probe development, since the physical properties of the imaging approach need to be closely linked with the biological application of the probe (i.e., nanoparticles and microbubbles). Various chemical strategies are discussed and related to the biological applications. Reporter-gene imaging is being addressed not only in experimental protocols but also first clinical applications are discussed. Finally, strategies of imaging to characterize apoptosis and angiogenesis are described and discussed in the context of possible clinical translation.

The editors thank all the authors for their contributions. We appreciate the extra effort preparing a book chapter during the already busy academic life. We hope this methodological discussion will increase the understanding of the reader with respect to established methods and generate new ideas for further improvement and for the design of new research protocols employing imaging. There is no question that this young field will further expand, stimulated by the rapid growth of biological knowledge and biomedical technologies. It is expected that the experimental work of today will become the clinical routine of tomorrow.

Heidelberg, Germany   *Wolfhard Semmler*
Munich, Germany   *Markus Schwaiger*

Contents

Contents of Companion Volume 185/II

Contributors

Silvio Aime
Dipartimento di Chimica I.F.M, Università degli Studi di Torino, V. P. Giuria
7 – 10125 Torino, Italy, silvio.aime@unito.it

Gunnar Antoni
GE Healthcare Uppsala Imanet AB P.O. Box 967 751 09 Uppsala, Sweden,
gunnar.antoni@ge.com

Carmen Burtea
Department of General, Organic and Biomedical Chemistry, NMR and Molecular
Imaging Laboratory, University of Mons-Hainaut, 24, Avenue du Champ de Mars,
7000 Mons, Belgium, carmen.burtea@umh.ac.be

Hannes Dahnke
Philips Research Hamburg, Röntgenstr. 24–26, 22335 Hamburg, Germany,
hannes.dahnke@philips.com

Walter Dastrù
Dipartimento di Chimica I.F.M. – Università degli Studi di Torino; V. P. Giuria
7 – 10125 Torino, Italy, walter.dastru@unito.it

Stuart Foster
Imaging Research, Sunnybrook and Women's Research Institute, Toronto, ON,
Canada, stuart.foster@sunnybrook.ca

Roberto Gobetto
Dipartimento di Chimica I.F.M. – Università degli Studi di Torino; V. P. Giuria
7 – 10125 Torino, Italy, roberto.gobetto@unito.it

Peter Hauff
Global Drug Discovery, Bayer Schering Pharma AG, 13342 Berlin, Germany,
peter.hauff@bayerhealthcare.com

Gavin Henry
Global Drug Discovery, Bayer Schering Pharma, 13342 Berlin, Germany,
gavin.henry@bayerhealthcare.com

Martin S. Judenhofer
Laboratory for Preclinical Imaging and Imaging Technology, University
of Tübingen – Department of Radiology, Röntgenweg 13, 72076 Tübingen, Germany,
martin.judenhofer@med.uni-tuebingen.de

Marc Kachelrieß
Institute of Medical Physics (IMP), Friedrich-Alexander-Universität
Erlangen-Nürnberg, Henkestraße 9, 91052 Erlangen, Germany,
marc.kachelriess@imp.uni-erlangen.de

Bengt Långström
Department of Biochemistry and Organic Chemistry BMC, Uppsala University,
Box 576, 751 23 Uppsala, Sweden
bengt.langstrom@biorg.uu.se

Sophie Laurent
Department of General, Organic and Biomedical Chemistry, NMR and Molecular
Imaging Laboratory, University of Mons-Hainaut, 24, Avenue du Champ de Mars,
7000 Mons, Belgium, sophie.laurent@umh.ac.be

Kai Licha
migenion GmbH, Robert-Koch-Platz 4-8, 10115 Berlin, Germany,
licha@migenion.com

Michael Schirner
migenion GmbH, Robert-Koch-Platz 4-8, 10115 Berlin, Germany,
schirner@migenion.com

Robert N. Muller
Department of General, Organic and Biomedical Chemistry, NMR and Molecular
Imaging Laboratory, University of Mons-Hainaut, 24, Avenue du Champ de Mars,
7000 Mons, Belgium, robert.muller@umh.ac.be

Christina Pfannenberg
Laboratory for Preclinical Imaging and Imaging Technology, University
of Tübingen – Department of Radiology, Röntgenweg 13, 72076 Tübingen, Germany,
christina.pfannenberg@med.uni-tuebingen.de

Bernd J. Pichler
Laboratory for Preclinical Imaging and Imaging Technology, University
of Tübingen – Department of Radiology, Röntgenweg 13, 72076 Tübingen, Germany,
bernd.pichler@med.uni-tuebingen.de

Michael Reinhardt
Global Drug Discovery, Bayer Schering Pharma, 13342 Berlin, Germany,
michael.reinhardt@bayerhealthcare.com

Daniela Santelia
Dipartimento di Chimica I.F.M. – Università degli Studi di Torino; V. P. Giuria
7 – 10125 Torino, Italy, daniela.santelia@unito.it

Tobias Schaeffter
Division of Imaging Sciences, King's College London, The Rayne Institute,
St Thomas' Hospital, London SE1 7EH, UK, tobias.schaeffter@kcl.ac.uk

Ralf Schulz
Helmholtz Zentrum München Institut für Biologische und Medizinische
Bildgebung, Ingolstädter Landstraße 1, 85764 Neuherberg, Germany,
ralf.schulz@helmholtz-muenchen.de

Wolfhard Semmler
Department of Medical Physics in Radiology, German Cancer Research
Center (DKFZ), Im Neuenheimer Feld 280, 69120 Heidelberg, Germany,
wolfhard.semmler@dkfz.de

Virginia C. Spanoudaki
Nuklearmedizinische Klinik und Poliklinik der TU München, Klinikum
rechts der Isar, Ismaninger Str. 22, 81675 München, Germany,
v.spanoudaki@lrz.tu-muenchen.de

Ulrich Speck
Institut für Radiologie, Universitätsklinikum Charité – Humboldt-Universität Schumannstraße 20/21, 10098 Berlin-Mitte, Germany, ulrich.speck@charite.de

Luce Vander Elst
Department of General, Organic and Biomedical Chemistry, NMR and Molecular
Imaging Laboratory, University of Mons-Hainaut, 24, Avenue du Champ de Mars,
7000 Mons, Belgium, luce.vanderelst@umh.ac.be

Alessandra Viale
Dipartimento di Chimica I.F.M. – Università degli Studi di Torino; V. P. Giuria
7 – 10125 Torino, Italy, alessandra.viale@unito.it

Sibylle I. Ziegler
Nuklearmedizinische Klinik und Poliklinik der TU München, Klinikum rechts der
Isar, Ismaninger Str. 22, 81675 München, Germany, sibylle.ziegler@tum.de

Glossary

Definition of the terms used in molecular imaging.

Allele The gene regarded as the carrier of either of a pair of alternative hereditary characters.

$\alpha_v\beta_3$ An integrin expressed by activated endothelial cells or tumor cells which plays an important role in angiogenesis and metastatic tumor spread ($\Rightarrow$ Integrins)

Amino acid An organic compound containing an amino and carboxyl group. Amino acids form the basis of protein synthesis.

Angiogenesis Formation of new blood vessels. May be triggered by physiological conditions, like during embryogenesis or certain pathological conditions, such as cancer, where the continuing growth of solid tumors requires nourishment from new blood vessels.

Annexin V A protein in blood which binds to phosphatidyl serine (PS) binding sites exposed on the cell surface by cells undergoing programmed cell death. $\Rightarrow$ Apoptosis.

Antibody A protein with a particular type of structure that binds to antigens in a target-specific manner.

Antigen Any substance which differs from substances normally present in the body, and can induce an immune response.

Antiangiogenesis The inhibition of new blood vessel growth and/or destruction of preformed blood vessels.

Antisense A strategy to block the synthesis of certain proteins by interacting with their messenger RNA (mRNA). A gene whose messenger RNA (mRNA) is complementary to the RNA of the target protein is inserted in the cell genome. The protein synthesis is blocked by interaction of the antisense mRNA and the protein-encoding RNA.

Apoptosis Programmed cell death. A process programmed into all cells as part of the normal life cycle of the cell. It allows the body to dispose of damaged, unwanted or superfluous cells.

Aptamer RNA or DNA-based ligand.

Asialoglycoproteins Endogenous glycoproteins from which sialic acid has been removed by the action of sialidases. They bind tightly to their cell surface receptor, which is located on hepatocyte plasma membranes. After internalization by adsorptive endocytosis, they are delivered to lysosomes for degradation.

Attenuation correction (AC) Methodology which corrects images for the differential absorption of photons in tissues with different densities.

Avidin A biotin-binding protein (68 kDa) obtained from egg white. Binding is so strong as to be effectively irreversible.

Bioinformatics The science of managing and analyzing biological data using advanced computing techniques. Especially important in analyzing genomic research data.

Biotechnology A set of biological techniques developed through basic research and now applied to research and product development. In particular, biotechnology refers to the industrial use of recombinant DNA, cell fusion, and new bioprocessing techniques.

Biotin A prosthetic group for carboxylase enzyme. Important in fatty acid biosynthesis and catabolism, biotin has found widespread use as a covalent label for macromolecules, which may then be detected by high-affinity binding of labeled avidin or streptavidin. Biotin is an essential growth factor for many cells.

Cancer Diseases in which abnormal cells divide and grow unchecked. Cancer can spread from its original site to other parts of the body and is often fatal.

Carrier An individual who carries the abnormal gene for a specific condition but has no symptoms.

Cavitation The sudden formation and collapse of low-pressure bubbles in liquids as a result of mechanical forces.

cDNA ⇒ Complementary DNA.

Cell The basic structural unit of all living organisms and the smallest structural unit of living tissue capable of functioning as an independent entity. It is surrounded by a membrane and contains a nucleus which carries genetic material.

Chromosome A rod-like structure present in the nucleus of all body cells (with the exception of the red blood cells) which stores genetic information. Normally, humans have 23 pairs, giving a total of 46 chromosomes.

Coincidence detection A process used to detect emissions from positron-emitting radioisotopes. The technology utilizes opposing detectors that simultaneously detect two 511 keV photons which are emitted at an angle of 180 degrees from one another as a result of the annihilation of the positron when it combines with an electron.

Complementary DNA (cDNA) DNA synthesized in the laboratory from a messenger RNA template by the action of RNA-dependent DNA polymerase.

Cytogenetics The study of the structure and physical appearance of chromosome material. It includes routine analysis of G-banded chromosomes, other cytogenetic banding techniques, as well as molecular cytogenetics such as fluorescent in situ hybridization (FISH) and comparative genomic hybridization (CGH).

Deoxyglucose $\Rightarrow$ 18 F-deoxyglucose.

DNA Deoxyribonucleic acid: the molecule or 'building block' that encodes genetic information.

DNA repair genes Genes encoding proteins that correct errors in DNA sequencing.

Enzyme A protein that acts as a catalyst to speed the rate at which a biochemical reaction proceeds.

Epistasis A gene that interferes with or prevents the expression of another gene located at a different locus.

Epitope The specific binding site for an antibody.

Expression $\Rightarrow$ Gene expression.

^{18}F-deoxyglucose The predominant PET imaging agent used in oncology. The deoxyglucose is 'trapped' in cells which have increased metabolic activity as a result of phosphorylation. The process results in an accumulation of fluorine-18 (^{18}F) in the cells, allowing the location of the cells and intensity of tumor metabolism to be determined using PET imaging.

Fluorine-18 (^{18}F) A positron-emitting radioisotope used to label deoxyglucose or other molecular probes for use as radiopharmaceuticals.

F(ab) fragment The shape of an antibody resembles the letter 'Y'. Antigen binding properties are on both short arms. Digestion by various enzymes yields different fragments. Fragments with one binding site are called F(ab).

F(ab')$_2$ fragment Antibody fragment with two binding sites ($\Rightarrow$ also F(ab) fragment).

Fc fragment (Crystallizable) antibody fragment which has no binding properties ($\Rightarrow$ also F(ab) fragment). The Fc fragment is used by the body's immune system to clear the antibody from the circulation.

Fibrin Fibrous protein that forms the meshwork necessary for forming of blood clots.

Fibroblast growth factor Acidic fibroblast growth factor (alpha-FGF, HBGF 1) and basic FGF (beta-FGF, HBGF-2) are the two founder members of a family of structurally related growth factors for mesodermal or neuroectodermal cells.

Fingerprinting In genetics, the identification of multiple specific alleles on a person's DNA to produce a unique identifier for that person.

Gadolinium A paramagnetic ion which changes the relaxivity of adjacent protons. It affects signal intensity in MR images ($\Rightarrow$ garamagnetism).

Ganciclovir An antiviral agent which is phosphorylated by thymidine kinase. As a phosphorylated substance it stops cell division by inhibiting DNA synthesis.

Gene The fundamental physical and functional unit of heredity. A gene is an ordered sequence of nucleotides located in a particular position on a particular chromosome that encodes a specific functional product (i.e., a protein or RNA molecule). The totality of genes present in an organism determines its characteristics.

Gene expression The process by which a gene's coded information is converted into the structures present and operating in the cell. Expressed genes include those that are transcribed into mRNAs and then translated into proteins, and those that are transcribed into RNAs but not translated into proteins (e.g., transfer and ribosomal RNAs).

Gene mapping Determination of the relative positions of genes on a DNA molecule (chromosome or plasmid) and of the distance, in linkage units or physical units, between them.

Gene prediction Predictions of possible genes made by a computer program based on how well a stretch of DNA sequence matches known gene sequences.

Gene sequence (full) The complete order of bases in a gene. This order determines which protein a gene will produce.

Gene, suicide $\Rightarrow$ Suicide gene.

Gene therapy An experimental procedure aimed at replacing, manipulating, or supplementing nonfunctional or misfunctioning genes with therapeutic genes.

Genetic code The sequence of nucleotides, coded in triplets (codons) along the mRNA, that determines the sequence of amino acids in protein synthesis. A gene's DNA sequence can be used to predict the mRNA sequence, and the genetic code can, in turn, be used to predict the amino acid sequence.

Genetic marker A gene or other identifiable portion of DNA whose inheritance can be followed.

Genetic susceptibility Susceptibility to a genetic disease. May or may not result in actual development of the disease.

Genome All the genetic material in the chromosomes of a particular organism; its size is generally given as its total number of base pairs.

Genomics The science aimed at sequencing and mapping the genetic code of a given organism.

Genotype The genetic constitution of an organism, as distinguished from its physical appearance (its phenotype).

ICAM Intercellular adhesion molecules: glycoproteins that are present on a wide range of human cells, essential to the mechanism by which cells recognize each other, and thus important in inflammatory responses.

Indium-111 (^{111}In) A single-photon-emitting radioisotope used to label various molecular probes for SPECT imaging.

Integrins A specific group of transmembrane proteins that act as receptor proteins. Different integrins consist of different numbers of alpha and beta subunits. Over 20 different integrin receptors are known.

Lectin Sugar-binding proteins which are highly specific for their sugar moieties. They bind to glycoproteins on the cell surface or to soluble gylcoproteins and play a role in biological recognition phenomena involving cells and proteins, e.g., during the immune response.

Liposome A spherical particle in an aqueous medium, formed by a lipid bilayer enclosing an aqueous compartment.

Locus The relative position of a gene on a chromosome.

Lysosome A minute intracellular body involved in intracellular digestion.

Messenger RNA (mRNA) RNA that serves as a template for protein synthesis.

Microarray Sets of miniaturized chemical reaction areas that may also be used to test DNA fragments, antibodies, or proteins.

Micronuclei Chromosome fragments that are not incorporated into the nucleus at cell division.

MID Molecular imaging and diagnostics.

Molecular biology The study of the structure, function, and makeup of biologically important molecules.

Molecular genetics The study of macromolecules important in biological inheritance.

Molecular medicine The treatment of injury or disease at the molecular level. Examples include the use of DNA-based diagnostic tests or medicine derived from a DNA sequence. It includes molecular diagnostics, molecular imaging and molecular therapy.

Monoclonal antibodies Antibodies made in cell cultures; these antibodies are all identical.

Monosaccharide A simple sugar that cannot be decomposed by hydrolysis.

Nucleic acid A nucleotide polymer. There are two types: DNA and RNA.

Nucleotide A subunit of DNA or RNA consisting of a nitrogenous molecule, a phosphate molecule, and a sugar molecule. Thousands of nucleotides are linked to form a DNA or RNA molecule.

Oligonucleotides Polymers made up of a few (2-20) nucleotides. In molecular genetics, they refer to a short sequence synthesized to match a region where a mutation is known to occur, and then used as a probe (oligonucleotide probes).

Operon Combination of a set of structural genes and the DNA sequences which control the expression of these genes.

Oncogene A gene, one or more forms of which is associated with cancer. Many oncogenes are directly or indirectly involved in controlling the rate of cell growth.

Paramagnetism Magnetism which occurs in paramagnetic material (e.g. $\Rightarrow$ gadolinium), but only in the presence of an externally applied magnetic field. Even in the presence of the field there is only a small induced magnetization because only a small fraction of the spins will be orientated by the field. This fraction is proportional to the field strength. The attraction experienced by ferromagnets is nonlinear and much stronger.

Peptide A short chain of amino acids. Most peptides act as chemical messengers, i.e., they bind to specific receptors.

Peptidomimetics Engineered compounds that have similar binding characteristics to those of naturally occurring proteins. The advantages are increased stability and prolonged presence in the bloodstream.

Perfluorocarbon A compound containing carbon and fluorine only.

PESDA Perfluorocarbon exposed sonicated dextrose albumin microbubbles.

PET Positron emission tomography. An imaging modality which utilizes opposing sets of detectors to record simultaneous emissions from a positron-emitting radioisotope throughout 360°. The image data are processed using reconstruction algorithms to create tomographic image sets of the distribution of the radioisotope in the patient.

PET/CT A combination technology which creates tomographic image sets of the metabolic activity from PET and the anatomical tomographic image sets from CT. CT $\Rightarrow$ computed tomography: An imaging modality employing a rotating x-ray tube and a detector as well producing numbers of projection imagings during its rotation around the object of interest. Specific reconstruction algorithms are used to generate three-dimensional image of the inside of an object. The two images sets are fused to form a single image, which is used to assign the PET abnormalities to specific anatomical locations.

Phage A virus for which the natural host is a bacterial cell.

Phagocytosis Endocytosis of particulate material, such as microorganisms or cell fragments. The material is taken into the cell in membrane-bound vesicles (phagosomes) that originate as pinched-off invaginations of the plasma membrane. Phagosomes fuse with lysosomes, forming phagolysosomes, in which the engulfed material is killed and digested.

Pharmacodynamics The study of what a drug does to the body and of its mode of action.

Pharmacogenomics The influence of genetic variations on drug response in patients. This is performed by correlating gene expression or single-nucleotide polymorphisms with a drug's efficacy or toxicity during therapy.

Pharmacokinetics The determination of the fate of substances administered externally to a living organism, e.g., the metabolism and half-life of drugs.

Phenotype The physical characteristics of an organism or the presence of a disease that may or may not be genetic.

Phosphorylation A metabolic process in which a phosphate group is introduced into an organic molecule.

Plasmid Autonomously replicating extrachromosomal circular DNA molecules.

Polymerase An enzyme that catalyzes polymerization, especially of nucleotides.

Polysaccharides Any of a class of carbohydrates, such as starch and cellulose, consisting of a number of monosaccharides joined by glycosidic bonds. Polysaccharides can be decomposed into the component monosaccharides by hydrolysis.

Polypeptide A peptide containing more than two amino acids.

Probe Single-stranded DNA or RNA molecules of specific base sequence, labeled either radioactively or immunologically, that are used to detect the complementary base sequence by hybridization.

Promoter A specific DNA sequence to which RNA polymerase binds in order to 'transcribe' the adjacent DNA sequence and produce an RNA copy. The action of RNA polymerase is the first step in the translation of genes, via mRNA, into proteins.

Protein A large molecule comprising one or more chains of amino acids in a specific order that is determined by the base sequence of nucleotides in the gene that codes for the protein. Proteins are required for the structure, function, and regulation of the body's cells, tissues, and organs. Each protein has unique functions. Examples are hormones, enzymes, and antibodies.

Proteomics The global analysis of gene expression in order to identify, quantify, and characterize proteins.

Receptor A molecular structure within a cell or on the cell surface that selectively binds a specific substance having a specific physiological effect.

Rhenium-188 (^{188}Re) A beta-emitting radioisotope used to label various molecular probes for targeted radiotherapy applications.

Reporter gene imaging Imaging of genetic or enzymatic products/events initiated by molecular therapies which have assigned specific reporter genes to express specific targets.

Ribosomal RNA (rRNA) A class of RNA found in the ribosomes of cells.

RNA Ribonucleic acid: a chemical found in the nucleus and cytoplasm of cells; it plays an important role in protein synthesis and other chemical activities of the cell. The structure of RNA is similar to that of DNA. There are several classes of RNA molecules, including messenger RNA, transfer RNA, ribosomal RNA, and other small RNAs, each serving a different purpose.

Selectins A family of cell adhesion molecules consisting of a lectin-like domain, an epidermal growth factor-like domain, and a variable number of domains that encode proteins homologous to complement-binding proteins. Selectins mediate the binding of leukocytes to the vascular endothelium.

Sequencing Determination of the order of nucleotides (base sequences) in a DNA or RNA molecule or the order of amino acids in a protein.

Sonothrombolysis Dissolving a thrombus using ultrasound, either alone or in conjunction with microbubbles.

SPECT Single photon emission computerized tomography: an imaging modality in which a detector is rotated about the patient, recording photon emissions throughout 360°. Reconstruction algorithms are used to convert the data into a set of tomographic images.

Stem cell Undifferentiated, primitive cells in the bone marrow that have the ability both to multiply and to differentiate into specific cells for the formation of specific tissues (hematopoetic, mesenchymal and neuronal stem cells).

Streptavidin A biotin-binding protein obtained from bacteria.

Structural genomics The study to determine the 3D structures of large numbers of proteins using both experimental techniques and computer simulation.

Suicide gene A protein-coding sequence that produces an enzyme capable of converting a nontoxic compound to a cytotoxic compound, used in cancer therapy.

Technetium-99m (^{99m}Tc) A single-photon-emitting radioisotope used to label various molecular probes for scintigraphic imaging, including SPECT imaging.

Theragnostics The application of MID for therapy guidance using genomic, proteomic and metabolomic data for predicting and assessing drug response.

Thymidine kinase (tk) The gene coding for the tk from the herpes simplex virus (HSV-tk) can be used as a 'suicide gene' or a reporter gene ($\Rightarrow$ Reporter gene imaging) in cancer therapy. $\Rightarrow$ also Ganciclovir.

Tissue factor An integral membrane glycoprotein of around 250 residues that initiates blood clotting after binding factors VII or VIIa.

Tracer principle The use of molecular probes labelled with radioisotopes to allow for nuclear imaging devices to detect the presence and location of the targeted structures by specific binding (e.g., to receptors, proteins, . . .) or trapping in cells.

Transfection The introduction of DNA into a recipient cell and its subsequent integration into the recipient cell's chromosomal DNA.

Transfer RNA Small RNA molecules with a function in translation. They carry specific amino acids to specified sites.

Transgene A gene transferred from one organism to another.

Translation The process by which polypeptide chains are synthesized, forming the structural elements of proteins.

Translational research Applying results obtained by basic research to answer scientific questions concerning human disease processes.

USPIO Ultrasmall particles of iron oxide. These particles have a high magnetic moment causing strong local susceptibility and field inhomogeneities, with strong effects in T2- and T2*-weighted MR imaging.

VEGF Vascular endothelial growth factor. VEGF is a protein secreted by a variety of tissues, when stimulated by triggers like hypoxia. VEGF stimulates endothelial cell growth, angiogenesis, and capillary permeability.

Virus A noncellular biological entity that can only reproduce within a host cell. Viruses consist of nucleic acid (DNA or RNA) covered by protein; some animal viruses are also surrounded by membrane. Inside the infected cell, the virus uses the synthetic capability of the host to produce progeny viruses.

Part I
Instrumentation

Fundamentals of Optical Imaging

Ralf B. Schulz(✉) and Wolfhard Semmler

Abstract Optical imaging techniques offer simplistic while highly sensitive modalities for molecular imaging research. In this chapter, the major instrumental necessities for microscopic and whole-animal imaging techniques are introduced. Subsequently, the resulting imaging modalities using visible or near-infrared light are presented and discussed. The aim is to show the current capabilities and application fields of optics.

Ralf B. Schulz

Helmholtz Zentrum München Institut für Biologische und Medizinische Bildgebung, Ingolstädter Landstraße 1, 85764 Neuherberg, Germany

ralf.schulz@helmholtz-muenchen.de

W. Semmler and M. Schwaiger (eds.), *Molecular Imaging I.*

Handbook of Experimental Pharmacology 185/I.

1 Introduction and Overview

Imaging techniques employing visible light have been a standard research tool for centuries: vision is usually our most developed sense, and thus the visual inspection of a specimen has always been a scientist's first choice. The development of lenses, telescopes, and microscopes has helped us visually explore large or small worlds previously not accessible. In biomedical research, with the discovery of fluorescence, fluorescence microscopy has become the technique of choice for single-cell imaging (Vo Dinh 2003a). Novel scanning techniques, as described further below, yield high resolution by overcoming the diffraction limit usually connected to lens-based systems. Thus, they allow tomographic imaging of individual cells without slicing them, as necessary for electron microscopy. This has led to a number of discoveries, including the tubular structure of mitochondria (Hell 2003).

The capabilities of fluorescence microscopes have in turn sparked further technological advances in fluorescent markers and probe systems. The discoveries of bioluminescent and fluorescent proteins have enabled biologists to produce cells that synthesize optically active markers by themselves, a fundamental simplification for gene expression imaging (Massoud and Gambhir 2003).

Compared with other types of contrast agents, optical probes offer unique imaging capabilities: not only can they be targeted to receptors, like radioactive tracers or MR-active substances, but fluorescent probes can also be activated due to enzymatic reactions (*activatable probes*), and they can be produced by cells themselves in the form of bioluminescent enzymes or fluorescent proteins (Hoffman 2005). Fluorescent proteins nowadays can be engineered to emit in the far red, necessary for in vivo applications (Shaner et al. 2005).

However, these advantages come with several caveats: compared with radiotracers, fluorescent molecules are big, relatively unstable (they are affected by photobleaching), and some of them are cytotoxic to some degree. Furthermore, biological tissues are highly diffuse; visible light is scattered within a few microns. Fluorescence-based imaging techniques are thus often either not applicable in vivo, only applicable to very superficial regions due to the scattering, nonquantitative, or highly experimental and not yet available for daily routine, as is the case for optical tomographic applications.

Over the past few years, optical imaging technologies for whole-animal imaging (or even patient-based imaging) have attracted more and more attention, the reason being that an abundance of highly specific optical probes is nowadays available for in vitro applications that would be of much help if applied in vivo (Weissleder and Ntziachristos 2003). Optical imaging is hoped to provide a reliable way of translating in vitro research to in vivo. Most of these techniques are planar [two-dimensional (2D)]. The advances in computer technology and mathematical modeling have also led to the development of optical tomographic (3D) techniques. For a current review of available techniques, please refer to Gibson et al. (2005) or Hielscher (2005).

This chapter will first introduce the basics of optical imaging and provide recommendations for further reading. While a couple of years ago, it was hard to find comprehensive summaries of optical imaging techniques, a number of complete books and reviews have now been published by various groups and are recommended to the interested reader, such as the books edited by Vo Dinh (2003a), Mycek and Pogue (2003), and Kraayenhof et al. (2002). Due to length constraints, this article can only concentrate on a few key points.

2 Biomedical Optics

2.1 Photon Propagation in Tissues

The fundamental limits for optical imaging in terms of either penetration depths or resolution are given by the optical properties of tissue; due to the many very small structures and boundaries in cells, tissue becomes highly scattering and absorbing for photons in the visible range. Absorption and scattering are measured in terms of the *absorption coefficient*, μ_a, and the *scattering coefficient*, μ_s, with physical units of cm^{-1} or mm^{-1}. The reciprocal value of these coefficients yields the mean free path.

While tissue is strongly absorbing for light having a short wavelength ($\mu_a \gg 1\,cm^{-1}$, resulting in a mean free path of much less than 1 cm) caused by the most common absorbers in cells, cytochromes and hemoglobin, light in the near infrared range (NIR) between 600 and 900 nm can penetrate several centimeters deep into tissue ($\mu_a < 0.5\,cm^{-1}$, even down to $\mu_a \approx 0.1\,cm^{-1}$; Fig. 1, yielding a mean free path of up to 10 cm if only absorption is taken into account). This wavelength region

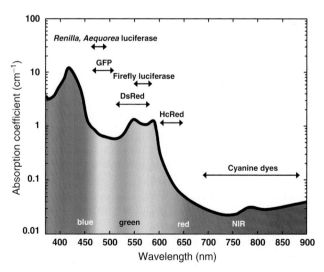

Fig. 1 Absorption and autofluorescence of tissue, depending on wavelength. The wavelength regions of important dyes are indicated by arrows. (Adapted from Weissleder and Ntziachristos 2003)

has been termed the "water window," as for longer wavelengths water absorption becomes the dominant term (Weissleder and Ntziachristos 2003).

The low absorption in the NIR wavelength range has led to the development of an abundance of NIR fluorescent molecules. However, in general, these fluorochromes are less efficient and less bright than their short-wavelength counterparts. This also implies that for a certain application the wavelength has to be chosen very carefully: in a more absorbing wavelength range, the increase in efficiency and stability of the molecules might outweigh the disadvantages of higher absorption.

The main problem when using visible photons, however, is not attenuation but scattering, with a scattering coefficient in the order of $\mu_s \approx 100\ \text{cm}^{-1}$, being about four orders of magnitude larger than absorption and thus leading to a total mean free path of only 0.1 mm. Scattering results from the many different diffracting interfaces present in the cells of which tissue is comprised. Scattering due to cells is largely anisotropic, with an average scatter angle of only $25°$.

Standard methods for scatter reduction, as known for example from nuclear imaging, will fail in these cases due to the extreme number of scattering events that detected photons have undergone. Scattering decreases with longer wavelengths, but otherwise it remains relatively constant over the visible range (contrary to the sharply peaked absorption spectra of biological chromophores, Fig. 1).

When choosing an appropriate fluorochrome or the optimal wavelength for a specific imaging purpose there is also another, counter-intuitive effect one might have to take into account: the choice of a wavelength in a strongly absorbing region will result in the preferential detection of photons that have undergone fewer scattering events, as scattering increases the length of the propagation path, and the higher absorption will constrain path lengths. Thus, scattering can be significantly reduced; however, signal intensities are decreased as well.

For a comprehensive list of tissue optical properties and according references, please refer to the review by Mobley and Vo-Dinh (2003).

2.2 Bioluminescence and Fluorescence

The term *fluorescence* refers to the emission of a photon caused by a molecule's transition from an excited electronic state to (usually) its ground state. Both states have the same spin multiplicity, which makes fluorescence a singlet-singlet transition. Fluorescent molecules often consist of a more or less a long chain of carbon atoms between two aromatic structures, which as a whole acts as an optical resonator. The length of the chain is related to the emission wavelength.

The excited state is reached by absorption of a photon with sufficient energy, i.e., of a photon of higher energy (shorter wavelength) than the energy difference between excited and ground state. The wavelength difference between the wavelength of maximum absorption and the emission wavelength is called *Stokes shift*. A large Stokes shift facilitates the creating of filters blocking the excitation light. Shifts range between less than 20 nm and several hundred nanometers. The lifetime of the excited state is termed the *fluorescence lifetime*, $\tau[\text{s}]$, and usually amounts to a time span between some 100 ps to several nanoseconds. For singlet-triplet transitions (phosphorescence) occurring for example in some lanthanides, even lifetimes of several milliseconds can be observed.

The probability that the transition from excited to ground state will occur by emission of a photon is called the *quantum yield*, γ, and is a measure for fluorochrome efficiency. The absorption efficiency is described by the *molar extinction coefficient*, ε [mol^{-1}cm^{-1}]. The total absorption created by the fluorochrome can be calculated using the relation $\mu_a = \varepsilon c$, where c [mol/l] is the fluorochrome concentration. It is important to notice that all these factors, including the emission and absorption spectra, are influenced by the chemical environment (pH value, etc). Please refer to Redmond (2003) or Lakowicz (2006) for details.

Bioluminescence is a special form of chemoluminescence. Photons are emitted when a bioluminescent enzyme (e.g., luciferase) metabolizes its specific substrate (e.g., luciferin). As in this case no excitation light is necessary to produce a signal, there is also no background, i.e., neither from autofluorescence nor from filter leakage. However, while it is relatively easy to guide light to fluorescent probes, it is hard to ensure that the substrate is transported to all possibly bioluminescent cells (Massoud and Gambhir 2003).

3 Imaging Requirements

Optical imaging of any kind requires three fundamental system parts: light sources to induce the desired signal, filters to eliminate background signal, and photon detectors to acquire the signal. These components will be discussed in the following. For a detailed overview please refer to Vo-Dinh (2003b) or Lakowicz (2006).

3.1 Light Sources

Light sources can generally be distinguished by their emission spectra, emission power, as well as their capabilities concerning pulsing or modulation. Fluorescence excitation is usually performed with one of the following:

- **High-pressure Arc Lamps:** They exhibit strong, nearly continuous emission between 200 nm (UV) and 1,000 nm (IR). These high intensity sources are of major interest in cell biology and spectroscopy but are less often used in whole animal imaging.
- **Light-emitting diodes:** Due to the recent developments of extremely luminous LEDs ("LumiLEDs") and the availability of all kinds of emission spectra between 300 nm and 700 nm, they have become a very cheap and stable alternative to lasers, if coherence is unimportant or even undesirable, e.g., due to speckle noise. To sharpen their emission spectrum, one usually combines LEDs with a filter system (Fig. 2).

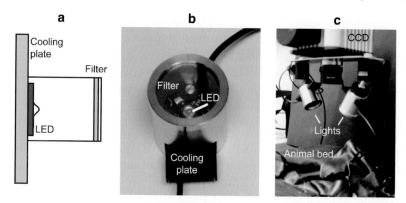

Fig. 2 a, b An LED light source for in vivo imaging. Light from a luminous LED, emitting isotropically in all directions, is filtered and can excite superficially located fluorochromes in mice. **a** Schematic drawing of the light source. **b** Close-up image of the source. **c** Application example

- **Lasers:** A standard tool in biomedical imaging. They are available in the form of solid state lasers (diodes), especially in the near infrared, red or green, but nowadays even blue; as gas lasers; as tunable dye lasers (usually pumped by gas lasers); or as nonlinear lasers that produce also IR output. The output of laser diodes can be continuous, pulsed, or modulated with frequencies of up to 100 MHz. Lasers exhibit a sharply peaked (monochromatic) spectrum, coherent and usually polarized light output. There are lasers available that can be tuned to different wavelengths.

3.2 Filters

Crucial for the signal-to-noise ratio of optical systems is the performance of the filters used. While optical signals are usually weak, one of the biggest issues is elimination of excitation light, as its wavelength is usually close to the emission, and at the same time, the signal is much stronger due to the limited quantum yield and the limited solid angle observable.

Filters are distinguished by their transmission spectra. *Neutral density filters* absorb a constant fraction of light, independent of wavelength. They are characterized by their *optical density* (OD), defined as $OD = \log_{10}(I_t/I_0)$, with (I_t/I_0) being the ratio of transmitted to original light intensity. *Longpass* and *shortpass filters* transmit light above and below a certain wavelength, respectively. *Bandpass filters* transmit a (narrow) light-band, characterized by its central wavelength and the full width half maximum of the transmission band. See Fig. 3 for examples of bandpass and longpass transmission spectra. *Notch filters* (sometimes called *band-rejection filters*) suppress the transmission of a narrow light band. They are characterized analogously to bandpass filters by central blocked wavelength, and the FWHM of the blocked band.

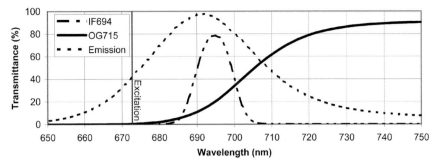

Fig. 3 Two possible filters for imaging of the Cy5.5 fluorochrome, a bandpass (IF694, Laser-Components, Germany) with peak transmission at 694 nm, and a long pass filter (OG715, Schott, Germany). Although the glass filter blocks significantly more light at the peak wavelength of the fluorochrome (695 nm), due to the red tail of the emission spectrum, total transmission is 30%, while for the interference filter, it is only 19%. The emission spectrum is shown as a *dotted line*. The usual excitation wavelength of 672 nm is indicated by a *vertical line*

Most of the available filters to date are based either on absorption, interference, or dispersion. The differences are described in the following.

3.2.1 Absorption-based Filters

In absorbing filters, light is either transmitted through the filter or absorbed in it. The filter itself consists of the absorber and a substrate, which is commonly either a gel or glass. The advantage is their low cost and the independence of transmission properties of the angle of incidence, contrary to interference-based filters (see below). Disadvantages are the relatively low specificity, i.e., these filters usually exhibit smooth transmission curves, which make it difficult to filter in the case of small Stokes shifts. Furthermore, as blocked light is absorbed, these filters are only suitable for low intensities. Gel filters additionally are prone to bleaching, and sensitive to heat or humidity.

Due to their smooth transmission spectra, absorption filters are mostly used as neutral density filters, or long- and shortpass filters. Absorption-based bandpasses do exist, but they have large FWHMs and are usually not suitable for fluorescence detection.

3.2.2 Interference-based Filters

Interference filters either transmit or reflect light. Thus, nearly no energy is absorbed by the filter, which makes them suitable for filtering very intense light. They consist of a number of dielectric layers that partially reflect incoming light. The distance between these layers is chosen such that interference occurs in a way that transmitted light constructively interferes in the forward direction, while destructively interfering in the backwards direction; blocked light needs to destructively interfere in the forward direction and constructively interfere in the backward direction.

Thus, these filters can be manufactured to be much more specific than absorbing filters, as can be seen in Fig. 3, where the transmission curves of the bandpass are much steeper than these of the absorbing longpass. However, the interference effects strongly depend on the angle of incidence; it is shortest for light rays incident at an angle of $0°$ (perpendicular to the surface), while the distances geometrically increase for larger angles. Thus, interference filters can only be used for parallel light as used in a fluorescence microscope (see below) but not in front of an objective.

3.2.3 Dispersive Elements

Dispersion is the wavelength-dependence of photon propagation speed in media. When light enters a dispersive medium, it is split into its spectral components as the diffraction angle will depend on wavelength. A typical example is an optical prism. Dispersive media can be used to filter out light if only parts of the resulting spectrum are used for illumination or detection, as in a photospectrometer. Typical examples of such dispersive media are *diffraction gratings*, which most often are comprised of a large number of grooves on a highly reflective surface. The distance between adjacent grooves determines the spectral properties of the grating.

Dispersive effects can also be used to create acoustically tunable bandpass filters (AOTFs) or liquid crystal tunable filters (LCTFs), novel types of devices that only recently found their way into biomedical imaging. In AOTFs, a standing acoustic wave is induced in a birefringent crystal to create spatially varying changes in refractive index via the acousto-optical effect. This wave pattern of changing refractive indices acts like a Bragg grating and thus can be used as a reflective monochromator. In LCTFs, a refractive index change is generated by alignment of the liquid crystal molecules in an externally applied electrical field.

The advantages of dispersive variable band-pass filters are their fast adjustment times (less than 100 ms) and narrow filtering possibilities (up to 1 nm FWHM). Filtering requires, however, exactly parallel light with normal incidence on the filter.

3.3 Photon Detectors

Characteristic properties of photon detectors are the number of measurement channels they provide (single channel or multichannel devices), their dynamics (for digitized signals commonly expressed in *bits*), sensitivity (in terms of the *quantum efficiency*, i.e., the probability that a single photon creates a signal), and time resolution.

In this section we distinguish between photon counting detectors—analog detectors that produce individual signals for each incoming photon as used in extreme low-light or time-resolved applications—and integrating detectors without inherent time resolution. Intensified imaging devices, consisting of a combination of the previous two types, are considered a third category. They allow for time-resolved acquisition of large-field images due to their gating capabilities.

3.3.1 Photon Counting Devices

In photon counting devices, an incident photon is absorbed and subsequently generates some kind of charge displacement via the photoelectric effect, which is then amplified by several orders of magnitude to result in a measurable current. Using suitable read-out electronics, this signal can be detected in real-time. The amplification can also be used to employ these devices as image intensifiers; see 3.3.3.

Two imaging modes are commonly applied. When a *pulsed light source* is used, counted photons can be related to the time of the source pulse, and thus provide information about the optical path length of these photons. The path length in turn is indirectly related to the amount of scattering photons have undergone. Scattering elongates the propagation path compared with a straight, unscattered propagation path. In this way, scattering and absorbing inclusions in tissue can be distinguished. This mode of operation is termed *time-domain detection*. If instead of a pulsed light source, a *modulated light source* is employed, the detection technique is termed *frequency-domain detection*. Here, the phase shift between light-source modulation and detected signal is examined, from which it is, for instance, related to the lifetime of a fluorochrome and the optical properties of tissue.

Single-channel photon-counting devices are commonly photomultiplier tubes (PMTs) (Fig. 4a), as known from nuclear imaging, and (avalanche) photodiodes.

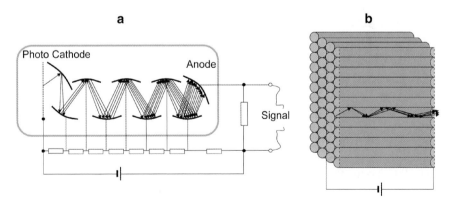

Fig. 4 a, b Light amplification via the photoelectric effect. **a** Schematic drawing of a PMT. Photons enter through a window on the left side and create free electrons when hitting the photo cathode. These electrons are accelerated due to an external field and consecutively hit different electrodes, where additional electrons are set free. In the end, a single photon entering the PMT creates a measurable signal at the anode. **b** Schematic drawing of an MCP. In a 2D grid of hollow tubes (channels), to which an electrical field is applied, entering photoelectrons are amplified when they hit the walls of one channel

Multichannel devices are usually either arrays of photodiodes, which can be fabricated on a single silicon waver, or *microchannel plates* (Fig. 4b). These provide a 2D grid of amplifying channels that each work similar to a PMT. The total amplification is lower, but unlike PMTs, the resulting information remains spatially resolved after amplification due to the 2D structure.

It must be noted that in order to operate one of these device in photon-counting mode, additional hardware is necessary to record and save all the acquired pulses with an accurate time stamp.

3.3.2 Integrating Detectors

Photon counting devices require very low light levels and expensive read-out electronics. For intense light fluxes, integrating detectors are used. In these, a capacitance is loaded via the photoelectric effect (integration). The charge stored in the capacitance is linearly related to the number of incident photons. It is sampled via an analog-digital converter after the exposure time.

To date, the most common integrating photon detector is the charge-coupled device (CCD), used for example in digital photo and video cameras. CCDs can be manufactured for high sensitivity, even in the NIR range, with up to 95% quantum efficiency. To obtain maximum sensitivity, they need to be cooled to reduce dark noise. Also, the CCD as a whole has limited dynamics due to the limited well capacities during image exposure.

Another type available nowadays is the CMOS array sensor. These are comprised essentially of a miniaturized photodiode array, including integrators, amplifiers, and readout electronics. CMOS arrays are integrating devices with high dynamics, but not yet as sensitive as CCDs.

Characteristic parameters of integrating detectors are:

- **Quantum Efficiency:** The probability that a single photon at a given wavelength will interact with the sensor and thus create a signal. For back-illuminated CCDs, this value can be in the order of 95%.
- **Full Well Capacity (FWC):** Only a limited number of electrons can be stored per pixel. If this number is reached, the detector is saturated. The full well capacity determines the maximum dynamics of the sensor.
- **Read Noise (RN):** The noise of the analog-to-digital (A/D)-converter. This effectively reduces the sensitivity of the sensor.
- **Dark Current (DC):** By heat dissipation, electrons are randomly stored in each pixel, thus limiting exposure times and sensitivity. Dark noise is effectively reduced by cooling. Sensitive CCD cameras are usually cooled to below $-50\,^{\circ}$C, reducing dark noise to about 0.001 electrons per pixel per second of exposure time.
- **Digitizing Accuracy (DA):** The A/D converters used can have different resolutions, ranging from 8 bits per pixel in simple cameras to 16 bits per pixel in highly sensitive CCDs.

The dynamic range (DR) of an array sensor is limited by the last four properties stated above, and can be calculated according to the formula:

$$DR = \min \left\{ \log_2 \frac{FWC}{DC \cdot EXP + RN}, DA \right\} \tag{1}$$

The unit of dynamic range, in this case, is bits per pixel. The unit of the full well capacity (FWC) is electrons per pixel, the dark current (DC) is expressed in electrons per pixel per second, the exposure time (EXP) in seconds, and the read noise (RN) in electrons per pixel.

3.3.3 Intensified and Time-Resolved Imaging

Due the limited bandwidth and sensitivity of A/D-converters, neither CCD nor CMOS sensors can be read out fast enough to yield a time resolution suitable for resolving photon propagation. However, if the process that is to be observed is repeatable, time-resolved imaging becomes possible by using image amplifiers that can be activated within a few picoseconds, so-called *gated imaging*. The combination of a light amplifier and a CCD is often called *intensified CCD* (ICCD).

Light amplification is usually performed using a micro-channel plate (MCP) with a scintillating material at the output which is imaged by the CCD. MCPs can be gated by modulating their operating voltage. The gate widths achievable to date are in the order of 100 ps.

Instead of using two separate units for light amplification and detection, both can also be combined on a single integrated circuit. These devices are called electron-bombardment (EB) or electron-multiplying (EM) CCDs, depending on the manufacturer. They do not yet achieve the high gain rates of current image intensifiers or ICCDs, nor the short gating times. However, they are much more cost-effective and easier to use.

A mechanical, time-resolved technique involving an integrating detector is the streak camera. It is usually based on a one-line CCD, sometimes also a complete 2D CCD. Incoming photons are swept over the pixels using a deflector, such that every column of the CCD corresponds to a certain time point after triggering. These devices offer very high temporal resolution below 1 ps, even for single shots, but cannot acquire complete 2D images over time.

4 Microscopic Imaging Techniques

The following techniques are termed "microscopic" as they offer high resolution (a few microns or less) but only limited depth penetration, so that their application to in vivo settings is limited. Generally, resolution is limited by Abbe's diffraction limit (Hell 2003):

$$d = \frac{\lambda}{2\,NA} \tag{2}$$

with d being the shortest distance at which two distinct objects can be separated, and NA is the numerical aperture of the lens used. While the aperture NA can be increased using oil immersion lenses, it is always less than 1. However, in this section we will also present new developments that overcome the limitations of Abbe's law.

4.1 Fluorescence Microscopy

In classical fluorescence microscopy, a single objective is used for illumination and detection at the same time. Excitation light is filtered out using a combination of a dielectric mirror and two (interference) filters (Fig. 5a). In acquired images, fluorescent structures located on the focal plane of the objective appear with high contrast and intensity. The intensity of structures at a distance r from the focal plane decays with r^2. As fluorochromes throughout the imaged object are excited, out-of-focus signals heavily disturb images, just as in ordinary light microscopy.

Adding temporal resolution to fluorescence microscopy leads to fluorescence lifetime imaging (microscopy) [FLI(M)]. Available as a microscopic as well as a macroscopic technique, lifetime imaging concentrates on the sensitivity of a fluorochrome (and of its lifetime) to the environment, e.g., pH value. As a source, either pulsed or modulated light is used. For pulsed light, the observed fluorescence decay is multi-exponential, with different exponents for the different lifetimes in the sample. For modulated light, phase shifts are observed.

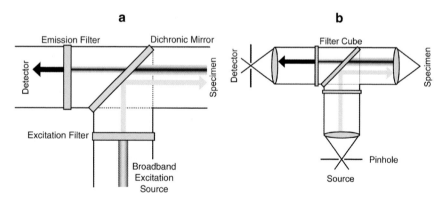

Fig. 5 a, b Principle of fluorescence and confocal microscope. **a** Schematic drawing of a filter cube as employed in fluorescence microscopes. Light from a source is filtered and reflected onto the sample by a dichroic mirror. Reflected fluorescence light is transmitted through the mirror and filtered, then guided onto the detector where a full image can be recorded. **b** In confocal scanning microscopy, the image of a point source is produced inside the sample. Only fluorescence light emitted from this focal spot is detected by the detector due to the presence of an additional pinhole aperture

4.2 Confocal Microscopy

To overcome the limitations of fluorescence microscopy, i.e., to limit detected signals to the focal plane (or to a focal spot) thus allowing full 3D scanning through the specimen, confocal microscopy was developed. Here, the specimen is not evenly illuminated. Instead, excitation light is focused onto a single point; detection is performed using basically the same optics as in standard fluorescence microscopy, including a pinhole aperture cutting away light originating from outside the focal spot (Fig. 5b). This single-point-illumination, single-point-detection technique allows scanning of the focal spot through the whole specimen, as long as there is only little scattering to disturb the appearance of the focus. Of course, necessary light intensities are high and scan times are long, so that photobleaching can become an issue when using fluorescent probes.

In order to further improve resolution, *two-photon microscopy* can be used. When two photons of approximately double the single-photon excitation wavelength interact with a fluorescent molecule within a very short time span, they can excite the molecule. The probability of two photons arriving simultaneously depends nonlinearly on light intensity. A laser beam of low photon flux is focused such that only in the focal spot the necessary photon density is reached to excite two-photon fluorescence (Helmchen and Denk, 2005) such that detected fluorescence signals originate exclusively from this small region. Three-dimensional images are obtained by scanning the focal spot over and into the specimen. In two-photon microscopy, light intensities are even stronger than in confocal microscopy, further increasing photobleaching and tissue damage issues.

4.3 4π Microscopy

The resolution in confocal microscopy is anisotropic: while it is about 250 nm in the focal plane, in axial direction it decreases to roughly half the resolution, about 500 nm. If, however, not one laser beam is focused, but if the beam is split and then focused from two sides, the focal spot will show an interference pattern (standing wave) with a strong central spot and smaller side lobes (Fig. 6). The central spot is much smaller than the original focal spot, thus increasing resolution if the side lobe signal is eliminated using deconvolution techniques. This technique can yield an isotropic resolution of about 100 nm (Hell 2003).

4.4 Stimulated Emission Depletion (STED)

An even higher resolution can be achieved using fluorescence depletion. Immediately following a very short excitation light pulse, another high-intensity light pulse at the emission wavelength is sent towards the sample. The time span between first

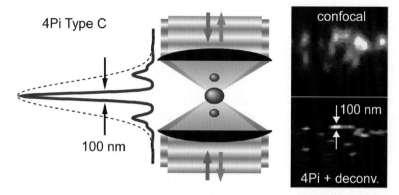

Fig. 6 Working principle of a 4π microscope and exemplary results. *Left*: Two lenses are used for focal spot creation from two opposing sides. As coherent light is used, a standing wave pattern evolves, having a small central maximum and several side lobes. The central lobe is significantly smaller than the size of the original focal spot in confocal microscopy. Side lobes have to be removed using deconvolution techniques. *Right*: Exemplary results, comparing cellular structures obtained with confocal and 4π microscopy, demonstrating the improved resolution. (Images kindly provided by Marion Lang, German Cancer Research Center, Heidelberg)

and second pulse needs to be shorter than the fluorescence lifetime. The second pulse is required to be sufficiently intense to force depletion of excited fluorescent molecules by *stimulated emission*. By use of a phase shifting plate, the shape of the focal region of the second pulse can be changed so that a very small central region is spared from depletion. Fluorescent signals originating from this region can still be detected after the depletion pulse. The size of this region can be less than 100 nm; a resolution of up to 50 nm seems realistic (Hell 2003). A schematic drawing of the instrument and the size of the source spot, which determines resolution, is depicted in Fig. 7.

4.5 Other Microscopic Techniques

Beside the techniques described in the paragraphs above, a couple of further microscopic imaging modalities are worth mentioning that try to overcome the diffraction limit. While the 4π or STED microscope use interference effects to reduce the size of the focal spot, structured illumination microscopy is a non-scanning, wide-field technique. Different excitation light patterns are used to excite fluorochromes; post-processing of the resulting images can yield highly resolved images. However, the spatial frequencies that can be contained in the excitation pattern are also band-limited due to Abbe's law. If again, as in STED or two-photon microscopy, non-linear effects exist in the excitation process, e.g., saturation effects, higher spatial frequencies will be contained in the emission and can be extracted in the post-processing (Gustafsson 2005).

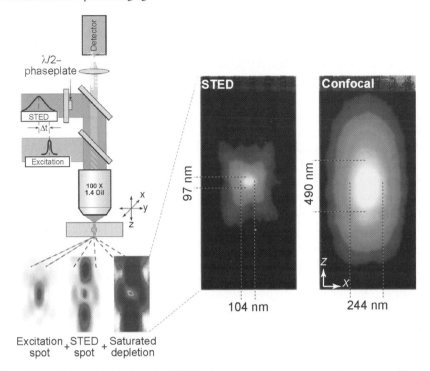

Fig. 7 *Left*: Schematic drawing of a STED microscope. The microscope is operated with two pulsed light sources, gated shortly after one another. The firs pulse excites the sample in the focal spot. The second pulse is directed through a phase plate to change appearance of the focal spot and depletes the excited fluorochromes in a region surrounding the focal spot. Only the remaining region can then spontaneously emit fluorescence photons. *Right*: Size and shape of the fluorescent spot in STED and confocal microscopy, showing significant resolution improvement. (Adapted from Hell 2003)

Microaxial tomography, as another candidate, extends confocal microscopy not to enhance resolution in the focal plane, but only axially, to get a more isotropic resolution. The imaged specimen, e.g., a cell, is fixed on the outside of a glass tube and rotated within the field of view of the confocal microscope. Thus, several sets of confocal 3D data are acquired, all having their own highly resolved focal plane; as those focal planes are not parallel to each other, tomographic reconstruction methods can be employed to reduce the size of the focal spot to the intersection of all focal spots. If images are acquired from 360°, the focal spot reduces to a sphere, yielding isotropic resolution (Heintzmann and Cremer 2002). A last technique to be mentioned is optoacoustic microscopy (Xu and Wang 2006). It is based on the photoacoustic effect, mentioned in more detail below.

5 Whole-Animal Imaging Techniques

5.1 Bioluminescence and Fluorescence Imaging

Acquiring bioluminescence signals in whole animals is rather trivial: all one needs, apart from suitable cell lines, is a light-tight chamber and a very sensitive CCD camera (Fig. 8). As no autofluorescence background or filter leakage from excitation light disturbs the actual signal, images are of rather good quality. It is possible to track very few cells even relatively deep inside the tissue (Massoud and Gambhir 2003).

Fluorescence reflectance imaging (FRI) requires additionally light sources to excite fluorochromes, and filters to eliminate the excitation light. Excitation and detection are performed on the same side of the imaged object, in reflectance geometry. As excitation light intensity as well as the sensitivity for fluorescence light decay exponentially with depth in tissue, this imaging modality is highly surface-weighted (Weissleder and Ntziachristos 2003). Filter leakage is a major problem, as a significant amount of excitation light is already reflected before entering the uppermost skin layer.

Yet another method to display fluorescent inclusions in tissue is to use *trans-illumination* instead of reflectance (Zacharakis et al. 2006). Here, excitation and detection are performed from opposite sides. Images are less surface-weighted as excitation light intensity decreases exponentially towards the detector while fluorescence sensitivity increases. Results can be further enhanced by "normalizing" acquired fluorescence images with images showing only excitation light. Thus, heterogeneities due to high absorption in tissue are reduced.

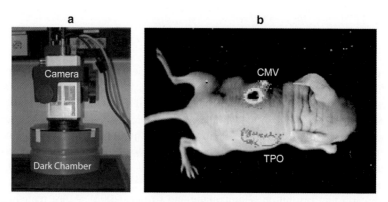

Fig. 8 a, b Bioluminescence imaging (BLI) of whole animals. **a** The necessary setup for BLI consists only of a dark chamber for animal placement and a sensitive CCD-camera; this setup is nowadays commercially available from a number of companies. **b** Sample result of bioluminescent tumors in a nude mouse. Modified Morris hepatoma cells were subcutaneously implanted as tumors on the left and right dorsal side of immunodeficient mice. Cells were modified to express firefly luciferase, tagged to different gene promoters (CMV and TPO, respectively)

5.2 Bioluminescence and Fluorescence Tomography

Tomographic imaging in optics requires a mathematical means of contributing a photon density distribution measured on the outer boundaries of the imaged object to absorbers, scatterers, or source inside the object; this is termed the *inverse problem*. Usually, the inverse problem is given via the direct problem: for a given propagation model, one tries to estimate a set of model parameters that give results fitting the actual measurements. The most common model used is the diffusion equation (Gibson et al. 2005):

$$\left[\nabla\frac{1}{3(1-g)\mu_s(\mathbf{r})}\nabla+\mu_a(\mathbf{r})\right]\Phi(\mathbf{r})=-q(\mathbf{r}) \tag{3}$$

In (3), $\mathbf{r}$ is the spatial coordinate, Φ is the photon density distribution, q is the photon source distribution, and μ_s and μ_a are scattering and absorption coefficients, respectively. The factor $(1-g)$, ranging between 0 and 2, accounts for the possibly anisotropic character of scattering. For purely isotropic scattering it is 1, for pure back-scattering it is 0, and for pure forward scattering, it is 2. Equation (3) models both, photon propagation from the excitation source as well as emitted photons. In the first case, q describes the light input and the model results in a photon distribution Φ_x that can excite fluorochromes. To model fluorescence, q is then replaced by Φ_x times the quantum efficiency and absorption (concentration times extinction) of the fluorochrome, i.e., $q_m(\mathbf{r})=\gamma\varepsilon c(\mathbf{r})\Phi_x(\mathbf{r})$.

Reconstruction is a process to estimate either μ_s and μ_a, or alternatively to calculate the concentration c. Usually, for fluorescence tomography μ_s and μ_a are assumed to be known and constant which simplifies the model dramatically. Nevertheless, reconstruction is mathematically challenging and time consuming. On the other hand, experimental acquisition of diffuse projections is a rather simple task, basically employing a laser diode source and a CCD coupled to the object either by an objective lens or by a number of fiber detectors mounted on some kind of gantry to enable transillumination of the object or animal from different directions, as shown in Fig. 9.

An important property of optical tomographic systems is whether light coupling is performed using fibers in contact with the imaged object, or whether contact-free detection via an objective lens is implemented (*noncontact imaging*; Schulz et al. 2004). While in fiber-based designs, complex shaped objects have to be embedded in some kind of optically matching fluid as the fiber ends usually cannot be positioned arbitrarily, this is unnecessary for non-contact designs. The embedding itself has another advantage as it simplifies the boundary conditions for the PDE and thus simplifies the reconstruction while attenuating the signal and making the mapping to anatomy more difficult in the end (when animals are imaged that have to be mounted floating in the matching fluids). Lens-coupled detection in turn offers much more channels, as every pixel of the CCD can be used, and enables imaging without matching fluid if and only if the object geometry is known (or can be acquired using a 3D scanning system) and thus appropriate boundary conditions can be applied.

a   b

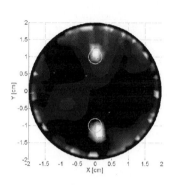

16bit cooled
CCD camera
with wide-angle
objective

Motor and gear

Phantom/Animal
in axis of rotation

Laser head, mounted
on linear stage

Fig. 9 **a** A typical non-contact optical tomography system, consisting of a sensitive CCD camera and a laser source, rotating around the imaged specimen. **b** Central transversal slice of a rat-sized diffuse phantom containing two fluorescent inclusions. Actual inclusion positions are denoted by *circles*. (Image courtesy of the authors)

For optical tomographic purposes, there exist also an abundance of techniques that employ time-resolved information for the location and quantization of fluorescence in vivo. The interested reader is referred to the review by Dunsby and French (2003).

In fluorescence tomography, usually several different source positions are chosen. For each position the fluorescent molecules located in the tissue are excited differently due to the different light distributions from different source positions. This change in excitation and thus emission pattern means additional information and in fact makes the whole problem of reconstructing concentrations tractable at all.

In bioluminescence tomography there is no excitation source. Therefore, one cannot acquire several different images from bioluminescence and then reconstruct based on the observed differences. Instead, what researchers try to perform is spectral imaging: light attenuation depends on wavelength. If the emission spectrum is known, the deviations of the observed light emissions from this original spectrum can be used to estimate the depth of the bioluminescent source in tissue (e.g., Dehghani et al. 2006). These techniques, however, are still under development; in vivo results are not yet available.

5.3 Optoacoustic Tomography

Another emerging imaging technique is optoacoustic tomography, which uses shortly pulsed laser sources for excitation but ultrasound detectors for detection (Xu and Wang 2006; Ntziachristos et al. 2005). The absorption of light by tissue or fluorochromes leads to local heating, which in turn leads to an expansion depending on the amount of energy absorbed. This expansion will create a pressure ($=$ sound) wave with a frequency in the ultrasound region.

This technique is advantageous over classical fluorescence tomography as ultrasonic reconstruction can be performed more easily than optical reconstruction, albeit it is more complex than standard ultrasound imaging as it is based on the diffusion equation as well, not on mere echo times. Optoacoustic tomography is capable of showing anatomic details, however, this might decrease its sensitivity for specific probes as probe signal and tissue signal have to be dissolved. For details on the technique, please refer to Wang (2003–2004).

6 Summary

Optical imaging offers unique possibilities for in vitro and in vivo imaging applications, especially in the context of molecular imaging. Understanding the fundamentals of optical imaging and grasping the pros and cons of available imaging techniques is a must for researchers interested in the field. This chapter reviewed the basic concepts of optical imaging instrumentation as well as state-of-the-art imaging techniques. For more detailed discussions of the subject, the reader is kindly referred to the articles below.

References

Dehghani H et al (2006) Spectrally resolved bioluminescence optical tomography. Opt Lett 31:365–367

Dunsby C, French PMW (2003) Techniques for depth-resolved imaging through turbid media including coherence-gated imaging. J Phys D: Appl Phys 36:R207–R227

Gibson AP, Hebden JC, Arridge SR (2005) Recent advances in diffuse optical imaging. Phys Med Biol 50:R1–R43

Gustafsson MGL (2005) Nonlinear structured-illumination microscopy: wide-field fluorescence imaging with theoretically unlimited resolution. Proc Natl Acad Sci USA 102:13081–13086

Heintzmann R, Cremer C (2002) Axial tomographic confocal fluorescence microscopy. J Microsc 206:7–23

Hell SW (2003) Toward fluorescence nanoscopy. Nat Biotechnol 21:1347–1355

Helmchen F, Denk W (2005) Deep tissue two-photon microscopy. Nat Methods 2:932–940

Hielscher AH (2005) Optical tomographic imaging of small animals. Curr Opin Biotechnol 16:79–88

Hoffman RM (2005) The multiple uses of fluorescent proteins to visualize cancer in vivo. Nat Rev Cancer 5:796–806

Kraayenhof R, Visser AJWG, Gerritsen HC (2002) Fluorescence spectroscopy, imaging and probes: new tools in chemical, physical and life sciences. Springer, Berlin Heidelberg New York

Lakowicz JR (2006) Principles of fluorescence spectroscopy, 3rd edn. Springer, New York

Massoud TF, Gambhir SS (2003) Molecular imaging in living subjects: seeing fundamental biological processes in a new light. Genes Dev 17:545–580

Mobley J, Vo-Dinh T (2003) Optical Properties of Tissue. In: Vo-Dinh T (2003) Biomedical photonics handbook. CRC Press, Boca Raton, pp 2/1–2/75

Mycek M-A, Pogue BW (2003) Handbook of biomedical fluorescence. Marcel Dekker, New York

Ntziachristos V et al (2005) Looking and listening to light: the evolution of whole-body photonic imaging. Nat Biotechnol 23:313–320

Redmond RW (2003) Introduction to fluorescence and photophysics. In: Mycek M-A, Pogue BW (eds) Handbook of biomedical fluorescence. Marcel Dekker, New York, pp 1–28

Schulz RB, Ripoll J, Ntziachristos V (2004) Experimental fluorescence tomography of tissues with non-contact measurements. IEEE Trans Med Imaging 23:492–500

Shaner NC, Steinbach PA, Tsien RY (2005) A guide to choosing fluorescent proteins. Nat Methods 2:905–909

Vo-Dinh T (2003a) Biomedical photonics handbook. CRC Press, Boca Raton

Vo-Dinh T (2003b) Basic instrumentation in photonics. In: Vo-Dinh T (2003) Biomedical photonics handbook, CRC Press, Boca Raton, pp 6/1–6/30

Wang LV (2003–2004) Ultrasound-mediated biophotonic imaging: a review of acousto-optical tomography and photo-acoustic tomography. Dis Markers 19:123–138

Weissleder R, Ntziachristos V (2003) Shedding light onto live molecular targets. Nat Med 9:123–128

Xu M, Wang LV (2006) Photoacoustic imaging in biomedicine. Rev Sci Instrum 77:41–101

Zacharakis G et al (2006) Normalized transillumination of fluorescent proteins in small animals. Mol Imaging 5:153–159

Micro-CT

Marc Kachelrieß

1 Introduction

Tomographic imaging started with clinical X-ray computed tomography (CT) in 1972 (Hounsfield 1973). Since then, CT technology has rapidly advanced and clinical CT became radiology's powerhouse. In addition to clinical CT imaging, there is increasing need for preclinical exams such as scans of tissue samples, organs or whole animals (in vitro or in vivo) that are used as models to evaluate human diseases and therapies (IEEE 2004). For example, noninvasive imaging of mice gains

Marc Kachelrieß

Institute of Medical Physics (IMP), Friedrich-Alexander-Universität Erlangen-Nürnberg, Henkestraße 9, 91052 Erlangen, Germany

marc.kachelriess@imp.uni-erlangen.de

W. Semmler and M. Schwaiger (eds.), *Molecular Imaging I.*   23
Handbook of Experimental Pharmacology 185/I.
© Springer-Verlag Berlin Heidelberg 2008

in importance due to recent advances in mouse genomics and the production of transgenic mouse models. Longitudinal studies that use a single animal population can provide internally consistent long-term data and help to reduce the number of animals used and to cut down the costs.

Since many of the objects of interest are far smaller than a human body, and since one is interested in imaging vessels, bone structures or other details of microscopic size, it turns out that clinical CT scanners are not suitable for many preclinical imaging tasks. For example, laboratory mice or rats have a body diameter of not more than 5 cm. Compared with the 50-cm diameter of a clinical CT scanner's field of measurement, this is 10% or less. Only one tenth of the detector elements would be used when scanning such a specimen in a clinical CT scanner and, evidently, small animal anatomy cannot be imaged in a clinical CT scanner with an image quality equivalent to human anatomy. This low efficiency calls for dedicated scanners that are specialized for small objects and have a high spatial resolution; this is the reason why all clinical imaging modalities have been scaled down in recent years.

Higher spatial resolution — in which clinical CT achieves 0.25 mm, sufficient for human diagnostics — is obtained by either using clinical flat-panel imaging systems that achieve in the order of 150–200 μm or by using dedicated micro-CT scanners, which are usually defined to achieve a spatial resolution of 100 μm or better (Kalender 2005). This chapter will not discuss flat-panel imaging systems such as C-arm CT scanners or conventional CT scanners equipped with a flat-panel detector, because these devices are a compromise, allowing for large object size whilst seeking for higher spatial resolution. Rather, we will consider micro-CT technology, where dedicated scanners enable the optimum in image quality to be achieved for a given application. Nevertheless, many considerations, such as the dependency of spatial resolution on object size and the number of detector pixels, apply to both categories.

This chapter will further be restricted to those widely used scanners that employ an area detector and therefore acquire the data in cone-beam geometry. Neither former generations of micro-CT scanners that use only a single detector row or even a single detector element nor scanners based on cyclotron radiation that require expensive electron accelerators and therefore are hardly available will be discussed here.

Basic CT principles are discussed at first. Then, we will detail today's micro-CT design followed by considerations about image noise, spatial resolution and dose. To become aware of potential pitfalls, the chapter finishes with discussing sources of image artifacts. Besides one image showing nondestructive material testing, our focus lies in small animal imaging and imaging of tissue samples.

2 CT Principles

From conventional radiography it is known that the information available from a single projection is limited, since it shows a superimposition of all the objects in the X-ray. The information can be increased by taking two projections, typically anteroposterior and lateral. However, the radiographic images still show a

Radiography   **Tomography**

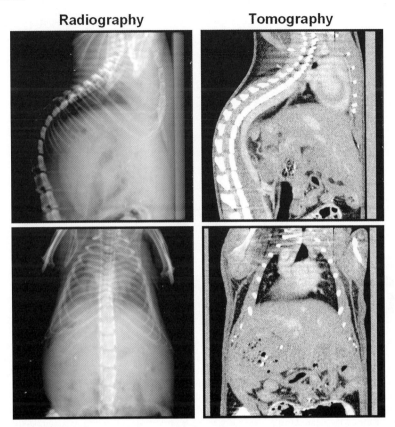

Fig. 1 Radiography provides only limited information due to the superimposed information of several objects. Typically, only one or two projections are acquired. CT, in contrast, allows complete volumetric information to be derived from a very large number of projections. The *left column* shows sagittal (*top*) and coronal (*bottom*) radiographic projections of a mouse in vivo. On the *right* we see multiplanar reformations (MPRs) of the reconstructed CT volume of the same mouse in the sagittal and coronal planes, respectively

superposition of all the objects that have been irradiated. Further, increasing the number of projection directions (views) is of little help because the observer is not able to mentally solve the superposition problem and to "reconstruct" the internal information of the object. The left column of Fig. 1 shows two such radiographic projections and we can clearly see the superposition of bone, tissue and lung. What we would rather like to see is a tomographic view of the object, as given in the right column.

2.1 Geometry

Fortunately it can be shown that a complete reconstruction of the object's interior is mathematically possible as long as a large number of views have been acquired over

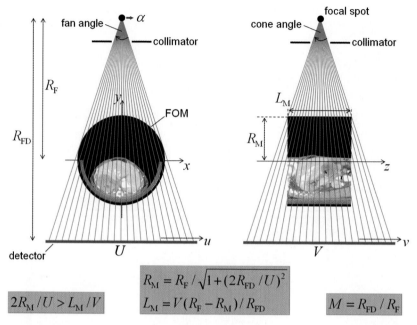

$$R_{\mathrm{M}} = R_{\mathrm{F}} / \sqrt{1 + (2R_{\mathrm{FD}} / U)^2}$$

$$2R_{\mathrm{M}} / U > L_{\mathrm{M}} / V \qquad L_{\mathrm{M}} = V(R_{\mathrm{F}} - R_{\mathrm{M}}) / R_{\mathrm{FD}} \qquad M = R_{\mathrm{FD}} / R_{\mathrm{F}}$$

Fig. 2 The principle of cone-beam micro-CT with flat-panel detectors. The object is illuminated by X-rays. Collimators shape the beam to match the rectangular shape of the detector. The gantry rotates about the z-axis to acquire a complete tomographic data set. Important relations for the radius R_{M} and the length L_{M} of the FOM are given in the *gray box* as a function of the distance of the focal spot to isocenter R_{F} and focal spot to detector R_{FD}, and the size $U \cdot V$ of the flat-panel detector. Note that the diameter of the FOM in relation to the detector size U is greater than the length of the FOM related to the detector size V. A ray or line integral is parameterized by the rotation angle α and the detector coordinates (u, v)

an angular range that covers at least 180° plus fan angle. This acquisition scheme is implemented in computed tomography scanners by using an X-ray tube together with a detector that rotate around the object or by using an object that rotates within the X-ray beam. On the opposing side of the X-ray tube, a flat area detector consisting of at least 1,000 by 1,000 detector pixels is mounted (Figs. 2, 3). Collimators are used to avoid radiation in those regions that are not covered by the detector. For today's rectangular flat-panel detectors, the shape of the X-ray ensemble is a pyramid; due to mathematical and historical reasons it is loosely called a cone-beam.

The rotation axis of the scanner defines the z-axis (longitudinal axis), the x- and y-axes are perpendicular thereto and define the axial plane. The opening angles of the cone are called the fan angle and cone angle, respectively (see Fig. 2). For square detectors that are perfectly aligned, the fan angle equals the cone angle. The distance of the focal spot to the isocenter (rotation center) R_{F} and the distance focus detector R_{FD} are important parameters in micro-CT imaging. Together with the radial size U and the longitudinal size V of the detector, they define the size of the cylinder that is measured in each projection during a 360° scan. This cylinder is called the field of

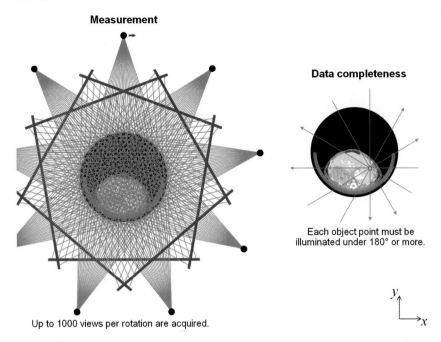

Measurement

Up to 1000 views per rotation are acquired.

Data completeness

Each object point must be illuminated under 180° or more.

Fig. 3 Micro-CT is the measurement of X-ray photon attenuation along straight lines. An object point can be reconstructed as long as it has been viewed by the X-rays under an angular interval of 180° or more. If this applies to all object points within the field of measurement, the data are said to be complete

measurement (FOM) and the object of interest must not exceed this volume laterally unless special techniques are used to enlarge the FOM (e.g., shifted detector, multiple scans or detruncation algorithms). For square detectors that are aligned with the z-axis, the cylinder's diameter always exceeds the cylinder's length. Objects that exceed the FOM longitudinally can be assessed by combining several circle scans or by performing a spiral scan.

In micro-CT, the typical scan trajectory is the circle scan. Here, the scanner performs a rotation about the stationary object. The rotation angle must be somewhat larger than a half circle, but to achieve good image quality it should be at least 360°. To scan objects longer than L_M, one can append the data from multiple circle scans. An alternative to this sequential, step-and-shoot or sequence scan is the spiral trajectory, where the scanner is rotating and acquiring continuously while the object is being translated through the isocenter along the z-direction (Kalender et al. 1990). Whereas the spiral trajectory is the most important trajectory in clinical CT, it has not yet received that much attention in micro-CT. Reasons may be dose due to the overscan problem and the requirement of slip-ring technology to allow for continuous scanning. We will, therefore, concentrate on the circle and sequence trajectories unless otherwise stated.

2.2 Measurement

During a full gantry rotation, in the order of 1,000 readouts of the detector are performed (Fig. 3). Altogether about 10^9 intensity measurements are taken per slice and rotation. Physically, X-ray CT is the measurement of the object's X-ray absorption along straight lines. For I_0 incident quanta, an object layer of thickness d and attenuation coefficient μ, the number I of quanta reaching the detector is given by the exponential attenuation law as

$$I = I_0 \, e^{-\mu d}.$$

The negative logarithm $p = -\ln I/I_0$ of each intensity measurement I gives us information about the product of the object attenuation and thickness. I_0 is the primary X-ray intensity and is needed for proper normalization. It is proportional to the tube current.

For nonhomogeneous objects, the attenuation coefficient is a function of x, y, and z. Then, the projection value p corresponds to the line integral along line L of the object's linear attenuation coefficient distribution $\mu(x,y,z)$:

$$p(L) = -\ln \frac{I(L)}{I_0} = \int_L dL \, \mu(x,y,z) \tag{1}$$

For flat-panel CT, the line L can be parameterized by the rotation angle α and the detector coordinates (u,v). Since $L = L(\alpha,u,v)$, one is free to abbreviate $p(L) = p(\alpha,u,v)$ whenever convenient. We are interested in gaining knowledge of $\mu(x,y,z)$ by reconstructing the acquired data $p(L)$. The process of computing the CT image $f(x,y,z)$ — the CT image is an accurate approximation to $\mu(x,y,z)$ — from the set of measured projection values $p(L)$ is called image reconstruction and is one of the key components of a CT scanner.

A more realistic description of the measurement process accounts for the polychromatic radiation that is emitted from the micro-focus X-ray tube's transmission or reflection anode. The attenuation coefficient is described as a function of the photon energy E and the coordinates (x,y,z) as $\mu(E,x,y,z)$. The spectrum as it is "seen" by the detector is given by the weight function $w(L,E)$, whose area is normalized to 1. Note that the spectrum depends on the ray position and orientation given by the line L. Then the observed attenuation is

$$p(L) = -\ln \int dE \, w(L,E) e^{-\int dL \mu(E,x,y,z)} \tag{2}$$

to which (1) is an adequate approximation whenever the polychromatic spectrum, and hence the integral over the energy, is replaced by a single effective energy E_{eff} that must be determined for a representative material and object, and that lies significantly below the electron charge tube voltage product eU. Errors that are introduced due to this polychromaticity and due to simply approximating it by (1) appear as cupping or capping artifacts and will be discussed in a separate section.

2.3 Reconstruction

For a moment, let us assume to have a single-slice CT scanner whose detector consists of one detector-row only. The raw data would be given by setting the longitudinal detector coordinate v to zero: $p(\alpha, u, 0)$. The easiest way to perform image reconstruction of these mid-plane data is to make a change of variables to obtain raw data in parallel-beam geometry: instead of describing the ray by the source position α and by the detector position u one can also describe the same mathematical line, $x\cos\vartheta + y\sin\vartheta = \xi$, using the ray's angle ϑ with respect to the coordinate system and the ray's distance ξ to the center of rotation by $\hat{p}(\vartheta, \xi) = p(\alpha, u, 0)$. The process of changing the variables to parallel geometry, which is also known as rebinning. Parallel beam image reconstruction consists of a filtering of the projection data with the reconstruction kernel, followed by a backprojection into image domain and can be formulated as

$$f(x,y) = \int_0^\pi d\vartheta \; \hat{p}(\vartheta, \xi) * k(\xi)|_{\xi = x\cos\vartheta + y\sin\vartheta}. \tag{3}$$

Here, $k(\xi)$ is the so-called reconstruction kernel. Usually, there are different convolution kernels available — e.g., smooth, standard, and sharp — to allow modifying image sharpness (spatial resolution) and image noise characteristics.

A historical derivation of this so-called filtered backprojection (FBP) is found in Shepp and Logan (1974). Formula (3) requires the projection data to be convolved with the reconstruction kernel $k(\xi)$. The filtered data are then backprojected into the image along the original ray direction for all ray angles ϑ. The extension to cone-beam data, where $v \neq 0$ in general, is straightforward and known as Feldkamp-type image reconstruction: simply ignore v during the filtering step (as done above), except for a length correction, but account for the true ray geometry during backprojection by using a three-dimensional backprojection. Feldkamp's original work did not perform a change of variables and used a true fan-beam filtered backprojection (Feldkamp et al. 1984). Today's micro-CT image reconstruction algorithms are mainly of the Feldkamp type. Whether there is rebinning involved or not does not significantly affect image quality and is often not disclosed by the manufacturers.

The discretization of the detector elements, the finite size of the active detector pixel area, the finite size focal spot and the discretization of the reconstructed volume, which is typically partitioned into cuboid voxels, imply a limited spatial resolution. The achievable spatial resolution of a given micro-CT scanner is mainly determined by the magnification factor, by the detector pixel size and by the size of the focal spot. A certain spatial resolution can only be achieved when it is not limited by the voxel size of the volume. Ideally, the voxel size should be half of the spatial resolution value or less. Achieving isotropic spatial resolution is desired. It allows the computation of arbitrarily oriented oblique multiplanar reformations (MPRs) with constant spatial resolution, and thus constant image quality.

Image reconstruction is a key component of the micro-CT scanner. Reconstruction times can range from some minutes up to 1 h, or even more, depending on the number of voxels used. Image reconstruction is an $O(N^4)$ process when N projections are backprojected into a volume of size N^3. The constant of proportionality lies in the range of 2–10 ns for today's micro-CT reconstruction engines, which means that a 512^3 reconstruction from 512 projections should be definitely finished in less than 5 min. Techniques that cut down this effort to $O(N^3 \log N)$ are described in the literature (Axelsson and Danielsson 1994; Basu and Bresler 2000; Bresler and Brokish 2003), but have probably not yet entered a product implementation for micro-CT cone-beam reconstruction.

2.4 Display

The image values $f(x, y, z)$ are usually converted into CT values prior to storage by passing them through the linear function

$$CT = \frac{f - \mu_{\text{water}}}{\mu_{\text{water}}} \cdot 1{,}000 \, \text{HU}$$

where HU stands for Hounsfield units. The relation is based on the demand that air (zero attenuation) has a CT value of $-1{,}000\,\text{HU}$ and water, the most common material CT scanners are calibrated for, has a value of $0\,\text{HU}$. The CT values have been introduced by Hounsfield to replace the handling with the rather inconvenient μ values by an integer-valued quantity. One can interpret the CT value of a pixel or voxel as being the density of the object relative to the density of water at the respective location. For example, $200\,\text{HU}$ means that the object density at that location is 1.2-times the density of water. This interpretation is only justified when polychromatic effects can be neglected. Otherwise the values are approximations to the density and to obtain the exact information an iterative beam hardening correction would have to be performed. An illustration of the CT scale is shown in Fig. 4. CT values typically range from $-1{,}000$ to $4{,}000\,\text{HU}$, except for very dense materials or for scans at very low energies.

Reconstructed CT data are usually displayed as grayscale images. To optimize contrast the mapping of CT numbers to gray values can be controlled by the user. In CT the display window is best parameterized by the two parameters, center C and width W. Values between $C - W/2$ and $C + W/2$ are linearly mapped to the gray values ranging from black to white, whereas values below and above that "window" are displayed in black and white, respectively (Fig. 5). For example, the window ($0\,\text{HU}/1{,}000\,\text{HU}$) means that it is centered at $0\,\text{HU}$ and has a width of $1{,}000\,\text{HU}$. Thus, values in the range from $-500\,\text{HU}$ to $500\,\text{HU}$ are mapped to the gray values; values below $-500\,\text{HU}$ are displayed black, and values above $500\,\text{HU}$ are displayed white.

It is understood that the micro-CT system needs to be calibrated against some typical object before any quantitative assessment of CT values is justified. In clinical CT, this calibration goes without saying and is done with respect to water. For

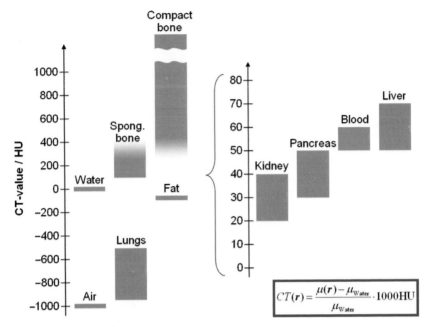

Fig. 4 Ranges of CT values of the most important organs (corresponding to humans at an effective energy of about 70 keV)

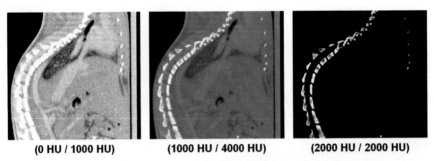

(0 HU / 1000 HU)   (1000 HU / 4000 HU)   (2000 HU / 2000 HU)

Fig. 5 In-vivo micro-CT image of a mouse displayed with three different window settings. The gray-scale windows are given in the format (center/width)

preclinical micro-CT imaging, adequate precorrection cannot be taken for granted and must be checked for explicitly. Typically, the system should be water-calibrated and a test image should show air at −1,000 HU and water at 0 HU. For nondestructive material, testing the base material may be chosen to be plastic, sand, or some other material of interest. The calibration is energy-dependent and must be carried out for the complete range of available tube voltages, prefiltrations, shaped filtration etc. Whenever quantitative analysis is required it is wise to scan a calibration phantom prior to the actual scans.

3 Micro-CT Design

Two basic design concepts are realized in micro-CT: the stationary tube-detector system with rotating object and the rotating gantry with stationary object.

3.1 Rotating Object Scanners

For in-vitro imaging, the design using a rotating object with a fixed focal-spot detector is the method of choice (Fig. 6). The design is robust and cost-efficient since the number of components moving during the scan — these must be of the highest precision to allow for high spatial resolution — is minimized to the rotation stage only. Furthermore, the scanner size is mainly determined by the distance of the focal spot to detector R_{FD}. For example, our self-made scanner shown in Fig. 6 requires an optical table of roughly 3 m by 1 m only. If the source and detector were to rotate about the object, a circular area of up to 3 m radius (6 m diameter) would be required, depending on the magnification used. The magnification itself can be easily adjusted with the help of automatic (or manual) translation stages that allow to

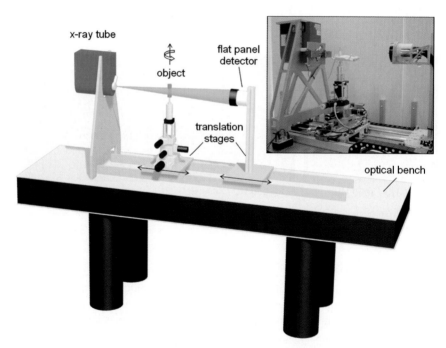

Fig. 6 Principle of in-vitro micro-CT (FORBILD scanner, self-made). The object rotates while the tube and detector are stationary. Translation stages allow the magnification of the scanner to vary over a wide range. When neither dose nor scan time is an issue, such scanners can achieve an extremely high spatial resolution (down to a few micrometers)

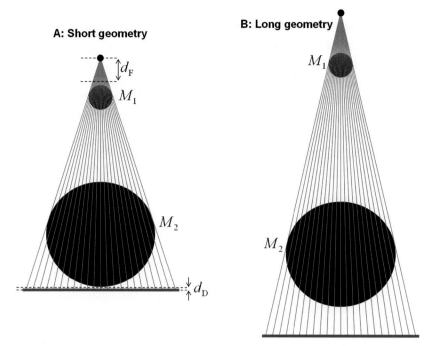

Fig. 7 The short cone-beam geometry has a larger fan and cone angle than the long cone-beam geometry. The wide cone yields a large X-ray flux but suffers from increased cone-beam artifacts. For the long geometry with the smaller solid angle, cone-beam artifacts are reduced, but one must cope with less quanta per time. Both geometries show identical small and large fields of measurement with identical magnification values and, consequently, identical spatial resolution

change R_F and R_{FD} over a wide range of values. The range itself is limited by the distance d_F of the exit window (that includes tube housing, prefiltration and shaped filtration) from the focal spot, by the distance d_D of the detector entrance window (that includes the detector housing and other protective gear) and by the radius of the field of measurement R_F such that the final inequality relating these parameters is $d_F + R_M < R_F < R_{FD} - d_D - R_M$.

Figure 7 illustrates two situations differing in the focus detector distance (short and long geometry). In both cases one may adjust R_F to achieve the same size of the field of measurement. A small and a large FOM are shown for the short and for the long geometry. The number of line integrals running through each of these FOMs is the same regardless of which geometry was chosen. Spatial resolution is merely a function of the mean distance of the rays, which is given by $2R_M/N_U$ and L_M/N_V. Thereby, N_U and N_V denote the number of detector pixels. Consequently, one may use the possibility to vary the magnification to balance between the size of the FOM and the spatial resolution.

But what is the difference between the short and the long geometry? There are negative effects of large cone angles. One disadvantage is that large angles usually imply a lower dose usage since parts of the object are irradiated which are not within

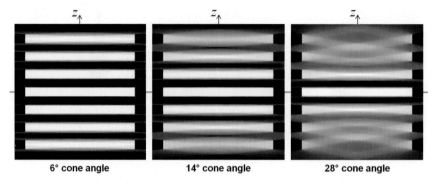

Fig. 8 Demonstration of cone-beam artifacts. The Defrise phantom consists of several disks centered about the z-axis. The cone-beam artifacts increase with increased distance to the midplane (*horizontal line*) and with increased cone angle

the longitudinal FOM (c.f. Fig. 2). Another disadvantage is that today's micro-CT image reconstruction algorithms are approximate and suffer from artifacts when the cone angle becomes large (Fig. 8). This requires small cone angles and therefore long geometries. However, the number of available X-ray photons is proportional to $1/R_{FD}^2$ will be low when the cone and fan angles are low. For example, doubling the focus detector distance will require a fourfold scan time (assuming the same tube power) to achieve the same image noise. Scan time, however, can become critical even for in-vitro scans. Figures 9 and 10 show some examples of in-vitro scans with very high resolution and a rather long scan time of 15 min.

A serious drawback of the rotating object scanners is the object placement. The rotation axis, and thus the object, is usually oriented vertically in these scanners. Regardless of what the actual orientation of the rotation axis is, be it vertical or horizontal, or something else, the object is subject to centrifugal or varying gravitational forces. Whereas this plays no role for rigid samples it can impair image quality when flexible objects or liquids are scanned. Prominent examples are vertically oriented small animals, where parts of the body tend to slide downwards due to released muscle tension during the scan; no fixation can completely avoid this kind of motion.

3.2 Rotating Gantry Scanners

Scanners with a rotating source-detector system are more complicated with respect to the mechanical setup but they provide far more comfort regarding the object placement. The rotating gantry is usually mounted with a horizontal rotation axis to allow the object to be supported by a simple table. Thereby, these scanners resemble the clinical CT scanners that also have a patient bed and a rotating gantry. Object fixation and immobilization is less tricky than with rotating object scanners. However, the mechanical design of rotating source-detector scanners is far more

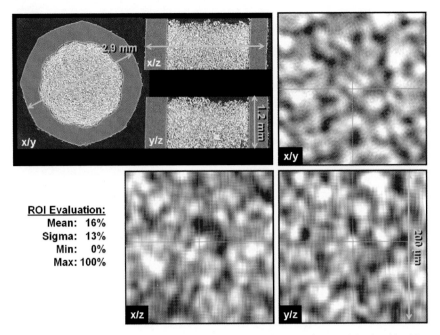

ROI Evaluation:
Mean: 16%
Sigma: 13%
Min: 0%
Max: 100%

Fig. 9 Scan of a butterfly catheter filled with chromatography gel (glass particles in air) with an average grid size of 35 µm. The high spatial resolution achieved with the FORBILD scanner allows each single glass particle (voxel size 1 µm) to be displayed

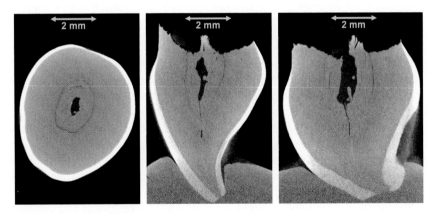

Fig. 10 Milk tooth fixed in plasticine scanned with a rotating object micro-CT scanner (FORBILD scanner) with 10-µm spatial resolution (5-µm voxel size) at 80 kV. The data are not corrected for beam hardening effects. Besides slight cupping, a seeming reduction of the enamel's density appears in the region where the tooth sticks inside the plasticine. Measurements outside that region yield $\rho_{enamel} \approx 2.3\rho_{dentine} \approx 2.8\rho_{plasticine}$

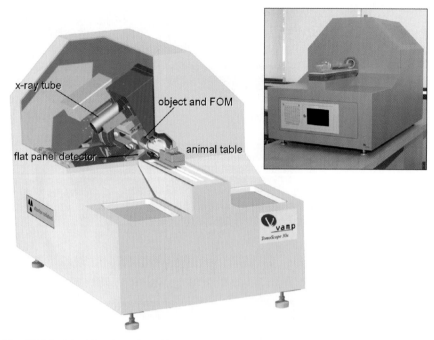

Fig. 11 Principle of in-vivo micro-CT. The object is placed on the animal table. During the scan the gantry rotates around the animal, just as in clinical CT scanners. Spiral scans are possible. Some in-vivo scanners allow the magnification to be changed. Desktop systems such as the one shown here (TomoScope 30s, VAMP, Möhrendorf, Germany) are often shipped with a fixed and optimized geometry (Karolczak 2005). Dose, scan time and interscan delay are critical issues that must be optimized by the manufacturers

demanding since high precision rotation components must be used and care must be taken that the varying gravitational forces do neither change the rotation speed nor change the mechanical alignment of the source and the detector relative to each other and relative to the rotation axis.

For dedicated imaging tasks, one can do without varying magnification. Then, compact cost-effective light-weight self-shielded desktop systems that even fit into small laboratories can be designed and, above all, be optimized (Fig. 11). In addition to such dedicated small animal scanners with a fixed FOM size, there are systems available with the possibility to mechanically change the magnification. Needless to say that the added flexibility requires a compromise in image quality and that these all-round systems are rather bulky and expensive.

Typical in-vivo images that are acquired with a rotating gantry micro-CT scanner are shown in Figs. 12 and 13 and in many of the other images of this chapter where cross-sections of mice are displayed. Figure 12 is a volume rendering (that actually resembles a shaded surface display) of the skeleton and only the high-contrast objects are shown. These kinds of bone images have been very popular in the past for several reasons. Besides the fact that displays of skeletons are spectacular and

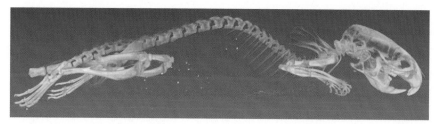

Fig. 12 Volume rendering of an in-vivo sequence scan with three table positions and 3 min per table position (TomoScope 30s scanner). Tube voltage 40 kV, tube current 0.8 mA, effective mAs product 144 mAs

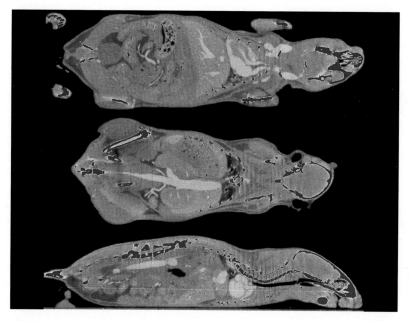

Fig. 13 Some cross-sections through the same data as shown in Fig. 12. The pixel values are mapped in color instead of using the usual gray scale

impressive, the main reason is that the past generation of micro-CT scanners was not able to show low contrast details, especially not for in-vivo scans. Low contrast details are easily obscured by image noise and it is a question of scan time, of X-ray power, of detector capacities (dynamic range) and, last but not least, of dose whether low contrast objects can be displayed or not.

Figure 13 and several other images in this chapter prove that today's technology allows to image low-contrast objects as well. Compared with clinical CT, which allows to distinguish between 10 HU contrast or less, micro-CT contrast is still slightly inferior and lies in the range of 20–100 HU.

Table 1 Essential parameters of CT-scanners

	In-vitro micro-CT	In-vivo micro-CT	C-arm CT	Clinical CT
Spatial resolution	$1\ldots200\,\mu$m	$50\ldots200\,\mu$m	$200\ldots400\,\mu$m	$250\ldots1000\,\mu$m
FOM diameter	$1\ldots200\,$mm	$30\ldots100\,$mm	$100\ldots250\,$mm	$500\ldots700\,$mm
Tube voltage	$10\ldots160\,$kV	$10\ldots160\,$kV	$50\ldots125\,$kV	$80\ldots140\,$kV
Tube current	$0.04\ldots2\,$mA	$0.04\ldots2\,$mA	$10\ldots800\,$mA	$10\ldots600\,$mA
Tube power	$1\ldots30\,$W	$1\ldots30\,$W	$20\ldots80\,$kW	$20\ldots100\,$kW
Scan time	$<1\,$h	$10\,$s$\ldots10\,$min	$5\ldots20\,$s	$0.3\ldots20\,$s
mAs$_{\text{eff}}$	$5\ldots200\,$mAs	$5\ldots200\,$mAs	$10\ldots750\,$mAs	$10\ldots750\,$mAs
Detector	$1024^2\ldots4096^2$	$1024^2\ldots4096^2$	$1024^2\ldots2048^2$	$\approx1000\times64$
Dose	$\leq1500\,$mGy	$50\ldots500\,$mGy	$1\ldots70\,$mGy	$1\ldots70\,$mGy
Acquisition rate	$\leq20\,$MB/s	$\leq20\,$MB/s	$\leq60\,$MB/s	$\leq600\,$MB/s

3.3 Typical Parameters

Table 1 lists important parameters as they are typically provided in today's flat-panel detector CT scanners and in today's clinical CT scanners. The values given should be understood as being orders of magnitude, and exact values as well as maximum and minimum values from specific systems will certainly differ from or exceed those given in the table. To differentiate between in-vitro and in-vivo scanners we mainly considered dose, low-contrast resolution and scan time. In-vivo small-animal imaging requires a good low-contrast resolution (i.e., low image noise) at dose values as low as reasonably achievable. In-vivo scans should be very short to simplify anesthesia and animal handling. These facts must be emphasized since they are not common practice in small animal imaging yet.

4 Dose and Image Quality

Dose and image quality are inherently related: less dose means higher image noise, which in turn implies inferior low contrast resolution. High spatial resolution demands for higher dose unless higher image noise can be accepted. Achieving a certain image quality within a given voxel requires a certain number of photons to be absorbed within that voxel.

4.1 Dose and Noise

Is dose an issue for micro-CT? Yes it is and there are reasons why it is of advantage to generate high image quality with as little photons as possible. The most obvious reason is potential radiation damage to the object. In particular, for in-vivo scans one may find that the animals can suffer from the radiation. Even if there is no deterministic risk to be expected — this is the case whenever dose levels are far below, say, 1 Gy — the measurement may influence those parameters that shall be observed in preclinical imaging. Tumor growth, for example, may be modified by a micro-CT scan with high dose levels. Cell populations may behave differently after having been irradiated. Functional parameters may change as a result of micro-CT radiation. Above all, longitudinal studies require multiple scans of the very same animal and the total dose to the subject must be kept as low as reasonably achievable.

Even if dose to the object does not have to be limited, there are technical restrictions that require to scan with low dose. One key component in micro-CT is the X-ray tube, whose maximum power is a function of the focal-spot size. A rule of thumb is that the maximum power per focal-spot area lies in the order of $1\,W/\mu m^2$. Values above that— some manufacturers offer tubes with up to $3\,W/\mu m^2$ — significantly decrease the tube's durability. High spatial resolution requires small focal-spot sizes and therefore reduced X-ray power. Low X-ray power means increased scan time. Any technology that allows scanning with less photons can be useful to decrease the scan time and thereby to improve throughput.

Another key component is the X-ray detector. Today, either direct or indirect converting detectors are used. The dose required to saturate the detector is determined by the absorption efficiency and by the detector pixel's capacity. A high absorption efficiency means a good dose usage and can reduce the total scan time. However, high absorption efficiencies require thick layers of scintillators, which in turn imply smoother presampling MTFs and thus a lower spatial resolution. The time required to read out the detector, the detector's frame rate, often determines the total scan time.

An important and basic parameter in CT imaging is the effective tube current time product mAs_{eff}, which is also called mAs product. It is defined as the tube current multiplied by the time a given voxel is irradiated. For $360°$-scans, the time of irradiation equals the rotation time of the scanner. The effective mAs value is proportional to the number of X-ray photons that contribute to the measurement and it is proportional to the number of X-ray photons that contribute to a certain projection voxel position, and thereby it is proportional to the dose. As an example, consider a tube that runs with 14 W of power at a voltage of 40 kV and thus delivers 0.35 mA. For an in-vivo scan of 20-s duration, this scanner would achieve an effective mAs value of 7 mAs. Typical effective mAs values range from 5 mAs to 200 mAs. Low values yield high image noise and vice versa. The pixel standard deviation σ is the typical measure of image noise. It is inversely proportional to the square of the effective mAs-value,

$$\sigma^2 \propto \frac{1}{mAs_{eff}}.$$

Reducing noise by 50% requires a fourfold increase of mAs_{eff}, for example.

4.2 Spatial Resolution

Another important parameter is spatial resolution. One has to distinguish between the in-plane spatial resolution Δr and the longitudinal resolution Δz. Ideally, one would expect isotropic spatial resolution, which means $\Delta r = \Delta z$. However, we have seen that the reconstruction process differs significantly in the way the axial and the longitudinal density distribution is reconstructed. The axial direction is the direction where filtering is applied and therefore in-plane resolution can be easily modified by choosing the reconstruction kernel. In the longitudinal direction there is no inherent possibility to modify the data, and the z-resolution is likely to be close to the detector pixel size projected to the isocenter $\Delta v R_F / R_{FD}$. Due to these differences in axial and longitudinal direction, $\Delta r \neq \Delta z$ is typical.

To find a quantitative relationship between image noise σ and spatial resolution, assume the linear attenuation of a resolution element of size Δr to be μ. Let I_0 be the number of photons incident on that voxel. Then the number of photons that leave the resolution element is given as

$$I = I_0 e^{-\mu \Delta r}.$$

Our aim is to estimate μ (which corresponds to the CT value). A good estimator is

$$\hat{\mu} = -\frac{1}{\Delta r} \ln \frac{I}{I_0}.$$

Since I and I_0 are random, the estimated value $\hat{\mu}$ is random, too. The error σ of the random variable $\hat{\mu}$ is the noise in that resolution element and can be estimated by error propagation as

$$\sigma^2 = \frac{1}{\Delta r^2} \left(\frac{\text{Var } I}{E^2 I} + \frac{\text{Var } I_0}{E^2 I_0} \right).$$

The number I_0 of incident photons is Poisson distributed and thus I is Poisson, too. This implies $\text{Var } I_0 = E I_0$ and $\text{Var } I = E I$. Further, one has the property $E I \propto E I_0$ due to the attenuation law and the property $E I_0 \propto \Delta r \Delta z \text{mAs}_{\text{eff}}$, where $\Delta r \Delta z$ is the beam cross-section and D is dose or flux. Using these, we obtain

$$\sigma^2 \propto \frac{1}{\text{mAs}_{\text{eff}} \cdot \Delta z \cdot \Delta r^3} \tag{4}$$

which relates spatial resolution, effective tube-current and image noise σ. Relation (4) is often derived under more special assumptions in Brooks and Di Chiro (1976b) and Ford et al. (2003), for example by assuming a filtered backprojection reconstruction.

The constant of proportionality in (4) depends in a complicated way on the object size and density, on the tube voltage, and on the prefiltration. (4) shows that a 16-fold increase of dose (or mAs_{eff}) is required when spatial resolution shall be improved by a factor of 2 in all three dimensions and pixel noise σ is to be held constant. Obviously it is impossible to significantly increase the spatial resolution in micro-CT without accepting more dose or higher image noise. Preclinical low-contrast imaging of small animals is possible with a spatial resolution in the order of 100 μm but not with a spatial resolution of 10 μm, where only high-contrast structures such as the skeleton can be imaged adequately and at acceptable dose.

4.3 Dose and Noise Reduction

Techniques to reduce image noise or, equivalently, to reduce object dose include adaptive filtering, statistical reconstruction techniques and automatic exposure control. Adaptive filtering is a raw data-based approach that selectively smoothes only a few raw data values using a three-dimensional smoothing kernel (both detector dimensions plus the rotation direction by accessing neighboring projections) (Kachelrieß et al. 2001; Kachelrieß and Kalender 2000a). In contrast to using smooth reconstruction kernels multidimensional adaptive filtering does not impair spatial resolution. Replacing the standard Feldkamp-type approximate micro-CT image reconstruction algorithms by statistical reconstruction techniques further promises to reduce image noise (Lange and Fessler 1995; Erdogan and Fessler 1999; Lange and Carson 1984; Beekman and Kamphuis 2001; Kachelrieß et al. 2005a). However, statistical reconstruction algorithms are iterative and too slow to be routinely used in micro-CT imaging. Adapting the exposure to the object shape is another option to improve dose usage. In clinical CT, such automatic exposure control (AEC) techniques are very successful already. To our knowledge there are no corresponding product implementations in micro-CT, yet.

Another parameter that plays a significant role in dose optimization is the total scan length or scan range. Although being trivial, it is worth mentioning that scan ranges which exceed the region of interest are a waste of dose. For example, consider a micro-CT scan where the organ of interest has a longitudinal extent of 1 cm, say. Let the size of the scanner's field of measurement be about 4 cm in diameter and length. A scan that acquires the full FOM would then apply three-times more dose than actually necessary. Therefore one must use the longitudinal collimators, if available, to reduce the length of the FOM as far as possible. Similarly, if a sequence or a spiral scan is performed to cover a very long region, it is of importance to keep the scan range as short as possible.

Tube voltage, target materials (e.g., tungsten or molybdenum), prefiltration and shaped filtration determine the X-ray spectrum $w(L,E)$ that is used for CT scanning. The image quality is a function of the X-ray spectrum, object size, shape and density (Sekihara et al. 1982; Gkanatsios and Huda 1997). There are no general guidelines of how to predict the optimal spectrum and how to choose the tube voltage as a function of the object. But it can be shown that the effective linear attenuation coefficient μ_{eff} multiplied by the object diameter d should be kept rather constant. The value of this constant depends on whether one optimizes the X-ray flux on the detector or optimizes the dose in the object, and it can be determined only under the highly restrictive assumption of homogeneous, circular cross-sections and monochromatic scatter-free radiation. Nevertheless, the rule $\mu_{\mathrm{eff}}d \approx const$ indicates that small objects require large attenuation coefficients. The attenuation coefficient becomes larger for lower energy photons, and consequently tube voltage should be decreased with decreasing object size and density. This dependency on object size is more significant for small objects than it is for large objects, since for low energies photon attenuation is dominated by the photo effect, which is strongly energy dependent. Therefore, there is a higher potential for dose reduction in micro-CT than in clinical CT. Note that tube voltages as low as 10 kV can be of interest for micro-CT imaging.

4.4 Quality Assessment

Dose and image quality can be easily assessed using dedicated micro-CT phantoms (Fig. 14). A convenient way to quantify spatial resolution is by bar patterns of various sizes (typically given in line pairs per millimeter). The spatial resolution of an image is defined to be the size of the smallest bar pattern whose bars are still separated. To find out whether two neighboring bars are separated reduce the CT image to a binary (i.e., black-and-white) image by setting the window width to 0 HU and then adjust the window center such that the bars appear white and

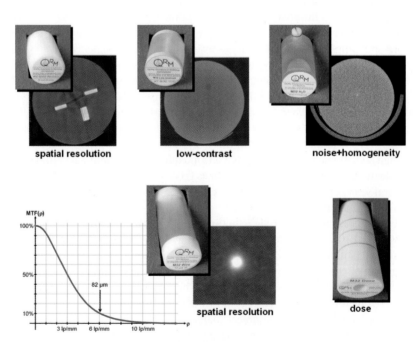

Fig. 14 Quality assurance phantoms (courtesy of QRM, Möhrendorf, Germany) are used to calibrate the scanner and to assess spatial resolution, low-contrast resolution, noise and dose

that the gap between the bars appears black — no white pixels must connect two bars. If this applies to a complete group of bars at once, this group is said to be resolved. Another possibility to measure the spatial resolution is to use wire phantoms such as the 10-μm wire phantom shown in Fig. 14. Reconstructions thereof allow the point spread function (PSF) and the modulation transfer function (MTF) to be determined. Typical figures of merit taken from there are the full width at half maximum (FWHM) of the PSF or the 10% value of the MTF.

The reader must be cautioned against mistaking spatial resolution with voxel size; the voxel size is merely a parameter of image reconstruction! Ideally, the voxels should be smaller than half of the desired spatial resolution. It is also worth noting that statements about a system's voxel size, as often provided by marketing departments, do not allow deduction of the scanner's resolution. For example, it is possible to perform reconstructions with a voxel size of 1 μm, although the spatial resolution of the system is only 5 μm (c.f. Fig. 9).

Low-contrast resolution can be estimated using phantoms with low-contrast inserts of different density levels and of different sizes. The phantom shown in Fig. 14 has four cylindrical inserts of −10-HU and −50-HU contrast and of 1-mm and 2.5-mm diameter.

Water phantoms are useful to control the system's homogeneity and to measure the pixel noise. Since the phantom is of homogeneous water the gray level of all voxels that lie in the phantom should be at 0 HU (plus minus noise). The surrounding air must show up at −1,000 HU. A region-of-interest (ROI) evaluation in the water gives the standard deviation of the pixel values which is a measure of image noise. Weekly automated quality check routines should test for homogeneity and they should ensure that the image noise meets the expectations (for a given effective mAs value and a given spatial resolution).

Dose D is measured by inserting an ionization chamber into a dedicated micro-CT dose phantom. Note that a separate dose assessment is necessary, although D is proportional to the effective mAs value. The constant of proportionality, however, is a function of tube voltage, of X-ray tube design, of detector type, of the phantom and of many more parameters. To obtain a complete dose distribution $D(\boldsymbol{r})$, a Monte Carlo-based dose calculation is required (Schmidt and Kalender 2002), which uses the central dose determined with the ionization chamber for normalization.

To compare different scan protocols and different scanners, given that the same set of phantoms is used and that the scanners are properly normalized to the Hounsfield scale, it is useful to boil down the parameters spatial resolution, noise and dose into a single image quality figure of merit Q. According to (2), and using the proportionality $D \propto \text{mAs}_{\text{eff}}$, we find

$$Q^2 = \frac{1}{\Delta z \cdot \Delta r^3 \cdot \sigma^2 \cdot D} \qquad (5)$$

where high values of Q are desired.

A recent study that compared in-vivo micro-CT scanners from four different vendors — the selected scan protocols were those dedicated to small animal imaging — found inter-vendor variations in Q by a factor of four (Kalender et al. 2005). From

(5), we find that this means that the best performing system is 16-times more dose efficient than the least performing system included in the said study. These differences among today's preclinical micro-CT systems should definitely alert the reader.

5 Artifacts

Our discussion of image quality did not include micro-CT artifacts so far. Similar to clinical CT, there are several sources of error that may propagate into the image. In contrast to clinical images, some of these artifacts are more pronounced and less easy to avoid in micro-CT. One source of artifacts, for example, is the geometric misalignment of the scanners. The position and orientation of the X-ray source, of the detector pixels and of the axis of rotation must be known much more accurately than the desired spatial resolution. For micro-CT applications, this means that the scanner must be aligned with micrometer precision or even better. Such a precise alignment is hardly possible; one difficulty is thermal expansion of the scanner, for example. Therefore, correction methods and methods to quantify the actual alignment of the components were developed. Most of these misalignment correction algorithms require to scan a phantom of known shape and/or density (Azevedo et al. 1990; Crawford et al. 1988; Hsieh 1999; Gullberg et al. 1987, 1990; Marquadt 1963; Bronnikov 1999; Noo et al. 2000; Rougee et al. 1993a, b; Wiesent et al. 1999, 2000; Stevens et al. 2001), which just passes on the alignment problem to the phantom manufacturer, but some correction methods are more flexible and allow for rather arbitrary calibration phantoms (von Smekal et al. 2004).

Defective detector pixels or completely defective detector columns or rows are another source of error in micro-CT. Here, every manufacturer uses their own correction algorithms. These may include some kind of interpolation to bridge the defect areas of the detectors. Advanced techniques to predict projection values falling into the range of defect detectors from previously acquired projections are considered too (Riess 2002). More subtle detector defects include a variation of the detector sensitivity as a function of scan time or detector age. In this case, the detector is not really defective but it rather reports a slightly shifted intensity value. The artifacts caused by these sensitivity variations are ring artifacts. These can be corrected by either analyzing and modifying the acquired CT raw data or by image-based methods (Riess 2002; Sijbers and Postnov 2004).

Given that a micro-CT scanner is well aligned and that defective detector pixels are corrected for there are still a number of other artifacts that can impair image quality in a qualitative or quantitative sense. One of these is cone-beam artifacts, which were discussed in Sect. 3 on micro-CT design and in Fig. 8. These cone-beam artifacts are inevitable as long as the scanner acquires from circular trajectories only. The circular trajectory is known to be incomplete with respect to image reconstruction. Other trajectories, such as the popular spiral trajectory, are complete, and given an exact image reconstruction algorithm, then cone-beam artifacts can be avoided. However, as long as efficient but approximate Feldkamp-type

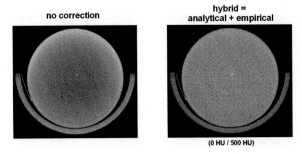

Fig. 15 Various levels of cupping correction are required to obtain a perfectly "flat" image of a homogeneous object. Only with cupping correction do the CT values become quantitative. For example, the table that has a density of 0.95-times the density of water shows up darker than the water phantom only in the precorreted data

cone-beam algorithms are used, one will encounter cone-beam artifacts, even for complete source trajectories.

X-ray polychromaticity is another source of artifacts. Physically, (2) reflects the measurement but technically (1) is assumed to be true. This approximation of polychromatic and thus nonlinear attenuation effects by a monochromatic situation (line integrals through the linear attenuation coefficient) is necessary since line integrals are required for analytic image reconstruction. Beam polychromaticity and X-ray scatter will result in cupping artifacts, which means that the gray values close to the center of the object will be artificially lowered compared with those values reconstructed at the edge of the objects (Fig. 15). These spectral effects, and especially the cupping effect, are a problem also for clinical CT and, consequently, there is a large amount of literature on helping to correct for the cupping (McDavid et al. 1975, 1977; Brooks and Di Chiro 1976a; Zatz and Alvarez 1977; Herman 1978, 1979a, 1979b; Kijewski and Bjarngard 1978; Reed, 1980; Imamura and Fujii 1981; Rao and Alfidi 1981; Rührnschopf an Kalender 1981; Herman and Trivedi 1983; Jackson and Hawkes 1983; Young et al. 1983; McLoughlin et al. 1991; Ruth and Joseph 1995; Goodsitt 1995). Instead of using the term cupping correction, one may speak of water precorrection. This reflects the fact that the cupping is corrected with respect to water, which resembles human or animal tissue very closely. In clinical CT, applying such a water precorrection algorithm is today's standard.

The effects of a novel cupping correction algorithm, which has the advantage over other existing approaches to require only very little knowledge about the calibration phantom (Sourbelle et al. 2004, 2006), are demonstrated in Figs. 15 and 16. It is interesting to note that the effect of the cupping correction is evident in the homogeneous phantom of Fig. 15, but it is not obvious in the mouse image of Fig. 16. Apparently, the gray values of Fig. 16 change from the noncorrected to the corrected images. But which images are better and which gray values are the true ones? This question cannot be answered from regarding the mouse images only, and the dilemma is that the unaware user is likely to apply quantitative evaluations to the noncorrected data (if his micro-CT scanner does not guarantee perfect calibration

no precorrection

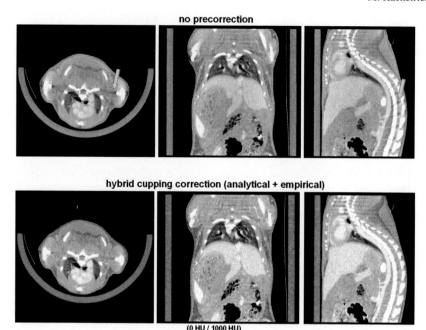

hybrid cupping correction (analytical + empirical)

(0 HU / 1000 HU)

Fig. 16 In-vivo scan of a mouse (TomoScope 30s scanner) with and without cupping correction. Whereas the cupping is not that apparent in inhomogeneous objects, we can clearly see the effects regarding the table and regarding the table's relative gray value compared with that within the mouse. Also note that second order beam-hardening effects, such as the dark streaks between bones (*arrows*), are far less pronounced in the bottom images, where first-order polychromatic effects were corrected

and homogeneity) and the invalid values will falsify the outcome of the study. Scans of a water phantom (Fig. 14) should be used to check for homogeneous and well-calibrated values before doing any quantitative analysis. In case of Fig. 16, we know that the density of the animal table is 5% lower than that of water. Consequently, the table must appear darker than the tissue and only the lower row of images can be the correct one.

Figure 16 also shows that dark streaks connecting high-density objects are greatly reduced by the water precorrection. The streaks cannot be completely removed because the precorrection assumes the object to be water equivalent and cannot perfectly correct for the effects caused by bones. For a better removal, second order beam hardening correction algorithms or even higher order approaches are required (Joseph and Spital 1978; Ruegsegger et al. 1978; Nalcioglu and Lou 1979; Stonestrom et al. 1981; Olson et al. 1981; Robertson and Huang 1986; Meagher et al. 1990; Hsieh et al. 2000). These are iterative; they slow down the reconstruction process and are not in routine use today. Beam hardening correction using dual-energy CT scans has been evaluated as an alternative (Coleman and Sinclair 1985).

In contrast to clinical CT, there are no scatter rejection methods, such as scatter grids, available in micro-CT. Scatter becomes more significant the larger the cone-angle becomes. X-ray scatter introduces cupping artifacts too, and scatter artifacts resemble first order beam hardening artifacts. Empirical precorrection algorithms that aim at reducing cupping in general do not discern between cupping due to spectral effects or due to scatter effects and thereby reduce both sources of errors (Figs. 15, 16). For higher order scatter removal, advanced correction algorithms must be used. To predict the scatter intensity, these either use raw data-based convolution approaches or image-based scatter prediction using Monte Carlo methods or deterministic calculations (Joseph and Spital 1982; Colijn and Beekman 2004; Johns and Yaffe 1982; Siewerdsen and Jaffray 2001; Ohnesorge et al. 1999; Ning et al. 2004; Seibert and Boone 1988). The image-based scatter correction algorithms are iterative. They require multiple reconstructions and are not in routine use yet.

Other sources of artifacts are object motion, dense objects and objects exceeding the field of measurement. Object motion can be minimized by adequate placement of the objects or by using prospective (Ford et al. 2005) or retrospective gating techniques (Kachelrieß and Kalender 1998; Kachelrieß et al. 2000b), the latter have the potential to be synchronized without acquiring external signals (Kachelrieß et al. 2002). Very dense objects, such as bones, pieces of metal (e.g. ECG leads) or very high concentration of contrast agent, tend to yield dark streaks in the image. In clinical CT, these artifacts are known as metal artifacts, since they most likely emerge from metal implants such as prostheses, dental fillings or surgical clips. These kinds of artifacts are reduced to some extent by cupping precorrection algorithms. Although there is a large amount of literature covering artifact removal from nearly radio-opaque objects (Watzke and Kalender 2004; Wang et al. 1999; De Man et al. 2000; Zhao et al. 2000; Glover and Pelc 1981; Kalender et al. 1987; Moseley et al. 2005), there is no optimal algorithm known yet. Data truncation by objects radially exceeding the field of measurement impairs image quality at the edge of the FOM. Empirical algorithms to correct for the data truncation are highly efficient to remove these truncation artifacts (Sourbelle et al. 2005; Hsieh et al. 2004; Ohnesorge et al. 2000).

6 Summary and Outlook

Modern micro-CT scanners achieve high image quality at high spatial resolution and moderate dose levels. There are dedicated systems for in-vitro imaging and for in-vivo imaging. These often differ in the system design, which is of rotating object type or of rotating source-detector type. The designs also differ in flexibility. Some scanners allow the magnification values to be varied, others are optimized with respect to predefined imaging tasks. An optimization should ensure the optimal balance between spatial resolution, image noise, low contrast resolution, tube voltage, dose and scan time. The optimization should distinguish between high contrast and low contrast imaging, between in-vitro and in-vivo scans, between small and large objects and it must account for the predominant object material. Scanner calibration and homogeneity is of utmost importance for quantitative studies.

   In particular for in-vivo small animal micro-CT imaging, it is of importance that the dose delivered to the animal is kept acceptably low (<100 mGy per scan), that the spatial resolution is high enough to image anatomical details (>500 pixels per object diameter), that signal to noise levels greater than 10 are achieved to image low-contrast details (<100 HU noise in soft tissue), that the time per scan is low enough to capture intravascular contrast agent before being absorbed by the kidneys and to allow for dynamic studies (<100 s), that there is no significant interscan delay (time between two successive scans) to cut down anesthesia times, and that the scanner delivers quantitative CT values and artifact-free images that lend themselves to quantitative evaluations such as the assessment of morphology or function.

   Temporal resolution is probably the most critical issue and must still be improved to allow for dynamic studies. Increased temporal resolution would open micro-CT to advanced assessment techniques of tissue kinematics. A recent study that has evaluated functional small animal imaging with CT indicated sufficient reproducibility. However, the scans were conducted with a clinical CT scanner with high temporal but low spatial resolution and high dose values (Krishnamurthi et al. 2005) and suggest a temporal resolution of 1 s or less should be achieved.

   Compared with clinical CT, micro-CT is still in its infancy. The above requirements and today's performance parameters will definitely continue to improve during the coming years. Advancements in tube and detector technology will allow for faster scanning and for better low-contrast imaging, increased detector dynamic range, higher absorption efficiency and faster read-out are to be expected. New target materials and optimized prefiltration will be of interest. Smaller detector pixels will allow for improved spatial resolution, even in compact desktop systems, or alternatively, increase dose efficiency if chosen adequately (Kachelrieß and Kalender 2005b, 2005c). Special reconstruction algorithms and precorrection methods, as well as special postprocessing and analysis tools will have to be adapted from clinical to micro-CT. Dual-energy CT techniques have the potential to enter preclinical imaging routinely. Above all, there is a great need for specialized and dedicated micro-CT scan protocols with respect to animal handling, contrast agent and others. Certainly, micro-CT will grow up to finally keep up with clinical CT standards.

Acknowledgements The author appreciates the discussions with and the assistance from Marek Karolczak, Katia Sourbelle, Elizaveta Stepina (Institute of Medical Physics, Erlangen, Germany), Ben Durkee (University of Wisconsin-Madison, Madison, USA), and Andreas Hess (Institute of Pharmacology and Toxicology and Core Unit IZKF, Erlangen, Germany).

References

Axelsson C, Danielsson PE (1994) Three-dimensional reconstruction from cone-beam data in O(N3 log N) time. Phys Med Biol 39(3):477–491

Azevedo S, Schneberk D, Fitch P, Martz H (1990) Calculation of the rotational centers in computed tomography sinograms. IEEE Trans Nucl Science 37(4):1525–1540

Basu S, Bresler Y (2000) An $O(N^2 \backslash \log_2 N)$ filtered backprojection reconstruction algorithm for tomography. IEEE Trans Image Process 9(10):1760–1773

Beekman FJ, Kamphuis C (2001) Ordered subset reconstruction for X-ray CT. Phys Med Biol. 46(7):1835–1844

Bresler Y, Brokish J (2003) Fast hierarchical backprojection for helical cone-beam tomography. In: ICIP 2003. Proc International Conference on Image Processing, ICIP-2003, Barcelona, Spain, pp 815–818

Bronnikov A (1999) Virtual alignment of X-ray cone-beam tomography system using two calibration aperture measurements. Opt Eng 38(2):381–386

Brooks, RA, Di Chiro G (1976a) Beam hardening in X-ray reconstructive tomography. Phys Med Biol 21(3):390–398

Brooks RA, Di Chiro G (1976b) Statistical limitations in X-ray reconstruction tomography. Med Phys 3:237–240

Coleman AJ, Sinclair M (1985) A beam-hardening correction using dual-energy computed tomography. Phys Med Biol. 30(11):1251–1256

Colijn AP, Beekman FJ (2004) Accelerated simulation of cone beam X-ray scatter projections. IEEE Trans Med Imaging 23(5):584–590

Crawford CR, Gullberg GT, Tsui BM (1988) Reconstruction for fan beam with an angular-dependent displaced center-of-rotation. Med Phys 15(1):67–71

De Man B, Nuyts J, Dupont P, Marchal G, Suetens P (2000) Reduction of metal streak artifacts in X-ray computed tomography using a transmission maximum a posteriori algorithm. IEEE Trans Nucl Sci 47: 997–981

Erdogan H, Fessler JA (1999) Ordered subsets algorithms for transmission tomography. Phys Med Biol 44(11):2835–2851

Feldkamp LA, Davis LC, Kress JW (1984) Practical cone-beam algorithm. J Opt Soc Am A 1(6):612–619

Ford NL, Thornton MM, Holdsworth DW (;2003) Fundamental image quality limits for micro-computed tomography in small animals. Med Phys 30(11):2869–2877

Ford NL, Nikolov HN, Thornton MM, Foster PJ (2005) Prospective respiratory-gated micro-CT of free breathing rodents. Med Phys 32(9):2888–2898

Gkanatsios NA, Huda W (1997) Computation of energy imparted in diagnostic radiology. Med Phys 24(4):571–579

Glover GH, Pelc NJ (1981) An algorithm for the reduction of metal clip artifacts in CT reconstructions. Med Phys 8(6):799–807

Goodsitt M (1995) Beam hardening errors in post-processing DE-QCT. Med Phys 22(7): 1039–1047

Gullberg GT, Tsui BM, Crawford CR, Edgerton E (1987) Estimation of geometrical parameters for fan beam tomography. Phys Med Biol. 32(12):1581–1594

Gullberg GT, Tsui BM, Crawford CR, Ballard JG, Hagius JT (1990) Estimation of geometrical parameters and collimator evaluation for cone beam tomography. Med Phys 17(2):264–272

Herman GT (1978) Demonstration of beam hardening correction in computerized tomography of head cross-sections. Technical Report MIPG5. Medical Image Processing Group. State University of New York, Buffalo

Herman GT (1979a) Correction for beam hardening in computed tomography. Phys Med Biol 24(1):81–106

Herman GT (1979b) Demonstration of beam hardening correction in computed tomography of the head. J Comput Assist Tomogr 3(3):373–378

Herman GT, Trivedi S (1983) A comparative study of two postreconstruction beam hardening correction methods. IEEE Trans Med Imaging MI-2(3):128–135

Hounsfield GN (1973) Computerized transverse axial scanning (tomography). Part I. Description of system. Br J Radiol 46:1016

Hsieh J (1999) Three-dimensional artifact induced by projection weighting and misalignment. IEEE Trans Med Imaging 18(4):364–368

Hsieh J, Molthen RC, Dawson CA, Johnson RH (2000) An iterative approach to the beam hardening correction in cone beam CT. Med Phys 27(1):23–29

Hsieh J, Chao E, Thibault J, Grekowicz B, Horst A, McOlash S, Myers TJ (2004) A novel reconstruction algorithm to extend the CT scan field-of-view. Med Phys 31(9):2385–2391

IEEE (2004) Special issue on molecular imaging. IEEE Trans Medi Imaging 24(7)

Imamura K, Fujii M (1981) Empirical beam hardening correction in the measurement of vertebral bone mineral content by computed tomography. Radiology 138(1):223–226

Jackson DF, Hawkes DJ (1983) Energy dependence in the spectral factor approach to computed tomography. Phys Med Biol 28(3):289–293

Johns PC, Yaffe M (1982) Scattered radiation in fan beam imaging systems. Med Phys 9(2): 231–239

Joseph PM, Spital RD (1978) A method for correcting bone induced artifacts in computed tomography scanners. J Comput Assist Tomogr 2(1):100–108

Joseph PM, Spital RD (1982) The effects of scatter in X-ray computed tomography. Med Phys 9(4):464–472

Kachelrieß M, Kalender WA (1998) Electrocardiogram-correlated image reconstruction from subsecond spiral CT scans of the heart. Med Phys 25(12):2417–2431

Kachelrieß M, Kalender WA (2000a) Computertomograph mit reduzierter Dosisbelastung bzw. reduziertem Bildpunktrauschen. Deutsches Patent- und Markenamt. Patent Specification DE 198 53 143

Kachelrieß M, Kalender WA (2005b) Presampling, algorithm factors, and noise: considerations for CT in particular and for medical imaging in general. Med Phys 32(5):1321–1334

Kachelrieß M, Kalender WA (2005c) Optimizing detector size in X-ray CT imaging. In: Proceedings of the ICMP and the BMT 2005, Nuremberg. Schiele & Schön, Berlin, pp 1160–1161

Kachelrieß M, Ulzheimer S, Kalender WA (2000) ECG-correlated image reconstruction from subsecond multi-slice spiral CT scans of the heart. Med. Phys 27(8):1881–1902

Kachelrieß M, Watzke O, Kalender WA (2001) Generalized multi-dimensional adaptive filtering for conventional and spiral single-slice, multi-slice, and cone-beam CT. Med Phys 28(4): 475–490

Kachelrieß M, Sennst D-A, Maxlmoser W, Kalender WA (2002) Kymogram detection and kymogram-correlated image reconstruction from sub-second spiral computed tomography scans of the heart. Med Phys 29(7):1489–1503

Kachelrieß M, Berkus T, Kalender WA (2005) Quality of statistical reconstruction in medical CT. Records of the 2003 IEEE Medical Imaging Conference. M10–325 (April)

Kalender WA (2005) Computed tomography. Fundamentals, system technology, image quality, applications, 2nd edn. Publicis, Erlangen

Kalender WA, Hebel R, Ebersberger J (1987) Reduction of CT artifacts caused by metallic implants. Radiology 164:576–577

Kalender WA, Seissler W, Klotz E, Vock P (1990) Spiral volumetric CT with single-breathhold technique, continuous transport, and continuous scanner rotation. Radiology 176(1):181–183

Kalender WA, Durkee B, Langner O, Stepina E, Karolczak M (2005) Comparative evaluation: acceptance testing and constancy testing for micro-CT scanners. In: Proceedings of the ICMP and the BMT 2005, Nuremberg. Schiele & Schön, Berlin, pp 1192–1193

Karolczak M, Kachelrieß M, Ott O, Engelke K, Kalender WA (2005) A high-speed micro-CT scanner with rotating gantry for in-vivo animal scanning. In: Proceedings of the ICMP and the BMT 2005, Nuremberg. Schiele & Schön, Berlin, pp 756–757

Kijewski PK, Bjarngard BE (1978) Correction for beam hardening in computed tomography. Med Phys 5(3):209–214

Krishnamurthi G, Stantz KM, Steinmetz R, Gattone VH, Cao M, Hutchins GD, Liang Y (2005) Functional imaging in small animals using X-ray computed tomography—study of physiologic measurement reproducibility. IEEE Trans Med Imaging 24(7):832–843

Lange K, Carson R (1984) EM reconstruction algorithms for emission and transmission tomography. J Comput Assist Tomogr 8(2):306–316

Lange K, Fessler JA (1995) Globally convergent algorithms for maximum a posteriori transmission tomography. IEEE Trans Med Imaging 4(10):1430–1438

Marquadt D (1963) An algorithm for least-squares estimation of nonlinear parameters. Soc Indust Appl Math 11:431–441

McDavid WD, Waggener RG, Payne WH, Dennis MJ (1975) Spectral effects on three-dimensional reconstruction from rays. Med Phys 2(6):321–324

McDavid WD, Waggener RG, Payne WH, Dennis MJ (1977) Correction for spectral artifacts in cross-sectional reconstruction from X-rays. Med Phys 4(1):54–57

McLoughlin R, Rayan M, Heuston P, McCoy C, Masterson J (1991) Quantitative analysis of CT brain images: a statistical model incorporating partial volume and beam hardening effects. Br J Radiol 65:425–430

Meagher J, Mote C, Skinner H (1990) CT image correction for beam hardening using simulated projection data. IEEE Trans Nuclear Sci 37(4):1520–1524

Moseley DJ, Siewerdsen JH, Jaffray DA (2005) High-contrast object localization and removal in cone-beam CT. In: Flynn MJ (ed) Medical imaging 2005. Physics of medical imaging. Proc SPIE 5745:40–50

Nalcioglu O, Lou RY (1979) Post-reconstruction method for beam hardening in computerised tomography. Phys Med Biol 24(2):330–340

Ning R, Tang X, Conover D (2004) X-ray scatter correction algorithm for cone beam CT imaging. Med Phys 31(5):1195–1202

Noo F, Clackdoyle R, Mennessier C, White TA, Roney TJ (2000) Analytic method based on identification of ellipse parameters for scanner calibration in cone-beam tomography. Phys Med Biol 45(11):3489–3508

Ohnesorge B, Flohr T, Klingenbeck-Regn K (1999) Efficient object scatter correction algorithm for third and fourth generation CT scanners. Eur Radiol 9(3):563–569

Ohnesorge B, Flohr T, Schwarz K, Heiken JP, Bae KT (2000) Efficient correction for CT image artifacts caused by objects extending outside the scan field of view. Med Phys 27(1):39–46

Olson EA, Han K, Pisano DJ (1981) CT reprojection polychromacity correction for three attenuators. IEEE Trans Nuclear Sci 28(4):3628–3640

Rao PS, Alfidi RJ (1981) The environmental density artifact: a beam-hardening effect in computed tomography. Radiology 141(1):223–227

Reed I, Truong T, Kwoh Y, Chang C (1980) X-ray reconstructionof the spinal cord, using bone suppression. IEEE Trans Biomed Eng BME-27(6):293–298

Riess T (2002) Beiträge zur Entwicklung von Flächendetektoren in der Röntgen-Computertomographie. Berichte aus dem Institut für Medizinische Physik. Bd 9. Shaker, Aachen

Robertson DD Jr, Huang HK (1986) Quantitative bone measurements using X-ray computed tomography with second-order correction. Med Phys 13(4):474–479

Rougee A, Picard C, Ponchut C, Trousset Y (1993a) Geometrical calibration of X-ray imaging chains for three-dimensional reconstruction. Comput Med Imaging Graph 17(4–5):295–300

Rougee A, Picard C, Trousset Y, Ponchut C (1993b) Geometrical calibration of 3D X-ray imaging. In: Kim Y (ed) Medical imaging 1993: image capture, formatting and display. Proc SPIE 1897:161–169

Ruegsegger P, Hangartner T, Keller HU, Hinderling T (1978) Standardization of computed tomography images by means of a material-selective beam hardening correction. J Comput Assist Tomogr 2(2):184–188

Rührnschopf EP, Kalender WA (1981) Artefakte durch nichtlineare Teilvolumen und Aufhärtungseffekte bei der Computertomographie. electromedica 49:96–105

Ruth C, Joseph PM (1995) A comparison of beam-hardening artifacts in X-ray computerized tomography with gadolinium and iodine contrast agents. Med Phys 22(12):1977–1982

Schmidt B, Kalender WA (2002) A fast voxel-based Monte Carlo method for scanner- and patient-specific dose calculations in computed tomography. Physica Medica XVIII(2):43–53

Seibert JA, Boone JM (1988) X-ray scatter removal by deconvolution. Med Phys 15(4):567–575

Sekihara K, Kohno H, Yamamoto S (1982) Theoretical prediction of X-ray CT image quality using contrast-detail diagrams. IEEE Trans Nuclear Sci NS-26(6):2115–2121

Shepp LA, Logan BF (1974) The Fourier reconstruction of a head section. IEEE Trans Nucl Sci NS-21:21–43

Siewerdsen JH, Jaffray DA (2001) Cone-beam computed tomography with a flat-panel imager: magnitude and effects of X-ray scatter. Med Phys 28(2):220–231

Sijbers J, Postnov A (2004) Reduction of ring artefacts in high resolution micro-CT reconstructions. Phys Med Biol 49(14):247–253

Sourbelle K, Kachelrieß M, Karolczak M, Kalender WA (2004) Hybrid cupping correction (HCC) for quantitative cone-beam CT. In: RSNA Scientific Assembly and Annual Meeting Program, p 293

Sourbelle K, Kachelriess M, Kalender WA (2005) Reconstruction from truncated projections in CT using adaptive detruncation. Eur Radiol 15(5):1008–1014

Sourbelle K, Kachelrieß M, Kalender WA (2006) Empirical water precorrection for cone-beam computed tomography. IEEE Medical Imaging ConferenceRecord, 2006 (in press)

Stevens GM, Saunders R, Pelc NJ (2001) Alignment of a volumetric tomography system. Med Phys 28(7):1472–1481

Stonestrom J, Alvarez R, Macovski A (1981) A framework for spectral artifact corrections in X-ray CT. IEEE Trans Biomed Eng BME-28(2):128–141

von Smekal L, Kachelrieß M, Stepina E, Kalender WA (2004) Geometric misalignment and calibration in cone-beam tomography. Med Phys 31(12):3242–3266

Wang G, Vannier MW, Cheng PC (1999) Iterative X-ray cone-beam tomography for metal artifact reduction and local region reconstruction. Microsc Microanal 5(1):58–65

Watzke O, Kalender WA (2004) A pragmatic approach to metal artifact reduction in CT: merging of metal artifact reduced images. Eur Radiol 14(5):849–856

Wiesent K, Barth K, Navab N, Brunner T, Seissler W (1999) Enhanced 3-D-reconstruction algorithm for C-arm systems based interventional procedures. Proc 1999 Int Meeting on Fully 3D Image Reconstruction, pp 167–170

Wiesent K, Barth K, Navab N, Durlak P, Brunner T, Schuetz O, Seissler W (2000) Enhanced 3-D-reconstruction algorithm for C-arm systems suitable for interventional procedures. IEEE Trans Med Imaging 19(5):391–403

Young SW, Muller HH, Marshall WH (1983) Computed tomography: beam hardening and environmental density artifact. Radiology 148(1):279–283

Zatz LM, Alvarez RE (1977) An inaccuracy in computed tomography: the energy dependence of CT values. Radiology 124(1):91–97

Zhao S, Robertson DD, Wang G, Whiting B, Bae KT (2000) X-ray CT metal artifact reduction using wavelets: an application for imaging total hip prostheses. IEEE Trans Med Imaging 19(12):1238–1247

PET & SPECT Instrumentation

Virginia C. Spanoudaki and Sibylle I. Ziegler(⊠)

Abstract The nuclear medical imaging methods, positron emission tomography (PET) and single photon emission computed tomography (SPECT), utilize the detection of gamma rays leaving the body after a radioactive tracer has been administered. The sensitivity of PET allows the detection of picomolar tracer amounts in vivo and current technology offers millimeter (PET) or submillimeter (SPECT) spatial resolution. These techniques are used in clinical and preclinical applications. The basic principles of gamma ray detection and image generation in PET and SPECT are summarized in this chapter. Furthermore, effects causing degradation of image quality are discussed.

Sibylle I. Ziegler

Nuklearmedizinische Klinik und Poliklinik der TU München, Klinikum rechts der Isar, Ismaninger Str. 22, 81675 München, Germany

sibylle.ziegler@tum.de

W. Semmler and M. Schwaiger (eds.), *Molecular Imaging I.*
Handbook of Experimental Pharmacology 185/I.
© Springer-Verlag Berlin Heidelberg 2008

1 Basic Detection Principles

Image formation in nuclear medicine is based on the detection of gamma radiation emitted from a radiopharmaceutical inserted into the patient's body. The detectors commonly used in positron emission tomography and single photon emission computed tomography (PET and SPECT, respectively) are a combination of a scintillation crystal, which converts the incident gamma radiation to visible scintillation light, and a photodetector, which collects the scintillation light and converts it into an electrical pulse.

1.1 Interaction of Photons with Matter

Gamma radiation passing through matter can lose energy via three different processes: photoelectric absorption, Compton scatter and pair production. During the first process, the gamma quantum is fully absorbed by a bound atomic electron, which in turn escapes from the atom, leaving it positively ionized. The second process is the scattering of the incident photon by a loosely bound atomic electron. In this process, the photon is not fully absorbed but only transfers a part of its energy to the electron, changing at the same time its direction of flight. The third process is the interaction of the incident radiation with the atomic nucleus during which the photon is fully absorbed and results in the production of an electron-positron pair. A minimum gamma energy of 1,022 keV is necessary for this process to happen.

The probability of each of the above processes depends on the gamma energy and the effective atomic number. This is summarized in Table 1.

The nuclides used to label pharmaceuticals in nuclear medicine emit photons of energies at which the photoelectric effect and Compton scatter are the most abundant. These interactions take place both within the object to be imaged as well as within the scintillation crystal, affecting in different ways the performance of the imaging device. Photoelectric absorption and Compton scatter within the object to be imaged contribute to reduced image quality, as will be discussed in the following sections. On the other hand, photoelectric absorption should be enhanced against Compton scatter within the scintillation crystal in order to improve detection efficiency (Hubbell 1999).

Table 1 Energy and material dependence of the three most important interaction modes of gamma radiation with matter

Photon interaction mode	Energy dependency	Atomic number dependency
Photoelectric	$\dfrac{1}{E^{3.5}}$	Z^{3-5}
Compton	$\dfrac{1}{E}$	Z
Pair production	$\log E$	Z^2

1.2 Properties of Scintillator-based Detectors

In all of the above-mentioned processes, the energy of the resulting electron will subsequently be converted to visible light within the scintillation crystal volume. Depending on the application, a scintillator should combine a number of properties that will guarantee optimum detector performance in terms of energy and time resolution. Defining the interaction of a gamma quantum with the scintillation crystal as an *event*, energy resolution is a quantity that indicates the detector's ability to discriminate between events of different deposited energies. Time resolution is a similar quantity indicative of the detector's ability to distinguish between events happening at different time points. Both of these properties depend on the scintillator's light yield and decay time. Typical values for energy resolution lie within the range 10–15% and a time resolution in the nanosecond or even sub-nanosecond range may be achieved by fast timing systems.

Since the detection of a gamma quantum is realized by the deposition of its full energy into the detector's sensitive volume, the scintillation crystal should be made from a material of high effective atomic number and high density in order to enhance the possibility of photoelectric effect and thus its stopping power, as seen in Table 1 from the Z-dependence of photoelectric effect. The light output, namely the number of optical photons produced from a specific amount of incident gamma ray energy deposited in the scintillator, determines the scintillator's energy resolution. For fast timing applications, such as required in PET, a small decay constant of the scintillator light pulse is essential.

The scintillators are divided into organic and inorganic materials with somehow complementary characteristics: organic scintillators usually exhibit poor light output but they are very fast, while inorganic scintillators are characterized by high light output and a slower decay constant. The effective atomic number of organic materials is much lower compared with inorganic scintillators. Table 2 summarizes the properties of the most commonly used scintillation crystals in nuclear medicine. Another important property shown in the table is the wavelength of maximum emission, λ_{max}, of the scintillator, which has to match the wavelength at which the photodetector is most sensitive in order to assure sufficient signal amplitude (Knoll 2000).

Table 2 Properties of the most common scintillation crystals in nuclear medicine

	Na(Tl)	BGO	LSO(Ce)	GSO(Ce)	CsI(Tl)	BaF$_2$	LaBr$_3$	Plastic
Density (g/cm^3)	3.67	7.13	7.40	6.71	4.51	4.89	5.29	1.03
Effective atomic number (Z)	50	74	66	59	54	54	46	12
Decay time (ns)	230	300	40	60	1,000	0.8, 620	26	2
Photon yield/keV	38	8	20–30	12–15	52	10	63	10
Index of refraction n	1.85	2.15	1.82	1.85	1.80	1.56	1.90	1.58
Hygroscopic	Yes	No	No	No	Slightly	No	Yes	No
Peak emission λ_{max} (nm)	415	480	420	430	540	225, 310	380	Various

1.3 Properties of Photodetectors

1.3.1 Photomultiplier Tubes (PMTs)

Photomultiplier Tubes (PMTs) have traditionally been used in order to convert scintillation light into an electrical pulse (Knoll 2000). The basic PMT architecture is constructed in a vacuum glass tube and consists of (1) a photocathode that emits photoelectrons when visible light is incident to its surface, (2) a number of dynodes that emit secondary electrons for every incident primary photoelectron, and (3) a single anode or an anode mesh that collects the secondary electron cloud and produces a current pulse which is proportional to the number of electrons in the cloud. A typical PMT architecture is shown in Fig. 1. The fast rise time in the order of

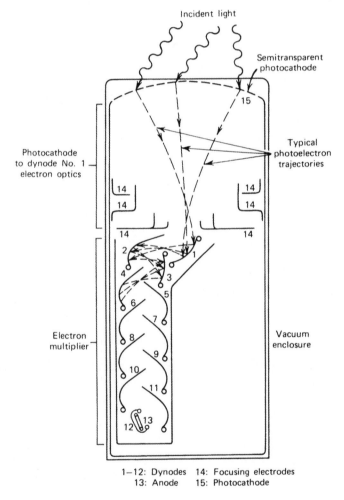

1–12: Dynodes   14: Focusing electrodes
13: Anode   15: Photocathode

Fig. 1 Basic elements of a photomultiplier tube. (Reproduced from Knoll 2000, with permission)

1 ns or less and the high gain in the order of 10^6 make the PMTs appropriate for fast timing applications and for gamma spectroscopy with good energy resolution. PMT performance is limited by the low quantum efficiency (QE); namely, the ratio of the number of photoelectrons produced at the photocathode to the number of incident photons at the photocathode surface (typically 25% at 420 nm). The performance of a PMT is highly degraded inside magnetic fields, making its use difficult for simultaneous MR/PET imaging (Christensen et al. 1995; Marsden et al. 2002).

1.3.2 Avalanche Photodiodes (APDs)

The use of semiconductor photodetectors, such as avalanche photodiodes (APDs), has largely evolved in recent years due to the increasing demand for multimodality imaging. The fact that APDs can be produced in various compact sizes and that their performance remains unchanged in magnetic fields makes them appropriate for PET devices that can be inserted to an MR scanner for simultaneous PET/MR imaging (see chapter by Pichler et al.). The main detector architecture consists of a p-to-n or n-to-p semiconductor junction operated at a reverse bias voltage; namely, negative voltage on the p-side relative to the n-side. Within the APD a depletion region is thus created, inside which no free charge can exist. When a photon is absorbed in the depletion region, the charge produced is swept out towards the respective electrodes. During its movement, the charge is accelerated by the electric field and moves towards the opposite polarity electrode, entering an avalanche region, where a number of secondary electrons is produced. The electron avalanche is collected by the anode, resulting in a current pulse. Compared with PMTs, APDs are characterized by low gain in the order of 100, by higher quantum efficiency (75% at 420 nm) and by slower rise times in the order of 5 ns. A photograph of the S8550 APD (Hamamatsu Photonics) is shown in Fig. 2 (Pichler et al. 2001).

1.3.3 Silicon Photomultipliers (SiPMs)

A new photodetector is currently considered to be one of the promising future trends in detector technology for multimodality imaging in nuclear medicine (Dolgoshein et al. 2006). Silicon photomultipliers (SiPMs) consist of an array of individual APDs working in Geiger discharge mode (cells). In this mode, above breakdown, every illuminated cell results in a fast (rise time $\sim$ 1 ns), well-defined, single-photoelectron pulse of very high gain of the order of 10^6. The individual cells are connected to each other through a polysilicon resistor and the resulting current pulse is proportional to the number of illuminated cells. The fast timing and the high gain of SiPMs are accompanied by their response to a small dynamic range of detected radiation energies due to the limited number of cells in an array, the low photon detection efficiency (PDE) and the high dark count rate. Currently, improvements on the SiPM design are well underway. Due to the well-defined SiPM output signal, the use of

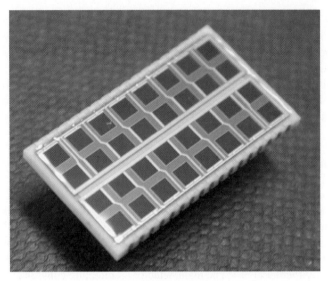

Fig. 2 Array of 32 avalanche photodiodes with each $1.6 \times 1.6\,mm^2$ sensitive area (Hamamatsu Photonics, Japan)

Table 3 Comparative table of the performance characteristics for three different photodetectors

	PMT	APD	SiPM
Photon detection efficiency (PDE) in blue	20%	50%	20–70%
Gain	10^6	100	10^6
Bias voltage (V)	$\sim$1,000	$\sim$400	<100
Sensitivity in magnetic field	Yes	No	No
Rise time (ns)	$\sim$1	$\sim$5	$\sim$1

sophisticated electronics, such as charge-sensitive preamplifiers, may be eliminated. This, in combination with their insensitivity to magnetic fields, may result in a potential simplified detector design for PET inserts in MR scanners. Table 3 compares the characteristics of PMTs, APDs and SiPMs.

Alternative detector technologies opt for elimination of the scintillation crystal and the direct detection of incident photons by the use of semiconductor detectors (Butler et al. 1998) or multiwire proportional chambers (Jeavons et al. 1999). These detector concepts can mainly be found in preclinical systems.

2 PET & SPECT Principles

2.1 Positron Emitters versus Single Photon Emitters

The radiopharmaceuticals used in SPECT contain long-lived radioisotopes emitting gamma rays with energy from $\sim$70 keV to 360 keV. The most commonly applied isotope is the metastable ^{99m}Tc. It decays through an isomeric transition (IT); namely, a nuclear deexcitation that results in the emission of a gamma ray or an electron through the process of internal conversion. The metastable radioisotopes are characterized by relatively long lifetimes, which make them appropriate for in vivo imaging.

On the contrary, the radiopharmaceuticals used in PET are labeled with beta emitters. The most probable deexcitation mode of the nucleus is through positron emission, according to which a proton of the nucleus is converted to a neutron with the simultaneous emission of a positron and a neutrino. The positron, depending on its initial energy, will travel a specific distance in the surrounding material, loosing energy until it annihilates with an electron, resulting in the emission of two photons. Supposing that both electron and positron are at rest, the energy and momentum conservation laws impose that the resulting two annihilation photons are emitted in opposing directions.

Some other radionuclides useful in nuclear medicine decay through electron capture (EC) followed by gamma deexcitation. EC is a process competitive to positron emission, during which a proton in the nucleus captures an electron and is transformed to a neutron. Table 4 summarizes the radioisotopes most commonly used in nuclear medicine.

Table 4 Characteristics of the most commonly used radionuclides in nuclear medicine

Radionuclide	Decay	Photon energy (keV)	Half life
^{11}C	β^+	511	20.3 min
^{13}N	β^+	511	10.0 min
^{15}O	β^+	511	2.07 min
^{18}F	β^+	511	110 min
^{67}Ga	EC	93, 183, 300	3.26 days
^{82}Rb	β^+	511	1.25 min
^{99m}Tc	IT	140	6.03 h
^{111}In	EC	172, 247	2.81 days
^{123}I	EC	159	13.0 h
^{201}Tl	EC	68–80	3.05 days

2.2 Electronic versus Mechanical Collimation

Collimation is defined as the hardware condition set to the detection of gamma rays in order to be able to localize the emission point of radiation. Although the detection principle of gamma radiation is the same for both PET and SPECT, the collimation principle is different.

2.2.1 Mechanical Collimation in SPECT

In SPECT, a collimator is defined as a mechanical structure made of a high-Z material which is placed in front of the detector head. Collimator geometries include the parallel hole, pinhole, converging and diverging with various hole geometries shown in Fig. 3 (Cherry et al. 2003). The high-Z material enhances absorption of the oblique gamma rays and will allow the passage of radiation only through the collimator openings. In this way, mechanical collimation allows for estimation of the trajectories of the detected gamma rays and thus for image reconstruction. In addition, the detection of gamma rays that have been subjected to Compton scattering inside the patient's body is reduced, hence limiting background in the reconstructed image. It is evident that mechanical collimation is the most critical hardware aspect in SPECT, since it sets a lower limit to the achieved spatial resolution and sensitivity.

2.2.2 Electronic Collimation in PET

PET imaging is based on the simultaneous detection of two annihilation photons by two opposing detectors. Since every pair of opposing detectors can be thought to define a line of response (LOR) along which the emission point of the two annihilation photons should be localized, an electronic collimation is imposed on the photon detection in PET, as illustrated in Fig. 4 (Cherry et al. 2003). Additional mechanical collimation (septa) is sometimes applied to reduce the detection of scattered radiation or radiation from parts of the object outside the tomograph's field of view (FOV). Septa may be inserted between the individual rings of crystals; thus, only direct or next-neighbor cross coincidences are recorded (2D acquisition) (Cherry et al. 2003). While scatter and random fraction is reduced significantly in 2D PET, sensitivity is low. PET without septa (3D acquisition) accepts all possible LORs, even with large axial opening angles for increased sensitivity (Cherry et al. 2003). Compared with 2D acquisition, the recorded scatter fraction is significantly higher and appropriate correction methods need to be applied. New detector developments, mainly fast and luminous scintillators, together with reconstruction and scatter correction algorithms have improved 3D PET performance significantly, such that today most scanners are 3D-only.

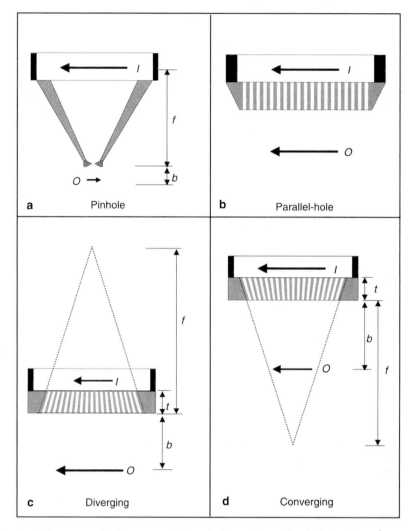

Fig. 3 a–d Four types of collimators used to project "γ-ray images" onto the detector of a gamma camera (*0* radioactive object, *I* its projected image). (Reproduced from Cherry et al. 2003, with permission)

2.3 Detector Design and Scanner Geometries

2.3.1 SPECT Imaging Devices

The main detector module of a SPECT imaging device is a gamma camera. A typical gamma camera consists of a collimator, a scintillation crystal, a light guide and a number of PMTs. The energy information is acquired by the sum of the PMT signals and the position information of the gamma ray interaction within the crystal is

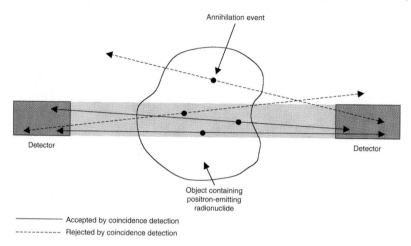

Fig. 4 Volume (*shaded area*) from which a pair of simultaneously emitted annihilation photons can be detected in coincidence by a pair of detectors. Not all decays in this volume will lead to recorded events, because it is necessary that both photons strike the detectors. Outside the shaded volume, it is impossible to detect annihilation photons in coincidence unless one or both undergo a Compton scatter in the tissue and change direction. (Reproduced from Cherry et al. 2003, with permission)

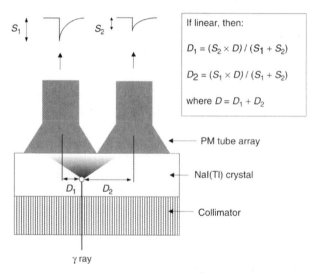

Fig. 5 Illustration of light sharing between photomultiplier (PM) tubes. The signal from a PM tube, S, is inversely related to the distance of the interaction site, D, from the center of the PM tube. Equations for a linear relationship are shown. (Reproduced from Cherry et al. 2003, with permission)

determined using a centroid algorithm (Anger 1958). An illustration of basic gamma camera design and the position and energy determination algorithms is shown in Fig. 5 (Cherry et al. 2003). A light guide is used in order to efficiently collect the scintillation light and distribute it among the PMTs. Segmented scintillation crystals

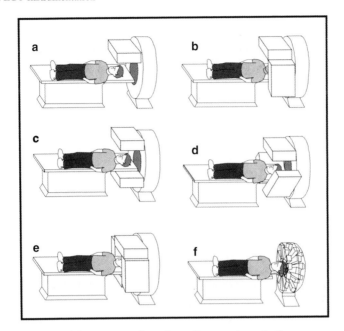

Fig. 6 a–f Several SPECT system configurations. Shown schematically are systems with **a** a single head, **b** two orthogonal heads, **c** two opposed heads, **d** three heads, **e** four heads, and **f** multiple small-FOV scintillation detectors. (Reproduced from Wernick and Aarsvold 2004, with permission)

and position-sensitive PMTs (PSPMTs) are also used in current systems in order to improve the spatial resolution for the preclinical application (Zeniya et al. 2006).

A typical SPECT device consists of one (single-headed), two (dual-headed) or more gamma cameras, which are able to rotate around the object. Figure 6 shows different configurations implemented in current SPECT systems (Wernick and Aarsvold 2004).

2.3.2 PET Imaging Devices

Block detectors are traditionally used in PET, and consist of a number of individual crystal elements read out by a small number of photomultiplier tubes (typically four). The four signals from the PMTs are used to determine the energy information, while the crystal where the interaction took place is determined by the four PMT signals using Anger logic (Casey and Nutt 1986). Another option is the readout of a large number of crystals with a continuous light guide and an array of PMTs, similar to a gamma camera (Surti and Karp 2004). Typical block detector designs are shown in Fig. 7.

A simplified PET scanner design would consist of two block detectors placed opposite each other, measuring in coincidence data acquisition mode. Tomographic acquisition requires scanning across and rotation of the two detector heads around

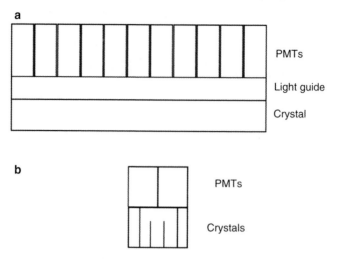

Fig. 7 a, b The major crystal-PMT decoding geometry options currently in use. **a** The continuous Anger-logic approach uses an array of PMTs to decode a large continuous crystal or an array of crystals. **b** The block detector uses four PMTs to decode an array of crystals with various combinations of reflectors and surface treatments between the crystals. (Reproduced from Wernick and Aarsvold 2004, with permission)

the object to be imaged. The number of steps can be minimized by increasing the number of detectors. Therefore, no rotation is required for scanner geometries with detectors covering the full 2π angle. Various PET scanner geometries are shown in Fig. 8 (Cherry et al. 2003).

Alternative to the block detector concept is the individual crystal readout which can be achieved by using more compact photodetectors such as APDs (Lecomte et al. 1996; Ziegler et al. 2001). The use of small size crystals is advantageous in PET, since the crystal size will determine a lower limit in the achieved spatial resolution. However, the need of a large number of electronic channels to individually process the large number of detector signals significantly increases the cost of such a design.

Measuring the difference in time-of-flight (TOF) of the two detected gamma rays can be used as a basis to limit the source position along the LOR. This technique had been introduced in the early 1980s but its success was limited owing to the materials and algorithms available at that time. With the availability of new luminous and very fast scintillation crystals and improvements in the readout electronics, TOF-PET has regained interest (Lewellen 1998; Surti et al. 2006) and has recently been implemented in a commercial product.

The thickness of the crystal is critical for both PET and SPECT imaging. A thick crystal increases the gamma detection efficiency and hence the sensitivity of the imaging device. However, in SPECT large thickness enhances the spread of the scintillation light before reaching the PMT; therefore, a larger uncertainty in the localization of the photon interaction is introduced. In PET, and especially in small

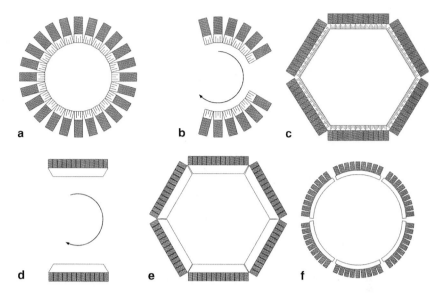

Fig. 8 a–f PET scanner geometries based on discrete scintillator elements *(top row)* or continuous scintillator plates *(bottom row)*. **a** Full ring of modular block detectors. **b** Partial ring of modular block detectors. **c** Hexagonal array of quadrant-sharing panel detectors. **d** Dual-headed gamma camera with coincidence circuitry. **e** Hexagonal array of gamma camera detectors. **f** Continuous detectors using curved plates of NaI(Tl). A complete set of profiles can be acquired without motion with systems **a**, **c**, **e**, and **f**, whereas detector motion is required with systems **b** and **d**. (Reproduced from Cherry and Sorenson 2003, with permission)

animal systems, making use of depth of interaction (DOI) information plays an important role in the improvement of the spatial resolution at the edges of the FOV when using long crystals. In order to minimize the crystal penetration effects and thus to determine the position along the crystal where the photon interaction took place, PET scanner geometries were suggested with two radial crystal layers of either the same or different material instead of a single scintillation radial crystal layer (Schmand et al. 1998; Seidel et al. 2003; Chung et al. 2004).

3 Image Reconstruction, Degradation and Corrections

3.1 Image Reconstruction Algorithms

Tomographic image reconstruction is based on measured estimation of the integral of radiotracer distribution as seen under different angles (projections). The reconstruction algorithms used for both SPECT and PET are the same, although, as previously described, the hardware and the principle of operation are different for the two modalities. These algorithms are used to produce a volume representation of

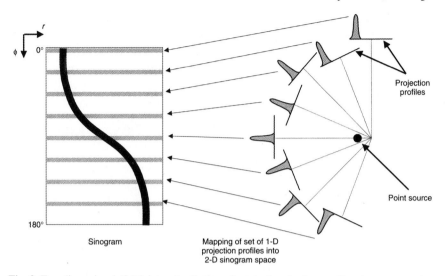

Fig. 9 Two-dimensional (2-D) intensity display of a set of projection profiles, known as a *sinogram*. Each row in the display corresponds to an individual projection profile, sequentially displayed from top to bottom. A point source of radioactivity traces out a sinusoidal path in the sonogram. (Reproduced from Cherry et al. 2003, with permission)

the radiotracer distribution inside the patient's body. The reconstruction algorithms can be divided into two groups: analytical and statistical.

For each projection the acquired data are organized as number of counts along each LOR. In SPECT, an LOR is defined as the radial extension of the collimator hole across the FOV; while in PET, an LOR is the line connecting a detector pair. For the total number of projections, it is convenient to reorganize the data into a 2D matrix called a sinogram, which contains the number of counts for every LOR at each angular view; namely, for every radial distance r and every angle θ, as illustrated in Fig. 9. Sinograms are then used as input to the reconstruction algorithms in order to generate the final image (Cherry et al. 2003).

Analytical reconstruction algorithms model the measurement of radiotracer distribution in a simplified way so that an exact solution may be calculated analytically. However, these algorithms ignore a number of physical effects during acquisition, such as limited sampling, Poisson statistics in photon counting, attenuation or radiotracer decay, resulting in reduced image accuracy. Filtered backprojection (FBP) has long been the most widely used analytical reconstruction algorithm. Data in each LOR are homogeneously backprojected and filtered. The filter introduces negative contributions, which cancel out the positive counts in areas of zero activity. The choice of filter and cut-off frequency determines resolution and noise level in the reconstructed image.

On the other hand, statistical, iterative reconstruction algorithms compensate for the inaccuracies introduced to the image by including in the initial estimate of the image the above-mentioned physical processes. Thus, the model becomes more complicated and an analytical solution is impossible to compute. An iterative calculation is thus needed which starts with an estimate of tracer distribution, computes the forward-projection and compares calculated and measured projections. The image is updated according to the differences found between calculated and measured projections until the estimate agrees with the measured data. The model used in the algorithm can account for geometrical and detector effects, yielding improved image quality especially in the case of low counting statistics. Maximum likelihood expectation maximization (MLEM) is most commonly used. Since convergence is slow, accelerated algorithms have become most important in clinical routine, such as ordered subsets expectation maximization (OSEM) (Hudson and Larkin 1994).

3.2 Attenuation and Scatter Effects

Since in nuclear medicine the radiopharmaceutical is injected into the patient's body (emission imaging), the emitted photons have a given probability of interacting within the body before being detected by the imaging device. This probability depends both on the energy of the emitted photons and on the composition of the material through which the photons are travelling. For the photon energies involved in PET and SPECT, the most probable interaction is Compton scatter; however, at energies below 100 keV photoelectric absorption is also a considerable effect. In the first case, the photon will be deflected from its initial trajectory and will either be still detected by a different detector than the expected one, or it will escape the FOV of the tomograph. In the latter case, the photon will never be detected by the imaging device. Attenuation correction applies in the case where the emitted photons are not detected by the imaging device; while scatter correction applies in the case where the photon is detected by the imaging device after being scattered, thus giving wrong information about the initial emission point within the patient's body. The presence of scatter and attenuation in the reconstructed image leads to reduced image contrast and distortions.

Assuming that N_0 photons are emitted from a point within the patient's body, the number of detected photons N will be given by the equation

$$N = N_0 \cdot e^{-\mu x} \tag{1}$$

where x is the distance travelled by the gamma ray within the body and μ is the linear attenuation coefficient of the material. In order to compensate for this effect in SPECT, several methods are being used. One method eliminates the distance-dependent attenuation by acquiring projection scans for a complete rotation ($360°$) of the detector head and combining the measurements of opposing projections. Another method is to calculate a patient-specific attenuation coefficient map, which is then be applied to the measured data. This is achieved by either using the measured data from a CT device or by performing a transmission scan using, for instance, gadolinium line sources (Bailey 1998). Since the attenuation factor depends on the source position relative to the body surface, this method can only be implemented in iterative algorithms with estimates of source distribution in the patient body.

The most commonly used method to correct for scatter in SPECT measurements is to acquire projections for two different energy windows: one around the photo-peak and one at the Compton continuum. The "scattered projections" are appropri-ately scaled and subtracted from the "photopeak projections" in order to compensate for scatter (Buvat et al. 1994).

PET imaging has the advantage that the attenuation effect does not depend on the position of the source to be imaged along a specific LOR, since the total length in the body defines the attenuation factor. Therefore, attenuation compensation can be derived from a direct measurement with rotating rod sources or from CT data.

The scatter fraction in clinical whole-body PET ranges between 50 and 60% in the case of 3D acquisition, making scatter correction essential for improved im-age quality and quantification. The scatter correction methods of different energy windows used in SPECT are not as successful in the case of PET, due to the signifi-cantly inferior energy resolution. Methods based on convolution-subtraction (Bailey and Meikle 1994) or single-scatter simulation (Ollinger 1996) are the most widely used. The use of CT information as input for the scatter estimate, especially, has improved the scatter correction in 3D PET.

3.3 Sensitivity

High sensitivity, thus high photon detection efficiency, is of utmost importance for clinical and preclinical SPECT or PET imaging. Sensitivity is strongly dependent on the material and the thickness of the scintillation crystal, as well as on the material and the geometry of mechanical collimation. Long crystals of high Z material will increase the scintillator's stopping power and consequently the number of detected events. On the other hand, a collimator of high Z material and long septa will tend to have a reduced acceptance of oblique incident photons, thus reducing the system's sensitivity. However, as it will be mentioned in the following section, there is a trade-off between sensitivity and spatial resolution which applies to both imaging modalities.

It should be mentioned that in PET or SPECT systems an additional correction for the geometry- and detector-dependent differences in efficiency must be per-formed (normalization).

3.4 Dead-time Losses and Pile-up Effects

In case of high injected dose, the tomograph's hardware may be subjected to dead-time losses. The dead time of a measuring system is defined as the minimum time interval between two separately detected events during which only one event may be processed and hence the system either is not sensitive to any other events occurring within the same interval or it considers all these events as one. Dead time depends on the system's detector and processing electronics. One effect of dead-time losses is underestimation of counts on the reconstructed image. Compensation for this effect can be realized by mathematically modeling the counting system's dead time, based on a count rate measurement covering the anticipated activity levels.

3.5 Distance Dependence of Spatial Resolution

Since collimation in SPECT is purely geometrical, spatial resolution strongly depends on the distance between source and detector head, as sketched in Fig. 10. This fact leads to distortions in the image if not taken into account in the reconstruction process. Some SPECT systems allow for elliptical rotation or for rotation along the patient's body contour in order to minimize the distance between the detector head and the patient.

Developments in SPECT reconstruction algorithms include descriptions of the resolution degradation, based on measurements, in order to minimize this effect (Liang et al. 1992).

In PET imaging, spatial resolution between two detector elements which define a certain LOR is independent of the position along the LOR. The so-called parallax error introduces spatially variable resolution, depending on the radial distance

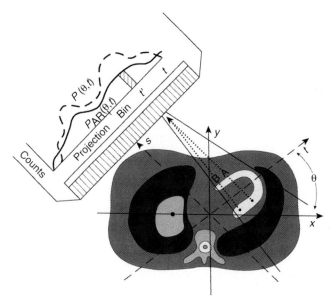

Fig. 10 Impact of system spatial resolution on SPECT imaging. Notice the distance-dependent enlargement of the region from which primary photons can contribute to the projections without penetrating the collimator. (Reproduced from Wernick and Aarsvold 2004, with permission)

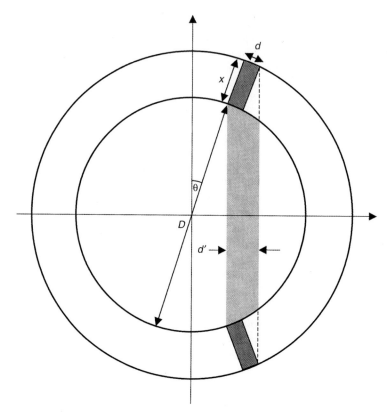

Fig. 11 Apparent width of a detector element, d', increases with increasing radial offset in a PET scanner consisting of a circular array of detector elements. Because the depths at which the γ rays interact within the scintillation crystal are unknown, the annihilation event for a pair of photons recorded in coincidence could have occurred anywhere within the shaded volume. The magnitude of the effect depends on the source location, the diameter of the scanner, D, the length of the crystal elements, x, and the width of the detector elements, d. (Reproduced from Cherry et al. 2003, with permission)

between the centre and the source within a ring tomograph. As depicted in Fig. 11, the larger the distance from the centre of the FOV, the wider the LOR due to oblique angles. Parallax error is more pronounced for small detector ring diameters, as it is the case in devices for small animal imaging. A number of depth detection methods are being investigated to reduce the resolution degradation in this situation.

3.6 Other Effects

The spatial resolution may be jeopardized by a number of other effects that are specific to the imaging modality or to the measurement conditions. In the case of PET, the detection of random coincidences may increase noise in the reconstructed image.

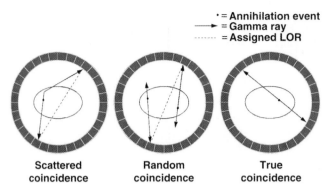

Fig. 12 The three types of coincidence events measured in a PET scanner. (Reproduced from Wernick and Aarsvold 2004, with permission)

As shown in Fig. 12, a random coincidence is the simultaneous detection by two opposing detectors of two photons that resulted from two independent positron annihilations. For comparison, the definition of scattered events (Sect. 3.2) and true coincidence events detected in PET are also depicted in the figure. In reality, due to statistical fluctuations and due to the finite time resolution of the detectors, a coincidence event is the detection of two photons by two opposing detectors within a specific time window. This window is usually chosen to be twice the system's time resolution. Since from theory, the random coincidence rate is proportional to the width of the time coincidence window, the number of randoms may be reduced by improving the detectors' time resolution; namely, by choosing fast scintillators, photodetectors and electronics. The detection and subtraction of random coincidences from measured data is performed by various methods, which may be software or hardware based (Brasse et al. 2005).

The partial volume effect is the bias introduced to the estimation of the radiotracer concentration due to the limited spatial resolution of the imaging device and is dependent on both the size and shape of the object (Hoffman et al. 1979) and on the relative radiotracer concentration with respect to the surroundings. An illustration of this effect is shown in Fig. 13 (Cherry et al. 2003). In general, the partial volume effect is minimized if the size of the object is relatively large in comparison with the system's spatial resolution. In order to acquire quantitative information about the radiotracer distribution, compensation for partial volume effects is a prerequisite (Chen et al. 1999).

Respiratory or cardiac movement of the patient during acquisition requires correction of the acquired data in order to compensate for artifacts in the reconstructed image. Usually a number of gated acquisitions are realized for every breathing or cardiac cycle. Thus, from several such cycles a reconstructed image corresponding to a specific time frame of the cycle is produced.

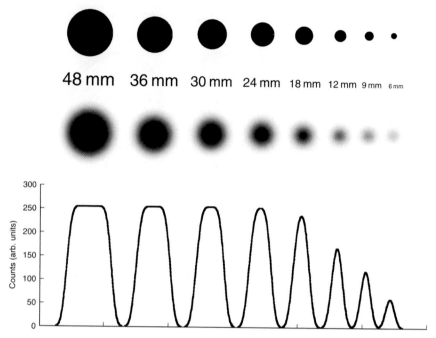

Fig. 13 Illustration of partial-volume effect. The cylinders shown in the *top row* have diameters ranging from 6 to 48 mm, and each contains the same concentration of radionuclide. The *middle row* shows a simulation of the images that would result from scanning these cylinders on a SPECT system with an in-plane spatial resolution of 12-mm full width at half maximum. The cylinders are assumed to have a height much greater than the axial resolution. The *bottom row* shows count profiles through the center of the images. Although each cylinder contains the same concentration of radionuclide, the intensity, and therefore the apparent concentration, appears to decrease when the cylinder size approaches and then becomes smaller than the resolution of the SPECT system. The integrated area under the count profiles does, however, accurately reflect the total amount of activity in the cylinders. (Reproduced from Cherry et al. 2003, with permission)

4 State of the Art Instrumentation

4.1 Preclinical

Small animals (mice and rats) are widely used in biological and medical research in order to model human diseases as well as in pharmacology in order to investigate and evaluate new radiopharmaceuticals. Obviously, spatial resolution is the primary requirement for these instruments. But sensitivity is as important since the amount of activity which can be injected may be limited by the specific activity (ratio of labeled tracer to nonlabeled substance) of the radiotracer.

Highest spatial resolution in preclinical SPECT in the range of a few hundred micrometers (μm) can be achieved with pinhole collimators, which on the other hand have a very low sensitivity (Meikle et al. 2005). In order to increase sensitivity, several detectors are used. The spatial resolution of commercial PET devices for imaging small animals has reached the 1.0–1.5 mm region (Tai et al. 2005), with sub-millimeter imaging possible (Schafers et al. 2005). The sensitivity of small animal PET scanners is increased by a long axial extent and 3D data acquisition.

4.2 Clinical

PET and SPECT devices are in routine clinical use. Most clinical SPECT systems are dual head cameras with application-specific collimators (low, medium, or high energy), yielding image resolution of 1–2 cm (distance dependent). Reconstruction methods, including attenuation and scatter correction as well as resolution recovery, are recent developments improving clinical SPECT imaging and potentially leading to quantitative SPECT (Song et al. 2005).

Current PET scanners are 3D devices with spatial resolution of 4–6 mm. Increasing sensitivity and further reducing the spatial resolution are goals of several innovations (Cherry 2006). Axial coverage, which is currently around 16 cm, needs to be expanded for higher sensitivity. The recent introduction of time-of-flight measurements is another step toward signal-to-noise improvements in whole-body PET imaging (Surti et al. 2006).

References

Anger HO (1958) Scintillation camera. Rev Sci Instr 29:27–33

Bailey DL (1998) Transmission scanning in emission tomography. Eur J Nucl Med 25:774–787

Bailey DL, Meikle SR (1994) A convolution-subtraction scatter correction method for 3D PET. Phys Med Biol 39:411–424

Brasse D, Kinahan PE, Lartizien C, Comtat C, Casey M, Michel C (2005) Correction methods for random coincidences in fully 3D whole-body PET: impact on data and image quality. J Nucl Med 46:859–867

Butler JF, Lingren CL, Friesenhahn SJ, Doty FP, Ashburn WL, Conwell RL, Augustine FL, Apotovsky B, Pi B, Collins T, Zhao S, Isaacson C (1998) CdZnTe Solid-state gamma camera. IEEE Trans Nucl Sci 45:359–363

Buvat I, Benali H, Todd-Pokropek A, Di Paola R (1994) Scatter correction in scintigraphy: the state of the art. Eur J Nucl Med 21:675–694

Casey ME, Nutt R (1986) Multicrystal two dimensional BGO detector system for positron emission tomography. IEEE Trans Nucl Sci 33:460–463

Chen CH, Muzic RF Jr, Nelson AD, Adler LP (1999) Simultaneous recovery of size and radioactivity concentration of small spheroids with PET data. J Nucl Med 40:118–130

Cherry SR (2006) The 2006 Henry N. Wagner Lecture: Of mice and men (and positrons)—advances in PET imaging technology. J Nucl Med 47:1735–1745

Cherry SR, Sorenson JA, Phelps ME (2003) Physics in nuclear medicine. Saunders, Philadelphia

Christensen NL, Hammer BE, Heil BG, Fetterly K (1995) Positron emission tomography within a magnetic field using photomultiplier tubes and lightguides. Phys Med Biol 40:691–697

Chung YH, Choi Y, Cho G, Choe YS, Lee KH, Kim BT (2004) Characterization of dual layer phoswich detector performance for small animal PET using Monte Carlo simulation. Phys Med Biol 49:2881–2890

Dolgoshein B, Balagura V, Buzhan P, Danilov M, Filatov L, Garutti E, Groll M, Ilyin A, Kantserov V, Kaplin V (2006) Status report on silicon photomultiplier development and its applications. Nucl Instr Methods Res A 563:368–376

Hoffman EJ, Huang SC, Phelps ME (1979) Quantitation in positron emission computed tomography: 1. Effect of object size. J Comput Assist Tomogr 3:299–308

Hubbell JH (1999) Review of photon interaction cross section data in the medical and biological context. Phys Med Biol 44:R1–R22

Hudson HM, Larkin RS (1994) Accelerated image reconstruction using ordered subsets of projection data. IEEE Trans Med Imag 13:601–609

Jeavons AP, Chandler RA, Dettmar CAR (1999) A 3D HIDAC-PET camera with sub-millimetre resolution for imaging small animals. IEEE Trans Nucl Sci 46:468–473

Knoll G (2000) Radiation detection and measurement. Wiley, New York

Lecomte R, Cadorette J, Rodrigue S, Lapointe D, Rouleau D, Bentourkia M, Yao R, Msaki P (1996) Initial results from the Sherbrooke avalanche photodiode positron tomograph. IEEE Trans Nucl Sci 43:1952–1957

Lewellen TK (1998) Time-of-flight PET. Semin Nucl Med 28:268–275

Liang Z, Turkington T, Gilland D, Jaszczak R, Coleman R (1992) Simultaneous compensation for attenuation, scatter and detector response for SPECT reconstruction in three dimensions. Phys Med Biol 37:587–603

Marsden PK, Strul D, Keevil SF, Williams SC, Cash D (2002) Simultaneous PET and NMR. Br J Radiol 75 Spec No:S53–S59

Meikle SR, Kench P, Kassiou M, Banati RB (2005) Small animal SPECT and its place in the matrix of molecular imaging technologies. Phys Med Biol 50:R45–R61

Ollinger JM (1996) Model-based scatter correction for fully 3D PET. Phys Med Biol 41:153–176

Pichler BJ, Bernecker F, Boening G, Rafecas M, Pimpl W, Schwaiger M, Lorenz E, Ziegler SI (2001) A 4×8 APD array, consisting of two monolithic silicon wafers, coupled to a 32-channel LSO matrix for high-resolution PET. IEEE Trans Nucl Sci 48:1391–1396

Schafers KP, Reader AJ, Kriens M, Knoess C, Schober O, Schafers M (2005) Performance evaluation of the 32-module quadHIDAC small-animal PET scanner. J Nucl Med 46:996–1004

Schmand M, Eriksson L, Casey ME, Andreaco MS, Melcher C, Wienhard K, Fluegge G, Nutt R (1998) Performance results of a new DOI detector block for a high resolution PET-LSO research tomograph: HRRT. IEEE Trans Nucl Sci 45:3000–3006

Seidel J, Vaquero JJ, Green MV (2003) Resolution uniformity and sensitivity of the NIH ATLAS small animal PET scanner: comparison to simulated LSO scanners without depth-of-interaction capability. IEEE Trans Nucl Sci 50:1347–1350

Song X, Segars WP, Du Y, Tsui BM, Frey EC (2005) Fast modelling of the collimator-detector response in Monte Carlo simulation of SPECT imaging using the angular response function. Phys Med Biol 50:1791–1804

Surti S, Karp JS (2004) Imaging characteristics of a 3-dimensional GSO whole-body PET camera. J Nucl Med 45:1040–1049

Surti S, Karp JS, Popescu LM, Daube-Witherspoon ME, Werner M (2006) Investigation of time-of-flight benefit for fully 3-D PET. IEEE Trans Med Imaging 25:529–538

Tai YC, Ruangma A, Rowland D, Siegel S, Newport DF, Chow PL, Laforest R (2005) Performance evaluation of the microPET focus: a third-generation microPET scanner dedicated to animal imaging. J Nucl Med 46:455–463

Wernick MN, Aarsvold JN (eds) (2004) Emission Tomography. The fundamentals of PET and SPECT. Elsevier, San Diego

Zeniya T, Watabe H, Aoi T, Kim KM, Teramoto N, Takeno T, Ohta Y, Hayashi T, Mashino H, Ota T, Yamamoto S, Iida H (2006) Use of a compact pixellated gamma camera for small animal pinhole SPECT imaging. Ann Nucl Med 20:409–416

Ziegler SI, Pichler BJ, Boening G, Rafecas M, Pimpl W, Lorenz E, Schmitz N, Schwaiger M (2001) A prototype high resolution animal positron tomograph with avalanche photodiode arrays and LSO crystals. Eur J Nucl Med 28:136–143

Magnetic Resonance Imaging and Spectroscopy

Tobias Schaeffter(✉) and Hannes Dahnke

Abstract Magnetic resonance imaging (MRI) and spectroscopy (MRS) are noninvasive techniques that allow the characterization of morphology, physiology and metabolism in vivo. MRI and MRS have become techniques of choice in many preclinical and clinical applications. In this chapter, the basic principles and the instrumentation of MRI and MRS are described. Furthermore, the factors that influence the sensitivity are discussed and examples for the limit of contrast agent detection are given.

1 NMR Basics

1.1 NMR Principle

Magnetic resonance imaging (MRI) and magnetic resonance spectroscopy (MRS) are based on the nuclear magnetic resonance (NMR) effect that was discovered in

Tobias Schaeffter

Division of Imaging Sciences, King's College London, The Rayne Institute, St Thomas' Hospital, London SE1 7EH, UK

tobias.schaeffter@kcl.ac.uk

W. Semmler and M. Schwaiger (eds.), *Molecular Imaging I.*

Handbook of Experimental Pharmacology 185/I.

ⓒ Springer-Verlag Berlin Heidelberg 2008

1946 independently by two groups at Stanford (Bloch et al. 1946) and at Harvard University (Purcell et al. 1946). In order to measure the NMR effect, three fundamental requirements have to be fulfilled. The first requirement is that the nucleus of interest possesses a nonzero magnetic moment. Typical nuclei used in NMR are, for instance, hydrogen (^{1}H), phosphorus (^{31}P), carbon (^{13}C), sodium (^{23}Na) or fluorine (^{19}F). The second requirement is the use of an external static magnetic field, B_0. In the absence of an external magnetic field, the individual magnetic moments of the atoms in the tissue being examined are randomly oriented and there is no net magnetization. In the presence of such a field, the magnetic moments align at a specific angle along with or opposed to the external field, as described by the Zeemann effect.

Therefore, a torque is produced that results in a precessional movement around the B_0 field (Fig. 1). The frequency of precession, also called the Larmor frequency, is proportional to B_0, and the constant called gyromagnetic ratio, which differs among nuclei (Table 1). Hydrogen plays an important role for biomedical applications, because its gyromagnetic ratio is the largest of all nuclei and it is abundantly present in biological tissue.

The sign of rotation depends on orientation of the spins; i.e., some spins are aligned along the B_0 field, whereas others opposed to it. Since an alignment along the B_0 field corresponds to a lower energy state, slightly more nuclei will align along the B_0 field rather than opposed to it. Consequently, the tissue will exhibit a

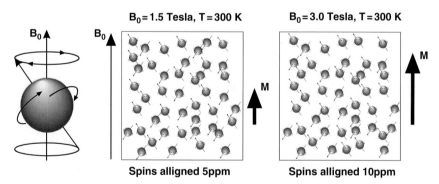

Fig. 1 *Left*: Larmor precession of a spinning nucleus about the axis of an applied magnetic field. *Right*: Influence of increased magnetic field strength on the net magnetization, *M*

Table 1 Properties of nuclei

Nucleus	Spin	γ (MHz/T)	Chemical shift range (ppm)
^1H	$^1/_2$	42.57	10
^{13}C	$^1/_2$	10.71	200
^{19}F	$^1/_2$	40.07	2,000
^{23}Na	$^3/_2$	11.26	70
^{31}P	$^1/_2$	17.25	30

net magnetization that is parallel to the external magnetic field and is called longitudinal magnetization (Fig. 1). The percentage is given by the Boltzmann distribution
and depends on the temperature and the field strength of the B_0 field. For an applied
field of 1.5 Tesla and at room temperature, the surplus of magnetic moments that
are aligned more along the magnetic field is about 5 parts per million (ppm). Therefore, the net magnetization, i.e., the inherent sensitivity of NMR, is rather small. By
using a higher magnetic field, a larger net magnetization is produced, increasing the
sensitivity of NMR.

The third requirement is the use of an additional time-varying magnetic field,
B_1, applied perpendicular to the static B_0 field and at the resonance condition (i.e.,
at Larmor frequency). For this, an additional RF coil is used to produce a B_1-field
pulse at a certain amplitude and duration. Such a B_1 pulse flips the longitudinal
magnetization to an arbitrary angle (also called the flip angle) with respect to the
external static field B_0. The transverse component of the flipped magnetization pre-
cesses around the static B_0 field at the Larmor frequency and induces a time-varying
voltage signal in the RF coil (Fig. 2).

The detected transverse magnetization does not remain forever, since two independent relaxation processes take place. First, the spin-lattice relaxation describes,
how fast the longitudinal magnetization recovers after applying the B_1 field. The
rate of the recovery process is determined by the relaxation time T_1. Second, the
spin-spin relaxation describes how fast the transverse magnetization loses its coherence and thus decays. The rate of dephasing is determined by the relaxation time
T_2. In addition to spin-spin interactions, dephasing between the coherently processing magnetic moments can also be caused by B_0-field inhomogeneities. As a result,
an apparently stronger relaxation process is visible, which is called T_2^* relaxation.
This T_2^* relaxation describes the decay envelope of the time-varying signal, which
is measured as time-varying voltage in the RF coil and thus is also called the free
induction decay (FID).

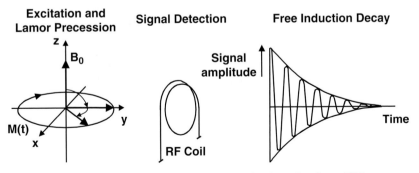

Fig. 2 Excitation of magnetization and measurement of a free induction decay (FID)

1.2 NMR Spectroscopy

As described above, nuclei of different elements resonate at different Larmor frequencies because they differ in gyromagnetic ratio. But even spins of the same isotope can resonate at different frequencies if they differ in their molecular environment, i.e., chemical structure. This frequency difference is called chemical shift and is commonly expressed as a relative measure in parts per million, which makes this parameter independent from the field strength. The range of the chemical shifts differs for the different nuclei (Table 1). In NMR spectroscopy, the chemical shift is exploited by acquiring the NMR signal from a defined volume within the body. Numerous techniques have been proposed for obtaining spectra from well-defined localized regions of the body by using methods like rotating frame (Hoult 1979) or PRESS (Ordige et al. 1985). The NMR signal is then Fourier transformed to yield an NMR spectrum. The comparison of the chemical shifts measured in a sample with values in reference tables allows the identification of chemical substances, while the signal intensity is proportional to their concentration. MRS provides a noninvasive window on the metabolism (Avison et al. 1986) with a wide range of preclinical and clinical applications (Evanochko et al. 1984; Prichard 1986). NMR is a relatively insensitive technique, i.e., tissue metabolites must be present in relatively high concentrations to be detectable. However, the sensitivity depends on the nucleus detected. Studies of tissue metabolism in vivo have generally made use of the ^{1}H, ^{31}P, ^{13}C and ^{19}F nuclei.

In in-vivo ^{1}H-NMR spectroscopy, the major signals come from water and lipids, since they are present in living tissue in very high concentrations. Therefore, these signals have to be suppressed by dedicated NMR techniques to see signals from much more dilute metabolites. In addition, the study of tissue metabolites is complicated by the large number of metabolites that produce signals in a relatively narrow chemical-shift range. Therefore, the use of higher magnetic field strengths is beneficial to avoid overlapping of corresponding peaks. The proton spectrum of the brain, for example, includes peaks from creatine (Cr), choline (Cho), *N*-acetylaspartate (NAA), lactate (Lac), myo-inositol (mI), glucose (Glx) and lipids (Fig. 3a). The relative levels of the corresponding spectral peaks can reflect the cellular status and health of the tissue. A wide range of spectroscopic imaging techniques has been developed to identify certain molecules and molecular pathways in vivo (Abraham et al. 1988).

The nucleus that has been used extensively for metabolic studies is ^{31}P. As can be seen from the gyromagnetic ratios (Table 1), phosphorus has a resonance frequency of about 40% that of protons. Therefore, the RF coil used to transmit and to receive must be tuned and matched at this lower frequency. While the ^{31}P-NMR is less sensitive than ^{1}H-NMR, the chemical-shift range is larger (about 30 ppm for biological phosphates). The major phosphorus-containing metabolites are adenosine triphosphate (ATP), phosphocreatine (PCr), phosphoryl choline (PC), phosphorylethanolamine (PE), glycerophosphophorylcholine(GPC) glycerophosphorylethanolamine (GPE) and inorganic phosphate (Pi) (Fig. 3b). NMR of ^{31}P is used to study

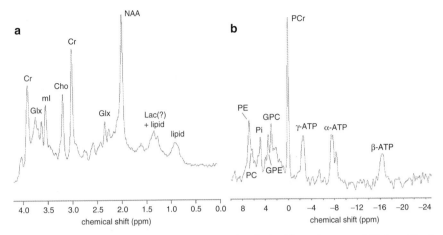

Fig. 3 a, b NMR spectroscopy obtained in the brain of a healthy volunteer at 3 Tesla. **a** Single voxel ^{1}H spectra (PRESS, TE = 35 ms, 15 ml) and **b** voxel (36 ml) of a proton-decoupled ^{31}P spectroscopic imaging experiment (Data Philips Medical Systems, Cleveland)

tissue energetics and allows the in-vivo measurement of pH value in tissue (Moon and Richards 1973).

NMR spectroscopy of ^{13}C has a much lower intrinsic sensitivity than ^{1}H-NMR. Therefore, in the absence of isotopic enrichment, ^{13}C signals are very weak. As a result, ^{13}C studies can be divided into the following categories: those in which compounds are present at high enough concentrations (e.g., glycogen in liver and muscle), and those in which ^{13}C-labeling is used to study metabolic pathways. Recently, a new technique was proposed to increase the sensitivity of ^{13}C-NMR by using hyperpolarization (Golman et al. 2001).

Fluorine-19 is one of the most sensitive of the NMR nuclei (about 80% of the gyromagnetic ratio of ^{1}H). However, there are no endogenous compounds that yield detectable ^{19}F signals in vivo. Therefore, exogenous ^{19}F-containing compounds have to be used. MRS of ^{19}F has been used to study the pharmacokinetics and metabolism of fluorinated drugs (Presant et al. 1994). Recently, ^{19}F-NMR has been performed using targeted perfluorcarbon nanoparticles for noninvasive dosimetry of restenosis therapy (Lanza et al. 2002).

1.3 NMR Imaging

The NMR signal described so far is simply the sum of individual signals from the nuclei. Assuming there is only one type of nucleus and only one chemical shift in the sample, all spins would resonate at the same frequency. In order to distinguish magnetization at different locations, magnetic field gradients are applied that cause a linear variation of the magnetic field strength in space. The spatially varying

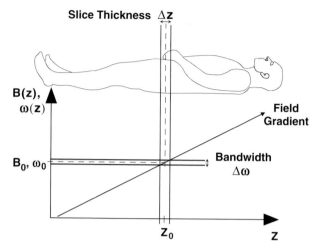

Fig. 4 Slice selective excitation. The slice thickness is determined by the steepness of the gradient and the radiofrequency (RF) bandwidth

gradient amplitudes determine the difference between the actual field strength at a certain location and the static field B_0, i.e., the precession frequency varies over space. Usually, for three-dimensional encoding, not all gradients are applied simultaneously and the image formation process can be separated into three phases: slice selection, phase encoding and frequency encoding.

Slice selection is accomplished using a frequency-selective B_1 pulse applied in the presence of a magnetic field gradient. The position of the slice is determined by the frequency of the B_1 pulse, whereas the slice thickness depends on its bandwidth and the gradient amplitude (Fig. 4). Having selected a slice, the signal has to be spatially encoded in the remaining two dimensions. One of these directions is encoded by producing a spatially varying phase shift of precessing transverse magnetization. This is achieved by applying a phase-encoding gradient for a short period before acquisition of the signal resulting in location-dependent phase shifts of the transverse magnetization. To achieve full spatial encoding, a number of experiments have to be carried out with stepwise variation of the phase-encoding gradient. The third spatial dimension is encoded by applying a frequency-encoding gradient during data acquisition. This gradient is changing the precession frequency over space and creates a one-to-one relation between the resonance frequency of the signal and the spatial location of its origin. Performing a two-dimensional Fourier transform of the acquired signal yields the position of the contributing magnetization.

The spatial resolution depends on the amplitude of the gradients and the acquisition bandwidth. Typical values of the spatial resolution of clinical scanners are in the order of millimeter. Dedicated animal scanners operating at a higher magnetic field strength and applying stronger gradients are able to obtain images with voxels smaller than 100 μm.

Spectroscopic imaging combines MR spectroscopy with spatial encoding in two or three directions, such that spectroscopic information can be displayed as an image: for each peak in the spectrum, the spatial distribution of the integrated peak intensity is displayed. Since the metabolite concentrations in living organisms are four to five orders of magnitude lower than the concentration of water, the voxel size in clinical MR spectroscopy and spectroscopic imaging is usually much larger, i.e., in the order of $1\,cm^3$.

2 Instrumentation: Magnet, Gradients, RF Coils

As described above, MRI and MRS studies use a combination of different hardware components: a magnet, a magnetic field gradient system and an RF transmit/receive system. Currently, magnets for clinical MRI systems range between 0.23 and 3 Tesla and most clinical systems operate at 1.5 Tesla. Recently, a number of research systems for human applications have been installed and work at 7 Tesla (Fig. 5) or higher. Most animal MRI systems use magnetic field strengths at 4.7 Tesla and 7 Tesla, but systems above 10 Tesla are also available. Although higher field strengths result in a higher signal, the use of such field strengths is hampered by a longer T_1 and increased RF heating due to RF losses in the body. All magnets for higher field strengths are made of superconducting coils that are immersed in cryogenic fluids (liquid helium). At this temperature the coil windings become superconducting, such that the static magnetic field, is maintained once an inductive current has been introduced. After installation, the magnet field homogeneity must be optimized either by applying correction fields. This procedure is also called shimming and can be achieved by placing pieces of iron into the magnet bore and by using additional shim coils.

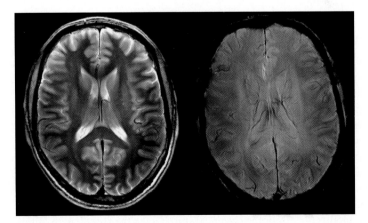

Fig. 5 MR images of the human brain obtained on a 7 Tesla whole-body scanner (Philips Medical Systems, Cleveland). *Left*: T2-weighted high-resolution image ($0.4 \times 0.4 \times 4\,mm$). *Right*: T1-weighted high-resolution image ($0.4 \times 0.4 \times 2\,mm$)

Spatial encoding requires the use of magnetic field gradients in three orthogonal directions. These weak magnetic field gradients are produced by three orthogonally positioned coils connected to independently controlled gradient amplifiers. The magnetic field gradients generated by these coils should be as linear as possible over the imaging volume. A complicating factor is the occurrence of eddy currents, which are generated inside conducting parts of the MR system due to fast switching of the magnetic field gradients. These eddy currents produce unwanted magnetic fields in the imaging volume resulting in artifacts. The effects of eddy currents are minimized by the design of actively shielded gradient coils. The applied currents through the gradient coils can be around several hundreds of amperes. Since these currents are flowing inside a static magnetic field, large forces act on the mechanical parts of the gradient coil causing acoustic noise during the MR measurement.

The RF coils in an MRI system are used for excitation and signal detection. The coils must be able to produce a uniform or well-defined B_1 field inside the imaging volume. The coils are tuned and matched to the resonance frequency of the type of nucleus being observed. The placement of an object inside the RF coil is equivalent to the addition of a resistance to the coil circuit, referred to as coil loading. At field strengths higher than 0.5 Tesla, the signal-noise introduced by the object dominates the inherent noise of coil circuit. Often separate coils are used for excitation and detection, i.e., a large volume coil (body coil) is used for excitation, whereas dedicated receive coils are used for detection. Usually, dedicated receive coils have a higher sensitivity, since they can be placed close to the region of interest and exhibit a better filling factor, i.e., obtain less noise. The concept of dedicated receive coils can be extended, if an array of receive coils is used. Each coil element covers a different part of the body and after acquisition the individual images of all coil elements can be combined to large field of view image. In addition, the spatial sensitivity of the array coil elements can also be used to speed up the acquisition by means of parallel imaging methods (Pruessmann et al. 1999).

3 Contrast Mechanisms

One of the most remarkable features of NMR is its superior soft-tissue contrast without the application of ionizing radiation. MRI is capable of measuring a wide range of endogenous contrast mechanisms that include the proton density, the spin-lattice relaxation time (T_1), the spin-spin relaxation time (T_2), the chemical shift, magnetization transfer (Mehta et al. 1996), temperature and different types of motion, like blood flow, perfusion or diffusion. The appropriate selection of measurement parameters results in a certain image contrast that allows the characterization of morphology, physiology, metabolism and molecular information in vivo. Some of these mechanisms can also be influenced by exogenous parameters, e.g., contrast agents to modify T_1, T_2 or the chemical shift. Given the short length of this chapter, this text is focusing on the description of the relaxation times only, whereas a detailed description of other mechanisms and related measurement techniques can be found in Haacke et al. (1999) and Vlaardingerbroek and den Boer (2002).

4 Relaxation Times

The contrast in MRI and the shapes of the spectral lines in MRS are strongly influenced by two relaxation processes. These processes can be described by exponential relationships characterized by the time constants T_1 and T_2, respectively. The relaxation times T_1 and T_2 depend on the specific molecular structure of the analyte, its physical state (liquid or solid) and the temperature; they vary among different tissues and are affected by pathologies.

The longitudinal relaxation time T_1 describes the statistical probability for energy transfer between the excited nuclei and the molecular framework, named the lattice: it is also termed spin-lattice relaxation time. The net magnetization returns to the equilibrium at a rate given by $R_1 = 1/T_1$. Typical T_1 values in biological tissue range from 20 ms to a few seconds. Efficient transfer of energy to the lattice is highly dependent on the molecular motion of the lattice causing fluctuations in the local magnetic fields and thus inducing transitions between the spin states of the nuclei. The motion modes, i.e., rotational, vibrational and translational motion, depend on the structure and the size of the molecules. The motion of large molecules is characterized by low frequencies, that of medium and small size molecules by higher frequencies. Efficient energy transfer (i.e., a short T_1) occurs when the frequency of the fluctuating fields, which is determined by the molecular motion, matches the Larmor frequency of the spins. Therefore, the T_1 relaxation time depends on the field strength. Finally, T_1 relaxation is affected by the presence of macromolecules that possess hydrophilic binding sites, i.e., water protons in tissue relaxing much faster than those in pure water. The T_1-relaxation time can be measured by the inversion recovery method (IR), which consists of two RF pulses (Fig. 6). The first RF pulse inverts the magnetization. After a time interval (TI) the second RF pulse flips all longitudinal magnetization into the transversal plane, which is then measured. In order to measure the T_1 decay, a number of inversion-recovery experiments have to be performed with different values of TI.

The transverse or spin-spin relaxation (T_2) relies on the transfer of energy between magnetic nuclei. Immediately after the excitation all spins precess coherently (i.e., in phase), but interactions between individual magnetic moments result in variations in the precession frequencies of the spins. As a result, a dephasing of the spins occurs, causing an exponential decay of the transverse magnetization. The transverse relaxation time T_2 is influenced by the physical state and the molecular size. Solids and large molecules are characterized by relatively short T_2 times, small molecules by long T_2 values. Therefore, the presence of macromolecules in solution shortens T_2, since the overall molecular motion is reduced leading to more effective

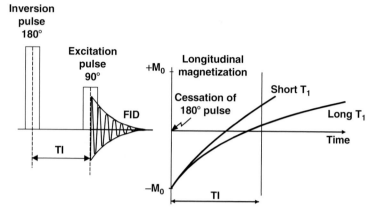

Fig. 6 Inversion recovery (IR) sequence. The combination of an inversion pulse followed by an excitation pulse allows strong T_1-weighting of the signal. For the measurement of the T_1-relaxation time a number of IR sequences with different inversion times have to be applied

spin-spin interactions. Typical T_2 relaxation times in biological tissue range from a few micro-seconds in solids to a few seconds in liquids. The T_2 relaxation process is nearly independent of the field strength. In addition to the spin-spin interaction, the phase coherence is also influenced by local field inhomogeneities in the applied magnetic field. The exponential decay resulting from the combination of T_2 relaxation and field inhomogeneities is referred to as the effective transverse relaxation time T_2^*. In order to measure the true T_2-relaxation, the influence of the B_0 inhomogeneity must be compensated by a spin-echo experiment (Fig. 7). In this experiment, two B_1 pulses are applied: the first pulse with a flip angle of 90° tilts all longitudinal magnetization into the transverse plane. The second pulse with a flip angle of 180° refocuses the dephasing caused by B_0 inhomogeneity. Both pulses are separated by a time period of $T_E/2$ and a signal is acquired after T_E (echo delay time). During the first $T_E/2$ period, i.e., between the 90° and 180° pulses, the individual magnetic moments precess at different Larmor frequencies due to the B_0 inhomogeneity. As a result, they obtain different phase shifts, which translate into a dephasing of the bulk magnetization. The 180° pulse applied at $T_E/2$ inverts the magnetic moments and correspondingly their phases; the phase shift acquired during the following delay $T_E/2$ exactly compensates the inverted phases shifts acquired during the period prior to the 180° pulse leading to the formation of a so-called spin echo. Its amplitude depends only on the relaxation time T_2 and the echo time (T_E). In order to measure the T_2 decay time a number of spin-echo experiments with different values of T_E have to be performed.

In some cases, the measurement of the effective relaxation time T_2^* is of interest. For instance, the oxygenation status of blood influences this relaxation time by local field inhomogeneities and the related contrast mechanism is termed blood-oxygen-level-dependent (BOLD) effect (Ogawa et al. 1990). The electron spin of iron center of blood hemoglobin changes from a diamagnetic to a paramagnetic

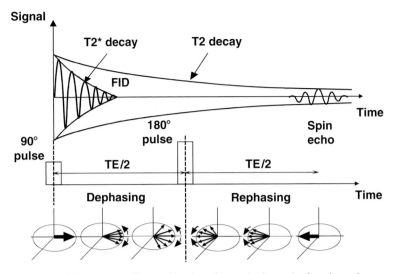

Fig. 7 Spin-echo (SE) sequence. The combination of an excitation and refocusing pulse generates an SE signal at the echo time (TE). For the measurement of T2-relaxation time a number of SE sequences with different TE have to be applied

state during deoxygenation. Therefore, blood deoxygenation results in a reduction of T_2^* relaxation time. This contrast mechanism is exploited in functional brain spectroscopy (Ernst and Hennig 1994) and imaging (Moonen and Bandettini 1999), which allows the visualization of activated brain areas. The quantification of T_2^* and the initial magnetization allows the separation of the BOLD effect from perfusion effects (Speck and Hennig 1998).

5 Sensitivity of NMR

The sensitivity of NMR can be described by the detection limit, which is defined as the smallest amount or concentration of a substance that can be reliably detected in a given type of sample by a specific measurement process. In biomedical imaging, the detection of two different types of substances has to be distinguished: tracers and contrast agents. A tracer is a distinguishable substance (typically with low natural abundance) that is administered to the body to determine the distribution of material. A contrast agent is a substance that improves the contrast of certain tissues and/or structures in diagnostic imaging. Tracers can be detected by a direct measurement and thus their detection limit is mainly by determined by the signal-to-noise ratio (SNR). Contrast agents are detected indirectly by measuring their influence on the image contrast. Therefore, the detection limit of contrast agents is mainly determined by the contrast-to-noise ratio (CNR). In the following, the factors will be discussed that affect the SNR and CNR and examples for the detection limits of NMR are given.

5.1 SNR

The SNR is given by the ratio of the signal amplitude and the noise deviation. The SNR is dependent on a wide range of factors, including the nucleus that is being studied, the concentration and the volume of the sample (i.e., the number of spins), the magnetic field strength, the design of the receive coil, and the measurement time (Macovski 1996). Because of the large number of variables, it is impossible to give anything other than an order of magnitude estimate for the number of spins that is required for detection. Bloembergen et al. (1948) stated that the detection limit of NMR at 1.5 Tesla is in the order of 10^{18} spins/voxel. However, for clinical MRI and MRS a much higher number of spins (approximately 6×10^{19} spins/voxel $= 10^{-4}$ mol) is required taking into account clinically relevant measurement times. The number of required spins becomes especially important if nuclei other than ^{1}H are investigated, e.g., ^{19}F, ^{13}C. For instance, the ^{19}F tracer perfluorooctylbromide (PFOB) contains 17 fluorine spins per molecule; therefore, approximately 6 μmol of PFOB per voxel will be required for detection. Assuming a voxel size of 1 cm^3, a concentration of 6 mM PFOB is needed for the detection by MRI or MRS. The sensitivity of ^{13}C is lower due to the lower gyromagnetic ratio (10.71 MHz/T). Recent studies show that a hyperpolarization (i.e., the polarization of a material far beyond thermal equilibrium conditions) of ^{13}C enables high detection sensitivity (Golman et al. 2003). The detection time is limited, since the T_1 time of the hyperpolarized ^{13}C is on the order of 40 s. The same applies for hyperpolarized gases like ^{3}He and ^{129}Xe, which are used, e.g., for lung imaging (Albert et al. 1994; Moller et al. 2002).

One straightforward approach for increasing the SNR is the use of higher magnetic field strengths. Figure 8 shows the comparison of a similar MRI sequence at different field strengths.

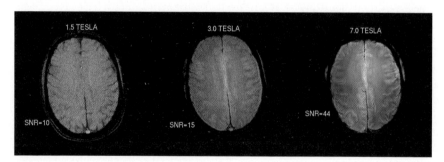

Fig. 8 SNR comparisons of three-dimensional gradient-echo sequence on 1.5-, 3.0-, and 7.0-Tesla (Philips Achieva) MR systems. ROIs located in same anatomical and background locations for measurements. The repetition time TR was adjusted: TR = 15 ms (1.5 Tesla), TR = 19 ms (3 Tesla), TR = 32 ms (7 Tesla) for optimum SNR at these field strengths

5.2 CNR

The contrast is defined as the difference of the signal intensity within two regions of interest. The CNR is, therefore, described by the contrast divided by the standard deviation of the noise. However, even if there is a high SNR within the image, it might not be possible to see the difference in contrast, since this is determined by the change in signal intensity.

Contrast agents change the relaxation rates $R_{1,2}(= 1/T_{1,2})$ of the surrounding spins (e.g., protons). Therefore, the detection limit does not depend on the number of spins per voxel but on the number of affected spins. The ability of an MR contrast medium to shorten the relaxation times of spins in its vicinity is described by their relaxivity. At the concentrations normally used in MR imaging, the effect of an MR contrast agent augments the relaxation rate proportionally to the concentration of the MR contrast medium. If $R_{\text{intrinsic\_1,2}}$ is the relaxation rate of tissue and $r_{1,2}$ is the relaxivity of the contrast agent, the $R_{1,2}$ relaxation rate in the presence of the contrast agent is given by $R_{1,2} = R_{\text{intrinsic\_1,2}} + r_{1,2}C$, where C is the concentration of the MR contrast agent. MR contrast agents consist of ions or molecules with one or more unpaired electrons. They are referred to as paramagnetic, superparamagnetic, or ferromagnetic, depending on their specific electrone configuration. Of widespread use in MR are paramagnetic, e.g., gadolinium (Gd^{3+}), and superparamagnetic, e.g., iron oxide particles (SPIOs), contrast agents.

Assuming the imaging parameters are optimized to generate the optimal CNR, then the MR contrast agent needs to change the relaxation rate $(R_{1,2})$ by a higher factor than the variation of the intrinsic relaxation rate among the tissues. These variations can be dominated by the SNR of the measurement if the tissue has a very homogeneous structure. But if the structure of the tissue is heterogeneous, the intrinsic relaxation rate varies spatially.

Paramagnetic agents influence mainly the relaxation rate R_1. Typical Gd-DTPA contrast agents have a relaxivity of $r_1 \approx 5$ (mM s^{-1}) (Toth et al. 2001). The intrinsic relaxation rates in tissue are in the order of $1\,\text{s}^{-1}$. Assuming that a change of the relaxation rate of $0.25\,\text{s}^{-1}$ results in a detectable CNR, a concentration of about $50\,\mu$M of a typical Gd-DTPA agent is required. Several ways of increasing the detectability of contrast agents have been proposed. For instance, the relaxivity can be increased by attaching a number of paramagnetic ions to carrier substances like dendrimers (Wiener et al. 1994), polymers (Schuhmann-Giampieri et al. 1991), liposomes (Unger et al. 1991), fullerenes (Mikawa et al. 2001) or perfluorcarbon nanoparticles (Lanza et al. 1996). It has been shown that a perfluorocarbon nanoparticle emulsion can be loaded with around 100,000 Gd-DTPA molecules per particle, resulting in a relaxivity of about 10^6 (mM s^{-1}). With this, only picomolar concentrations of paramagnetic perfluorocarbon nanoparticles are required for the detection and quantification at clinical field strengths (Morawski et al. 2004).

Superparamagnetic agents affect the $R_2^{(*)}$ as well as R_1 relaxation rate. Typically, superparamagnetic iron oxide particles (SPIOs) show a relaxivity of $r_1 = 20$ (mM s^{-1}) and $r_2 = 100{-}190$ (mM s^{-1}) (Wang et al. 2001; Lawaczeck et al. 1997), i.e., those agents shorten strongly the T_2 relaxation time. The intrinsic relaxation rates in tissue are on the order of $R_2 = 10$–$20\,\mathrm{s}^{-1}$ and also the variations of the intrinsic relaxation are in the same order as the relaxation rates. Therefore, a much higher effect on the relaxation rate R_2 needs to be achieved by the SPIO contrast agents in order to result in an appropriate CNR.

Another way to detect contrast agents directly is to measure the spatial distribution (map) of the relaxation rates. In order to detect a contrast agent, the change in relaxation rate due to the contrast agent must be 3- to 5-times higher than the standard deviation of the intrinsic relaxation rate of the tissue (which results in an appropriate CNR in the relaxation rate map). It has been shown that relaxation rate mapping allows sensitive detection of SPIO agents (Dahnke and Schaeffter 2005). In particular, the necessary concentration for detection of a typical SPIO agent (Resovist, Schering) was calculated to be $43\,\mu M$ [Fe] in brain.

In some cases, the spatial resolution is also influencing the sensitivity. For instance, a low image resolution can attenuate the relaxation effects through the partial volume effect, e.g., if labeled cells only account for a small fraction of the voxel volume. It was recently shown in ex-vivo studies that single iron oxide labeled cells can be detected by lowering the voxel volume down to $100\,\mu m^3$. In the special case of having highly localized contrast agent concentrations as well as a very homogeneous background, a reasonable CNR can be generated to image single labeled cells. Lowering the resolution only enhances the sensitivity if the contrast agent is highly localized.

6 Conclusion

MRI is a nonionizing imaging technique with superior soft-tissue contrast, high spatial resolution and good temporal resolution. MRI is capable of measuring a wide range of endogenous contrast mechanisms that allow the characterization of morphology and physiology in vivo. MRS provides a noninvasive window on the metabolism. NMR spectroscopy, which was originally developed as an analytical technique to study the composition of chemical compounds, is an essential tool for studying various aspects of the biochemistry, physiology, and pathophysiology. Therefore, MRI and MRS have become the techniques of choice in many preclinical and clinical applications. With ongoing developments to improve the acquisition speed and quantitative accuracy of MRI and MRS, the range of applications continues to expand.

References

Abraham RJ, Fisher J, Loftus P (1988) Introduction to NMR spectroscopy. Wiley, Chichester
Albert MS, Cates GD, Driehuys B et al (1994) Biological magnetic resonance imaging using laser-polarized 129Xe. Nature 370:199–201
Avison MJ, Hetherington HP, Shulman RG (1986) Applications of NMR to studies of tissue metabolism. Annu Rev Biophys Biophys Chem 15:377–402

Bloch F, Hansen WW, Packard ME (1946) Nuclear induction. Phys Rev 69:127
Bloembergen N, Purcell EM, Pound RV (1948) Relaxation effects in nuclear magnetic resonance absorption. Phys Rev 73:679–712
Dahnke H, Schaeffter T (2005) Limits of detection of SPIO at 3.0 T using T2 relaxometry. Magn Reson Med 53(5):1202–1206
Ernst T, Hennig J (1994) Observation of a fast response in functional MR. Magn Reson Med 32(1):146–149
Evanochko WT, Ng TC, Glickson JD (1984) Application of in vivo NMR spectroscopy to cancer. Magn Reson Med 1(4):508–534
Golman K, Axelsson O, Johannesson H et al (2001) Parahydrogen-induced polarization in imaging: subsecond (13)C angiography. Magn Reson Med 46(1):1–5
Golman K, Olsson LE, Axelsson O et al (2003) Molecular imaging using hyperpolarized 13C. Br J Radiol 76(2):118–127
Haacke EM, Brown RW, Thomson MR et al (1999) Magnetic resonance imaging, physical principles and sequence design. Wiley-Liss, New York
Heyn C, Bowen CV, Rutt BK et al (2005) Detection threshold of single SPIO-labeled cells with FIESTA.Magn Reson Med 53(2):312–320
Hoult DI (1979) Rotating frame zeugmatography. J Magn Reson 33:183–197
Lanza GM, Wallace KD, Scott MJ et al (1996) A novel site-targeted ultrasonic contrast agent with broad biomedical application. Circulation 95:3334–3340
Lanza GM, Yu X, Winter PM et al (2002) Targeted antiproliferative drug delivery to vascular smooth muscle cells with a magnetic resonance imaging nanoparticle contrast agent: implications for rational therapy of restenosis. Circulation 106(22):2842–2847
Lawaczeck R, Bauer H, Frenzel T et al (1997) Magnetic iron oxide particles coated with carboxydextran for parenteral administration and liver contrasting. Pre-clinical profile of SH U555A. Acta Radiol 38(4):584–597
Macovski A (1996). Noise in MRI. Magn Reson Med 36(3):494–497
Mehta RC, Pike GB, Enzmann DR (1996) Magnetization transfer magnetic resonance imaging: a clinical review. Top Magn Reson Imaging 8(4):214–230
Mikawa M, Kato H, Okumura M et al (2001) Paramagnetic water-soluble metallofullerenes having the highest relaxivity for MRI contrast agents. Bioconjug Chem 12:510–514
Moller HE, Chen XJ, Saam B et al (2002) MRI of the lungs using hyperpolarized noble gases. Magn Reson Med 47(6):1029–1051
Moon RB, Richards JH (1973) Determination of Intracellular pH by 31P Magnetic Resonance. J Biol Chem 248:7276–7278
Moonen CTW, Bandettini PA (1999) Functional MRI. Springer, Berlin Heidelberg New York
Morawski AM, Winter PM, Crowder KC et al (2004) Targeted nanoparticles for quantitative imaging of sparse molecular epitopes with MRI. Magn Reson Med 51(3):480–486
Ogawa S, Lee TM, Kay AR et al (1990). Brain magnetic resonance imaging with contrast dependent on blood oxygenation. Proc Natl Acad Sci USA 87(24):9868–9872
Ordige RJ, Bendall MR, Gordon RE et al (1985) Volume selection for in-vivo biological spectroscopy. In: Govil G, Khetrapal CL, Saran A (eds) Magnetic resonance in biology and medicine. Tata McGraw Hill, New Delhi, pp 387–397
Presant CA, Wolf W, Waluch V et al (1994) Association of intratumoral pharmacokinetics of fluorouracil with clinical response. Lancet 343(8907):1184–1187
Prichard JW, Shulman RG (1986) NMR spectroscopy of brain metabolism in vivo. Annu Rev Neurosci 9:61–85
Pruessmann KP, Weiger M, Scheidegger MB et al (1999) SENSE: sensitivity encoding for fast MRI. Magn Reson Med 42(5):952–962
Purcell EM, Torrey HC, Pound RV (1946) Resonance absorption by nuclear magnetic moments in a solid. Phys Rev 69:37–38
Schuhmann-Giampieri G, Schmitt-Willich H, Frenzel T (1991) In vivo and in vitro evaluation of Gd-DTPA-polylysine as a macromolecular contrast agent for magnetic resonance imaging. Invest Radiol 26:969–974

Speck O, Hennig J (1998) Functional imaging by I_0- and T_2^*-parameter mapping using multi-image EPI. J Magn Reson Med 40(2):243–248

Toth E, Helm L, Merbach AE (2001) Relaxivity of gadolinium(III) complexes: theory and mechanism. In: Toth E, Merbach AE (eds) The chemistry of contrast agents in medical magnetic resonance imaging. Wiley, New York

Unger E, Shen DK, Wu GL et al (1991) Liposomes as MR contrast agents: pros and cons. Magn Reson Med 22:304–308

Vlaardingerbroek MT, den Boer JA (2002) Magnetic resonance imaging, theory and practice, 3rd edn. Springer, Berlin Heidelberg New York

Wang YX, Hussain SM, Krestin GP (2001) Superparamagnetic iron oxide contrast agents: physicochemical characteristics and applications in MR imaging. Eur Radiol 11(11):2319–2331

Wiener EC, Brechbiel MW, Brothers H et al (1994) Dendrimer-based metal chelates: a new class of magnetic resonance imaging contrast agents. Magn Reson Med 31:1–8

Ultrasound Basics

Peter Hauff(✉), Michael Reinhardt, and Stuart Foster

Abstract Imaging technologies for in vivo functional and molecular imaging in small animals have undergone a very fast development in the last years with very intense competition to further develop resolution and molecular sensitivity. Among the imaging technologies available, ultrasound-based molecular imaging methods are of particular interest, since the use of ultrasound contrast agents allows specific and sensitive depiction of molecular targets. Together with new developments in quantification methods of targeted microbubbles, sonography represents a dynamic and seminal tool for molecular imaging.

1 Introduction

Diagnostic ultrasound is one of the most common techniques used in diagnostic investigations today. It's a safe, noninvasive, inexpensive technology compared with other diagnostic modalities and causes minimum inconvenience and stress to the patient. In recent years, advances in sonographic equipment and techniques and the introduction of commercially produced echo-enhancing agents have led to substantial

Peter Hauff
Global Drug Discovery, Bayer Schering Pharma AG, 13342 Berlin, Germany
peter.hauff@bayerhealthcare.com

W. Semmler and M. Schwaiger (eds.), *Molecular Imaging I.*
Handbook of Experimental Pharmacology 185/I.
© Springer-Verlag Berlin Heidelberg 2008

improvements in the image quality obtained and widened the scope of sonography. Furthermore, new ultrasound technologies, such as µ-ultrasound and the feasibility for creating target-specific ultrasound contrast agents (USCAs) for molecular imaging, offers new possibilities in the field of experimental pharmacology in small rodents. They allow biological processes in living animals to be visualized noninvasively and the tracking in real time of the spread of disease, and the effects of a drug candidate throughout the system.

2 Technical Aspects

2.1 Basics

The ultrasonic waves employed for medical purposes are generated by piezoelectric elements. These are tiny chips of vibrating quartz, which produce elastic vibrations that are transmitted to the material being investigated. The transmission of sound waves from the sound source — known as the transducer — to the material takes place on the basis of elastic vibrations. The elastic vibrations emanate from the transducer in the direction of propagation of the waves (longitudinal waves) (cf. Fig. 1).

A sound wave is made up of a series of compressions and rarefactions. The unit, made up of one compression and one rarefaction, comprises a wave. The distance between the start (maximum compression) of a wave and the next comprises one wavelength (λ).

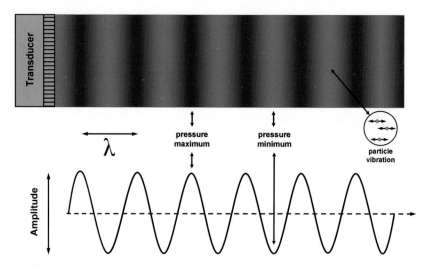

Fig. 1 Principle of the propagation of ultrasound

The individual molecules of the irradiated material vibrate in such a manner that regions of compression and regions of rarefaction periodically alternate in space, as illustrated in Fig. 1. The reflected vibrations of the irradiated material are received again by the transducer and are analyzed in the ultrasound equipment. It is this double function that is the reason for the use of the term "transducer".

The deflection in space of the particles making up the material is known as the amplitude of vibration. The distance between two regions of the same vibrational state (e.g., two pressure maxima) is a wavelength (λ). The number of vibrations a point makes per second is the frequency [1 vibration per second = 1 Hertz (Hz)].

The following simple relationship between the wavelength (λ), frequency (f) and the velocity of propagation (v) (here the speeds of wavelength are dependent on sound) applies generally to the other propagation of waves:

$$\lambda = \frac{v}{f}$$

e.g., $$\lambda = \frac{1,500\,m/s}{1.5\,MHz} = \frac{1.5 \cdot 10^6\,mm/s}{1.5 \cdot 10^6\,vibrations/s} = 1\,mm\,(per\,vibration)$$

For water ($v \approx 1,500\,\mathrm{m/s}$), the calculation given above shows that a frequency of 1.5 MHz corresponds to a wavelength of 1 mm. Other substances yield other results specific for them, because the speed of sound is material-specific. In media with low density and a low amount of mass particles, as for example in gases, a relatively long period passes before the neighboring mass particle becomes excited. In such cases, the propagation speed of sound is relatively slow compared with media of higher density and a larger mass of mass particles, e.g., in liquids or solids (cf. Table 1).

The phenomena of reflection and refraction, which take place on transition between materials with differing propagation velocities known from light waves, also take place with sound waves (cf. Fig. 2).

Here the reflected portion of the ultrasonic energy depends on both the difference between the velocity of sound in the two media (impedance difference) and on the angle between the ray beam and the interface (angle of incidence).

Moving through the tissue, the energy of the wave weakens continuously due to internal loss of friction, which is called absorption. In air, for example, there is a marked absorption, while liquids weaken sound only a little. The specific absorption rate is not the same for all frequencies: low frequencies have a relatively low absorption rate compared with high frequencies. From that point of view, transducers with low frequencies would always be the best choice. Unfortunately, low

Table 1 Propagation speed of ultrasound in various media

Media	Density (g/cm^3)	Propagation speed (m/s)
Air	1.2×10^{-3}	330
Water (37 °C)	1.0	1,520
Soft tissue	1.026	1,540 (mean)
Bone	1.9	3,800

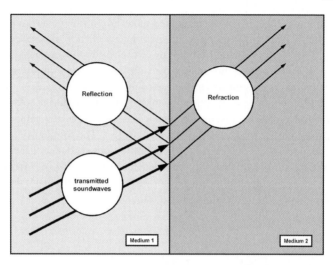

Fig. 2 Ultrasound divides at the interface between media with differing sound velocities into a portion which is refracted and continues and a portion which is reflected

frequencies have also the decisive disadvantage of having a low spatial resolution, which increases with frequency. Therefore, different types of transducers with different frequencies are available, depending on different diagnostic targets and the different penetration depths needed.

2.2 Conventional Techniques

Although the phenomenon of sound waves has been observed and described since antiquity, the view generally prevails that the discovery of the piezoelectric effect by the brothers Pierre and Jacques Curie in 1880 form the basis for the medical use of ultrasound. This effect is a characteristic of crystals (e.g., quartz, tourmaline) or ceramic materials (e.g., barium titanate, barium zirconate), which become electrically polarized under physical pressure. On the other hand, these materials begin to vibrate and emit high-frequency acoustic waves when charged with alternating electrical voltage. All ultrasonic probes (transducers) used with medical ultrasound devices are equipped with so-called piezo elements and function according to the principle of the piezoelectric effect. The high frequency ultrasonic waves are induced by creating an electrical voltage and are emitted by the transducer. The ultrasonic waves reflected by the body are collected by the transducer and converted by piezo elements into electrical signals, which are then processed by the ultrasound machine and represented as pixels. Nonetheless, over 60 years elapsed from discovery to the first use of the piezoelectric effect in medical ultrasound diagnostics. As in many other technical fields, the selective use of high-frequency acoustic waves was developed for military detection of submarines during the First

World War. This resulted in the development of SONAR (sonar = sound navigation and ranging) by Lewis F. Richardson from the UK and Reginald A. Fessenden from Canada, nearly in the same time. Based on that, in 1916 Paul Langevin and Constantin Chilowsky developed a high-performance sonar, a so-called hydrophone, which enabled the detection of submarines. This hydrophone is also regarded as the "first ultrasound machine". Besides military application, the possibilities for the nonmilitary use of ultrasound were also investigated. Here, the Russian, Sergei Y. Sokolov carried out pioneer work in 1929 with for the development of the first ultrasound machine for the examination of material defects in metals. Also, in other countries of Europe and in America, researchers developed similar devices. Experiments were conducted with ever higher frequencies and shorter pulse widths and, as a result, better spatial resolution was attained. The devices developed for this purpose were called reflectoscopes and work in the so-called A mode.

In the A mode ("A" for amplitude), the backscattered signal intensities that are received are represented oscillographically as amplitude over time. The height of the amplitudes reflects the intensity of the backscattered ultrasonic signals and the distances between the amplitudes, which is the running time. Both the distance of the reflecting structures from the transducer, as well as the distance between the individual structures can be determined via the running time. The first physician to use ultrasound successfully for diagnostic purposes was the Austrian neurologist, K. Th. Dussik. He described in 1942 and 1949 a new method for brain examination and the cerebral ventricles using the A mode: *hyperphonography*. Colleagues critically discussed these examinations at that time, particularly with regard to the complex accessibility to the brain, due to it being surrounded by bone. John Wild at the beginning of the 1950s, carried out much promising research for differentiating between healthy and tumorous intestine and breast tissue. Apart from the improvement in linear sonography (A mode), there was intensive work carried out on two-dimensional (2D) sonography. As a result, John Weid and John Reid developed a B-mode contact scanner for clinical use and they were, thereby, capable of producing so-called real-time images.

The B mode ("B" for brightness) is a modified representation of the A mode, whereby many neighboring A-mode lines are used here. The amplitudes of the A-mode lines are translated into gray tones. Usually, the highest amplitude is assigned the brightness value *white*, whereas the zero line of the amplitude scale is assigned the brightness value *black*. The intermediate amplitudes are assigned certain gray tones on an appropriate gray-tone scale (maximum 256).

During the same period, a further gray-scale technique, i.e., the M (motion)-mode procedure, was developed by Edler and Hertz for cardiological indications. Here, the same part of the body is constantly exposed to ultrasound. The ultrasonic lines are, however, located temporarily next to each other on the monitor, although they belong to the same part of the body. This procedure allows for a dynamic representation of bodily processes and is predominantly used in cardiology for the assessment of cardiac valve function and myocardial contraction.

The next qualitative leap in medical ultrasound diagnostics took place through the use of the Doppler effect for the measurement of blood flow. This effect was named after the physicist Christian Johann Doppler (1803–1853). Doppler's acoustic law states that frequency changes occur in the sound field if transmitters and receivers move in relation to each other. A frequent example used to explain Doppler's principle is the acoustic perception of a bystander/listener (= receiver) of a moving car (= transmitter). The acoustic waves produced by the car transmit in all directions. For the listener, the frequency rises as a car approaches and decreases as it departs. For determining blood flow, the transducer emits ultrasonic waves of a known frequency, which are reflected (backscattered) by the blood cells and are received again by the transducer. The frequencies, now being received, differ according to the direction of the flowing blood cells. Higher frequencies are received from blood cells moving towards the transducer and lower frequencies when they move away. We can, therefore, deduce the rate and direction of motion of objects relative to each other from the measured frequency. First examinations of transcutaneous blood flow measurements were described as early as 1959 by Satomura. The first implementation of the Doppler principle in sonography was the continuous wave Doppler mode (CW-Doppler), which allowed for the measurement of blood-flow by use of a transducer, which contained one crystal for transmit and another for receive, which operated simultaneously. Such transducers provided a flow-spectrum over time, whereby the depth of the measurement could be chosen by controlling the time between transmission and reception (range gating). A further improvement was made by the development of pulse Doppler (PW-Doppler). This mode was already possible by using a 2D-array transducer, enabling to set a sample volume precisely into the vessel aided by the B-mode image (= duplex sonography). In contrast to the CW-Doppler mode, the PW-Doppler allowed to depict the "systolic window" and to distinguish between normal and tourbulent flow. The rapid development of computer performance in the late 1980th finally allowed color coding of blood-flow within a two dimensional image and also the combination of this functional image with the anatomical B-mode image by superimposing both. This procedure is also known as *color-flow mapping* (CFM), or in the countries where German is spoken as *farbkodierte Duplexsonographie* (color-coded duplex sonography, CCDS). The CCDS technique color-codes the areas of the image in which movement is detected, e.g., the blood flow. Today's ultrasonic diagnostic units usually code the color *red* for movements on the transducer and *blue* if these move away from the transducer, whereby the color adjustment is left up to the user. With the introduction of a further Doppler method, i.e., power-Doppler sonography, a higher sensitivity was obtained in the representation of low flow rates and volumes. With this procedure, which is also known as intensity Doppler, the energy of the Doppler signal, which is calculated mathematically from the integral via the signal amplitudes, is represented as being color-coded in superposition to the B-image (Lorenz and Betsch 1995; Frentzel-Beyme 1994, 2005; Paulsen Nautrup and Tobisa 2001; Edler and Lindström 2004; Baker 2005).

Further conventional ultrasonic procedures, such as B-flow, tissue harmonic imaging, SieFlow, SieScape, coherent image formation or 3D and 4D imaging will not be discussed at any length here, as these do not play any or only a subordinate role in contrast-agent-enhanced sonography.

2.3 Contrast-specific Techniques

The beginnings of diagnostic ultrasound were characterized by USCA-free examinations for the morphological characterization of tissue, which was soon followed
by functional examinations through the introduction of Doppler technologies. On
the other hand, USCA-dependent examinations were introduced and established
initially in the area of functional diagnostics. The clinical use of USCA for mor-
phologic diagnostics was developed later.

Various physical interactions between ultrasonic waves and USCA, as well as
USCA-specific imaging technologies, will be discussed in this section. Details regarding the morphology of USCA microbubbles and their clinical and preclinical
use are described by us later in this volume (see Part II Imaging Probes in the chapter by Peter Hauff et al.).

Gas-filled microbubbles (MBs) are particularly well suited for enhancing the
contrast (to increase the ratio between the target and the surrounding tissue), due
to their special physical and acoustic characteristics. Their contrast characteristics
can be induced and employed as a function of the used frequency and sound intensity (= amplitude or sound pressure) of the irradiated ultrasonic wave both without
destruction and with destruction of these MBs. Ultrasonic waves of very low sound
intensity lead to a resonant oscillation of the MBs (= linear), i.e., the MBs contract
and expand symmetrically to the rhythm of the positive and negative pressure phases
of the applied acoustic wave. In doing so, acoustic waves of the same frequency to
which these MBs were exposed are reflected and converted into an image by the
ultrasound device, as illustrated in Fig. 3 (Schrope et al. 1992; de Jong 1997).

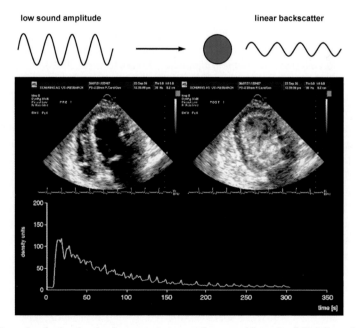

Fig. 3 Example of echo signal enhancement at a very low sound intensity (MBs' linear behavior)
after administration of Levovist in the left ventricle of a dog's heart

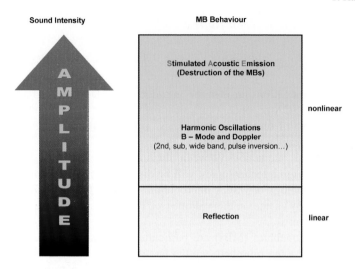

Fig. 4 Diagram of the linear and nonlinear performance of USCA bubbles at different sound intensities

Greater sound amplitudes cause asymmetrical oscillation of the MBs, since the encapsulated gas bubbles oppose compression with a greater resistance than they do expansion (cf. Fig. 4). During this process, which is also called nonlinear performance, other frequencies besides the output frequency are also emitted during the signal response. These other frequencies are the so-called harmonic frequencies, or overtones and undertones. The frequency components that are harmonic overtones are multiples of (i.e., double, triple, quadruple, etc.) the fundamental frequency used and/or its half, third, quarter, etc. in the case of undertone frequency component. The latter are also called subharmonic frequencies (Forsberg et al. 2000).

Among the harmonic overtone frequencies, the second harmonic overtone frequency is of special importance in contrast-agent-specific sonography, due to its high amplitude. For example, the basic frequency received from tissue and the contrast-agent bubbles, is suppressed by special filtering techniques during signal processing. Only the contrast-agent-specific parts of the second harmonic frequency are used to generate the image. This procedure results in a clear reduction of the tissue signal portion, resulting in a more intensive representation of the contrast signal in relation to the tissue (improvement of the signal-to-noise ratio). On the other hand, for the effective separation of the basic frequency signals from the harmonic frequencies, a narrow-band transmission frequency has to be selected, and a narrow-band pass filter has to be used with the receiver, which results in the serious disadvantage of reduced spatial resolution and less contrast. The technique, known as *second-harmonic imaging* has, in the meantime, been integrated into the ultrasound equipment of all manufacturers as a contrast-agent-specific mode (Burns et al. 1992; Schrope et al. 1992; Schrope and Newhouse 1993; de Jong et al. 1994, 2002).

As opposed to second-harmonic imaging, for which an additional specific filter is necessary for the selective use of the second-harmonic frequency of the contrast-agent bubbles, another technology, *wideband harmonic imaging* (= phase or pulse-inversion technique), makes use of the entire frequency spectrum for the representation of contrast-agent-specific signals. The decisive advantages are found in the fact that the signal intensity of the contrast-agent bubbles is higher, on the whole, and the use of a wideband transducer results in a better spatial resolution when compared with second harmonic imaging. To simplify this technology, which is also known as the pulse-subtraction procedure, two successive ultrasonic pulses are emitted, whereby the phase of the second pulse is inverted with the phase of the first. Now, from the received (backscattered) signals the two sequential waves (positive and negative wave) are subtracted from each other, whereby mathematically, the results cancel each other out with linear signals. The nonlinear signals of the contrast-agent bubbles have not, on the other hand, been cancelled and are represented. This procedure is offered by the various ultrasound equipment manufacturers under a number of synonyms (Chapman and Lazenby 1997; Eckersley et al. 2005; Zheng et al. 2005).

Both procedures are used in combination with the B mode and with Doppler technologies.

While the described procedures in the nondestructive mode for contrast-agent bubbles (also known as *low MI* = low mechanical index) are predominantly used, there are other technologies, which use the destructibility of the contrast-agent bubbles (*high MI* mode = high mechanical index). The MI, which is today usually displayed on the screen of the ultrasonic equipment, is the respective transmitting power, calculated from the maximum negative sound pressure divided by the square root of the sonic frequency.

At very high sound intensities, the MBs are destroyed by mechanical force. Sound pressure can, however, vary in intensity, due to the different type of morphology presented by the various USCA. With the possibility of visualizing the destruction process by using high speed cameras, different mechanisms were identified, which have been summarized in the overview by Postema et al. (2004). Three of the phenomena specified therein are the fragmenting of gas bubbles, the destruction of the bubble shell and the radiation effect (synonyms: jetting, microstreaming, microjets). Examinations have shown that the wall thickness and elasticity of the material encapsulating gas MBs are crucial for triggering a fragmentation or a destruction of the encapsulation. While fragmenting was provable mainly in USCA bubbles with thin and flexible encapsulation (8–20 nm), thick-walled (200–300 nm) and rather inelastic encapsulation caused their destruction. Fragmentation causes one gas MB to create many smaller bubbles. The destruction of the encapsulation causes the gas to escape through a tear in the encapsulating material and dissolve in the blood (Postema et al. 2005).

One very interesting and indicative observation, concerning the future of ultrasound diagnostics, was the emergence of color pixels on the monitor of the ultrasound device in color Doppler during the destruction process of polymer-coated air MBs after their accumulation in the livers of rabbits. This USCA consists of

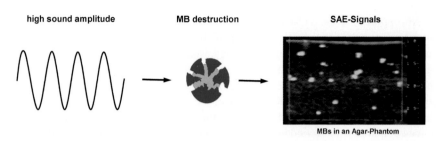

high sound amplitude   **MB destruction**   **SAE-Signals**

MBs in an Agar-Phantom

Fig. 5 Example of nonlinear signals of USCA bubbles during the application of very high sound pressure. On the right side of the illustration are SAE signals recognizable in the color Doppler mode, which were received by immobile USCA bubbles during destruction

rather thick (approximately 200 nm) and not very flexible bubble shell (Olbrich et al. 2006). There are two explanations for this phenomenon:

1. At the time of the destruction process of this USCA, a short-lived wideband, nonlinear frequency signal is emitted, which differs clearly from the signals of the MBs in the nondestructive mode, which is called *stimulated acoustic emission* (SAE).
2. A significantly shorter pulse length is reflected during the extremely fast bubble destruction process compared with the emitted one, which can not be clearly interpreted by the software of the ultrasound machines. This process is also known as *loss of correlation* (LOC).

However, both explanations describe the same process. In this chapter as well as in the chapter by Peter Hauff et al. of this volume, we use the term "SAE" for describing some characteristics and applications of this process in molecular ultrasound imaging.

It could also be shown that the SAE signal is also generated by stationary, immobile MBs and is (incorrectly) interpreted as movement by the color Doppler mode of the ultrasound device. The received signal is represented in the color Doppler image as colored pixels on the monitor of the ultrasound device due to this misinterpretation.

The discovery of the SAE signal generated by stationary MBs represents a crucial basis for the new field of research in diagnostic molecular imaging with ultrasound (cf. Fig. 5). The strength of these SAE signals is sufficiently high to detect individual USCA bubbles, even at depths of several centimeters within the tissue (Reinhardt et al. 1993; Uhlendorf and Hoffmann 1994).

3 Techniques for Molecular Ultrasound Imaging

Various procedures for the quantification of echo signals have been established in functional sonography. The simplest measuring procedures are conducted by providing a time-echo signal-intensity curve. The echo signal intensity is either determined directly by digital registration of the ultrasonic signals (B mode, spectral or color Doppler) or indirectly by measuring the volume of the spectral Doppler sound signal or respectively by measuring the film density in B mode or by recording color changes in color Doppler (video densitometry) (Cosgrove 1996). Ellegala et al. (2003) conducted the first examinations of in-vivo specific quantification of bound MBs in intracerebral tumors of mice. In another examination, Thiemann et al. (2000) showed the possibility of quantifying stationery MBs in large concentrations, however with poor spatial resolution.

However, new ultrasound technologies have been recently developed for qualitative and quantitative molecular ultrasound imaging in preclinical settings. One, *microultrasound*, is a high resolution ultrasound technique specifically developed for investigations in small rodents; the other technique, *sensitive particle acoustic quantification*, works on another principle and can be also used for larger lab animals. Both techniques will be described in more detail due to their importance for the experimental pharmacology field.

3.1 High-resolution Imaging: Microultrasound

In recent years, high-frequency ultrasound between 20 and 60 MHz has emerged as an important tool in the clinical imaging of the eye and skin (Foster et al. 2000) and especially as a means of preclinical imaging of the mouse and other small animal models of disease (Foster et al. 2002; Zhou et al. 2002). In this frequency range, resolution between 30 and 150 μm is possible, offering the potential to perform both targeted molecular and untargeted MB imaging with unprecedented resolution. This technology, referred to as ultrasound biomicroscopy or microultrasound, has enabled the quantitative assessment of anatomy and functional analysis of normal tissue development and disease models to be studied under reproducible conditions in mice and other small animals. The imaging equipment and scanning method for mouse imaging are shown in Fig. 6.

The scanner (VisualSonics Vevo 770, Toronto) controls an imaging scanhead that is held in proximity to the mouse by means of a "rail" system to maintain a rigid frame of reference. The mouse lies anesthetized on a heated stage instrumented for ECG, temperature and if necessary blood pressure and breathing cycle. A thin layer of gel is used to couple the ultrasound beam to the mouse. Applications of microultrasound have focused studies of development, cardiovascular disease, cancer and inflammation (Franco et al. 2006; Kulandavelu et al. 2006; Zhou et al. 2004). Functional imaging of blood flow hemodynamics and morphology has been central to the work performed. The spontaneous contrast of blood has been used to image two- and three-dimensional flow in tumor micro vasculature in mice (Foster et al. 2000; Goertz et al. 2000, 2002, 2003). This has allowed the effects of different anticancer therapeutic agents to be assessed in preclinical studies (Goertz et al. 2002; Shaked et al. 2006). The process of image gathering, segmentation and visualization

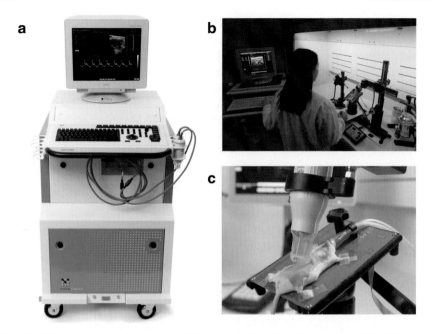

Fig. 6 a High-frequency micro-ultrasound instrumentation (VisualSonics Vevo 770). **b** Laboratory configuration in a laminar flow hood showing rail system for image stabilization and three-dimensional imaging. **c** Configuration for freehand imaging of a mouse

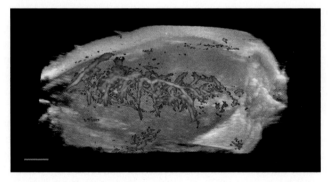

Fig. 7 Three-dimensional image of a KHT fibrosarcoma showing natural contrast of the blood at high frequencies (30 MHz). *Bar* ~ 1 mm

has now been automated in commercially available instrumentation, with the result that tumors like the KHT sarcoma, shown in Fig. 7, can be imaged in three dimensions, analyzed, and rapidly segmented into vascular and tissue compartments.

The above studies rely solely on the natural contrast of blood flowing in the microcirculation and reflect flow down to the level of the terminal arterioles (vessel diameters of about 50 μm). To penetrate deeper into the true microcirculation,

MB contrast agents are needed to enhance the signal from the capillary blood pool. Probing molecular targets in the capillary microcirculation of tumors and other targets requires that the MBs be labeled with an appropriate ligand, as described by us later in this volume (Part II Imaging Probes in the chapter by Peter Hauff et al.).

The choice of MB shell and gas has an important influence on how microbubbles respond at high frequencies. Two principal mechanisms of contrast exist. The first is based on the large acoustical impedance discontinuity that exists between the gas inside the bubble and the adjacent tissues. Rayleigh scatter that results from the interaction of an ultrasound beam with such a particle is proportional to the 6th power of the radius and the 4th power of frequency. Another and even stronger mechanism for contrast arises from the driven oscillation of the microbubble in the ultrasound field that can result in significant nonlinearities (Leighton 1994). In this case the microbubble resonates in the ultrasound field expanding during periods of negative pressure and contracting during positive pressure. The combination of Rayleigh and resonant scatter provides an enhancement of many orders of magnitude for bubbles in the low MHz range with the result that low frequency clinical imaging is very successful using nonlinear processing schemes (Becher and Burns 2000). It is not clear that currently approved agents or the previously developed nonlinear processing methods are suitable for imaging of mice at frequencies greater than 20 MHz. Several companies, such as Targeson (Charlottesville, Va.) and VisualSonics (Toronto, Canada), now provide MB kits that can be targeted to endothelial cell surface markers and are well suited to small animal imaging. Although high frequency nonlinear processing has shown promise (Goertz et al. 2005, 2006), current implementations of high-frequency contrast imaging rely on subtraction schemes in which reference data sets are subtracted from a contrast-enhanced images.

3.2 Sensitive Particle Acoustic Quantification (SPAQ)

Reinhardt et al. (2005) recently described a totally new type of ultrasonic procedure allowing the quantification of approximately 100-fold more targeted MBs than possible with the conventional ultrasound techniques using the SAE effect. This procedure, called SPAQ (sensitive particle acoustic quantification) makes it possible to obtain a highly sensitive quantification of target-specific bound MBs in concentrations >100,000 MB/ml volume in three-dimensional structures. Due to its novelty, this technology will be described in greater detail in the following section.

With the SPAQ technology, the characteristic SAE signals of MBs in the color Doppler are counted, which occur during their ultrasonically induced destruction. The SAE signal strength is so high that even individual MBs can be detected. The individual SAE signal, however, is represented on the monitor dimensioned in millimeters (cf. Fig. 8a) (according to the unit, transducer and settings), which is substantially larger than the actual size of the undestroyed MBs ($\leq 5\,\mu m$). This

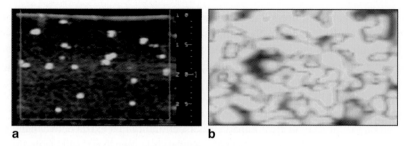

a   **b**

Fig. 8 a, b Destruction of air-filled MBs in two agar phantoms with different MB concentrations. **a** Separate SAE signals are visible in the left phantom (100 MBs/ml), each of them representing the destruction of one single MB. Thereby, the size of one individual SAE-signal is up to one mm. **b** In the right phantom, which contains 3,000 MBs/ml, no individual SAE-signals are detectable, due to a complete signal overlay based on the size of the SAEs, which is again dependent on the spatial resolution of the transducer. Any higher MB concentration would yield the same result in the image and MBs could therefore not be quantified

results from the simple fact that the spatial resolution of diagnostic ultrasound is also given in the millimeter range (the smallest volumes that can be displayed by the ultrasound unit: 1 voxel is approximately $1\,mm^3$).

Under these conditions, with conventional ultrasonic methods, above a concentration of approximately 1,000 MB/ml tissue there is a complete saturation of the ultrasonic image with SEA effects (= saturation bubble concentration), which no longer permits any reliable quantification of individual signals (cf. Fig. 8b).

It is to be strongly assumed, however, that a specific MB enhancement is mostly above 1,000/ml with regard to the target density. Therefore, an accurate quantification of targeted microbubbles will be impossible in many cases. With present-day SPAQ technology, even MBs in concentrations $>100,000/ml$ tissue can be quantified; that is more than 100-fold. The principle of SPAQ is based on generating defined overlaps (shifts) between consecutive ultrasonic (cross-) sectional views and the use of SAE signals that are linked to the complete destruction of the appropriate MBs.

The functionality of SPAQ, as it is schematically represented in Fig. 9, shows different stages of the overlapping of consecutive ultrasonic (cross-) sectional views at the same MB concentration with the different number of SAE signals resulting from it. Here, it has to be recognized that a small overlapping (= large advance) of the ultrasonic sectional views result in a high SAE image layer thickness with complete color saturation of the ultrasonic image with SEA signals (cf. Fig. 9 *upper part*) and does not allow any quantification of the signals (high SAE image layer thickness). In contrast, an increase in overlapping (middle SAE image layer thickness) results in a thinner SAE image layer thickness, which now also makes it possible to recognize individual SAE signals alongside large-surface signals (cf. Fig. 9 *middle part*). A further increase in overlapping (= small advance) now enables us to quantify individually represented SAE signals (thin SAE image layer thickness) (cf. Fig. 9 *lower part*). In order to assure the predefined overlapping advance of an object against the

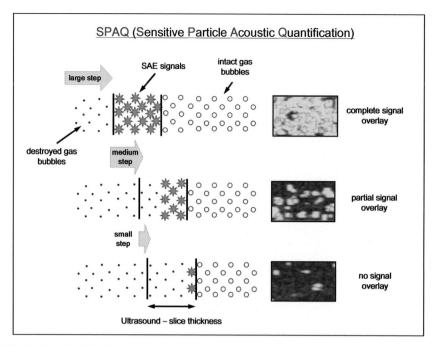

Fig. 9 The principle of SPAQ. If an object moves toward a transducer, the ultrasound beam destroys the MPs within the acoustic field (*black dots*). Further movement results only in the destruction of those MPs (*red stars*), which are additionally reached by the ultrasound beam, whereby the step size of the transducer determines the SPAQ resolution independently of the slice thickness of the ultrasound beam. A low step-size corresponds to a high SPAQ resolution and vice versa. All ultrasound images in the *right column* show the same agar-phantom with the same high MB concentration. Depending on the used SPAQ resolution, the ultrasound image can show a complete or partial signal overlay or individual SEAs in the case of a high SPAQ resolution

transducer, the object to be investigated is affixed to a highly precise positioning device, which makes it possible to advance within the range of micrometers and which is synchronized with the image repetition rate of the ultrasound device. It is also of particular importance to recognize that each MB is capable of emitting an SAE signal once only, since its emission is resulting from the destruction of the MB. Consequently, new SAE signals can only result from those MBs that have newly arrived in the ultrasound field during a further advance of the object being examined. If, for example, the advance between two sequential images is 10 μm (= high overlapping of the ultrasound images), then the SAE signals represented in this image can only come from this 10-μm thick layer. Therefore, the width of the advancement defines the resolution of the SPAQ method (SAE layer thickness) (Reinhardt et al. 2005). Application examples for microultrasound and SPAQ are given in Part II Imaging Probes in the chapter by Peter Hauff et al. of this volume.

References

Baker JP (2005) The history of sonographers. J Ultrasound Med 24:1–14

Becher, Burns PN (2000) Handbook of contrast echocardiography. Springer, Berlin Heidelberg New York

Burns PN, Powers JE, Fritzsch T (1992) Harmonic imaging: a new imaging and Doppler method for contrast enhanced ultrasound. Radiology 185:142

Chapman CS, Lazenby JC (1997) Ultrasound imaging system employing phase inversion substraction to enhance the image. US Patent No. 5,632,2777

Cosgrove D (1996) Warum brauchen wir Kontrastmittel für den Ultraschall? Clin Radiol 51 Suppl. 1, 1–4.

De Jong N, Cornet R, Lancee CT (1994) Higher harmonics of vibrating gas-filled microspheres. Part one: Simulations. Ultrasonics 32:447–453

DeJong N (1997) Physics of microbubble scattering. In: Nanda NC, Schlief R, Goldberg BB (eds) Advances in echo imaging using contrast enhancement, 2nd edn. Kluwer, Dordrecht, pp 39–64

De Jong N, Bouakaz A, Ten Cate FJ (2002) Contrast harmonic imaging. Ultrasonics 40: 567–573

Eckersley RJ, Chin CT, Burns PN (2005) Optimising phase and amplitude modulation schemes for imaging microbubble contrast agents at low acoustic power. Ultrasound Med Biol 31:213–212

Edler I, Lindström K (2004) The history of echocardiography. Ultrasound Med Biol 30:1565–1644

Ellegala DB, Leong-Poi H, Carpenter JE et al (2003) Imaging tumor angiogenesis with contrast ultrasound and microbubbles targeted to $\alpha_v\beta_3$. Circulation 108:336–341

Forsberg F, Shi WT, Goldberg BB (2000) Subharmonic imaging of contrats agents. Ultrasonics 38:93–98

Foster FS, Burns PN, Simpson DH et al (2000) Ultrasound for the visualization and quantification of tumour microcirculation. Cancer Metastasis Rev 19:131–138

Foster FS, Pavlin CJ, Harasiewicz KA et al (2000) Advances in ultrasound biomicroscopy. Ultrasound Med Biol 26:1–27

Foster FS, Zhang MY, Zhou YQ (2002) A new ultrasound instrument for in vivo microimaging of mice. Ultrasound Med Biol 28:1165

Franco M, Man S, Chen L (2006) Targeted anti-vascular endothelial growth factor receptor-2 therapy leads to short-term and long-term impairment of vascular function and increase in tumor hypoxia. Cancer Res 66:3639–3648

Frentzel-Beyme B (1994) Als die Bilder laufen lernten oder die Geschichte der Ultraschalldiagnostik [When the pictures started moving — history of diagnostic ultrasound]. Ultraschall Klein Prax 8:265–275

Frentzel-Beyme B (2005) Vom Echolot zur Farbdopplersonographie – Die Geschichte der Ultraschalldiagnostik. Radiologe 45:363–370

Goertz DE, Christopher DA, Yu JL et al (2000) High-frequency color flow imaging of the microcirculation. Ultrasound Med Biol 26:63–71

Goertz DE, Yu JL, Kerbel RS et al (2002) High-frequency Doppler ultrasound monitors the effects of antivascular therapy on tumor blood flow. Cancer Res 62:6371–6375

Goertz DE, Yu JL, Kerbel RS et al (2003) High-frequency 3-D color-flow imaging of the microcirculation. Ultrasound Med Biol 29:39–51

Goertz DE, Needles A, Burns PN et al (2005) High Frequency Nonlinear Color Flow Imaging of Microbubble Contrast Agents. IEEE Trans Ultrason, Ferroelect, Freq Contr 52:495–502

Goertz DE, Frijlink ME, de Jong N et al (2006) High frequency nonlinear scattering from a micrometer to submicrometer sized lipid encapsulated contrast agent. Ultrasound Med Biol 32:569–77

Kulandavelu S, Qu D, Sunn N et al (2006) Embryonic and neonatal phenotyping of genetically engineered mice. Ilar J 47:103–17

Lorenz A, Betsch B (1995) Zur Geschichte der Ultraschalldiagnostik - von der Compoundtechnik zur Realtimesonographie. Ultraschall Klin Prax 10:41–49

Olbrich C, Hauff P, Scholle F et al (2006) The in vitro stability of air-filled polybutylcyanoacrylate microparticles. Biomaterials 27:3549–3559

Postema M, van Wamel A, Lancee CT et al (2004) Ultrasound-induced encapsulated microbubble phenomena. Ultrasound Med Biol 30: 827–840

Postema M, Boukaz A, Versluis M et al (2005) Ultrasound-induced gas release from contrast agent microbubbles. IEEE Trans Ultrason, Ferroelect, Freq Contr 52:1035–1041

Poulsen Nautrup C, Tobias R (2001) Atlas und Lehrbuch der Ultraschalldiagnostik bei Hund und Katze, 3rd edn. Schlütersche, Hannover

Reinhardt M, Fritzsch T, Heldmann D et al (1993) Use of microcapsules as contrasting agents in colour Doppler sonography. WO 93/25241

Reinhardt M, Hauff P, Briel A et al (2005) Sensitive particle acoustic quantification (SPAQ): a new ultrasound-based approach for the quantification of ultrasound contrast media in high concentrations. Invest Radiol 40:2–7

Schrope V, Newhouse VL, Uhlendorf V (1992) Simulated capillary blood flow measurement using a non-linear ultrasonic contrast agent. Ultrasonic Imag 14:134–158

Schrope V, Newhouse VL (1993) Second harmonic ultrasonic blood perfusion measurement. Ultrasound Med Biol 19:567–579

Shaked Y, Ciarrochi A, Franco M et al (2006) Therapy induced acute recruitment of circulating endothelial progenitor cells to tumors. Science 313:1785–1787

Uhlendorf V, Hoffmann C (1994) Nonlinear acoustic response of coated microbubbles in diagnostic ultrasound. In: Ultrasonics Symposium, Cannes, France, pp 1559–1562

Tiemann K, Pohl C, Schlosser T et al (2000) Stimulated acoustic emission: pseudo-Doppler shifts seen during the destruction of non-moving microbubbles. Ultrasound Med Biol 26:1161–1167

Zheng H, Mukdadi O, Kim H et al (2005) Advantages in using multifrequency excitation of contrast microbubbles for enhancing echo particle image velocity techniques: initial numerical studies using rectangular and triangular waves. Ultrasound Med Biol 32:99–108

Zhou YQ, Foster FS, Qu DW et al (2002) Applications for multi-frequency ultrasound biomicroscopy in mice from implantation to adulthood. Physiol Genomics 10:113–126

Zhou YQ, Foster FS, Nieman BJ et al (2004) Comprehensive transthoracic cardiac imaging in mice using ultrasound biomicroscopy with anatomical confirmation by magnetic resonance imaging. Physiol Genomics 18:232–244

Multimodal Imaging Approaches: PET/CT and PET/MRI

Bernd J. Pichler(✉), Martin S. Judenhofer, and Christina Pfannenberg

Abstract Multimodality imaging, specifically PET/CT, brought a new perspective into the fields of clinical and preclinical imaging. Clinical cases have shown, that the combination of anatomical structures, revealed from CT, and the functional information from PET into one image, with high fusion accuracy, provides an advanced diagnostic tool and research platform. Although PET/CT is already an established clinical tool it still bears some limitations. A major drawback is that CT provides only limited soft tissue contrast and exposes the patient or animal, being studied, to a significant radiation dose. Since PET and CT scanner are hard-wired back to back and share a common patient bed, PET/CT does not allow simultaneous data acquisition. This temporal mismatch causes image artefacts by patient movement between the two scans or by respiration motion. To overcome these limitations, recent research concentrates on the combination of PET and MRI into one single machine. The goal of this development is to integrate the PET detectors into the MRI scanner

Bernd J. Pichler
Laboratory for Preclinical Imaging and Imaging Technology, University of Tübingen – Department of Radiology, Röntgenweg 13, 72076 Tübingen, Germany
bernd.pichler@med.uni-tuebingen.de

W. Semmler and M. Schwaiger (eds.), *Molecular Imaging I.*
Handbook of Experimental Pharmacology 185/I.
© Springer-Verlag Berlin Heidelberg 2008

which would allow simultaneous data acquisition, resulting in combined functional and morphological images with an excellent soft tissue contrast, very good spatial resolution of the anatomy and very accurate temporal and spatial image fusion. Additionally, since MRI provides also functional information such as blood oxygenation level dependant (BOLD) imaging or spectroscopy, PET/MRI could even provide multi-functional information of physiological processes in vivo. First experiments with PET/MRI prototypes showed very promising results, indicating its great potential for clinical and preclinical imaging.

1 Combining Functional and Morphological Information

The early detection of a disease at the vascular, cellular, or genomic rather than at the systematic or symptomatic level, in order to positively influence the course of the disease, is the utmost goal in clinical diagnosis. Noninvasive functional and morphological imaging increases the chances of accomplishing this aim. The strength of new imaging approaches lies in the combination of several methods providing complementary information about morphology and different functional processes in vivo.

Image Fusion by Software or Hardware?
There are several ways to fuse and analyze acquired morphological and functional image data. For visual fusion, images originated from two independent acquisitions are displayed and analyzed side by side. The fusion is carried out by the observer who is reviewing corresponding image slices and who correlates findings from one to the other modality. The visual fusion is very time-consuming and the success of revealing additional information of the two independently acquired images depends very much on the experience and skill of the observer. Nevertheless, this type of fusion is very widespread since it does not require technical infrastructure and it is cost effective.

The use of software fusion becomes more and more attractive since very advanced and fully automated algorithms, as well as the necessary computing power for a time effective workflow, are nowadays available (Slomka 2004). The software-based fusion usually uses fiducial markers or contour-finding algorithms to determine landmarks within both image data sets and find a "best fit" with least discrepancies. Basic approaches are mostly limited to rigid fusion, meaning that the applied transformation matrix has six degrees of freedom, three space directions and three rotational directions; there is no warping of the image data. These software tools produce very good results for rigid body regions such as the head. However, for abdominal or thoracic regions, where distortion due to the patient repositioning or movement of internal organs can not be avoided, more advanced algorithms are used to accurately fuse the images by applying additional linear transformations to the image data (Shekhar et al. 2005). These more advanced nonrigid transformation techniques very often require manual user assistance and are therefore more time-consuming.

To reduce the probability of patient or organ movement during scans, multi-modality imaging is the favorable choice (Beyer et al. 2000). Here, both imaging modalities are physically mounted next to each other or they are fully integrated into one device and have a fixed and known transformation matrix. Since the patient bed transfers from one to the other modality, the movement of the patient is minimized. Nevertheless, the movement of the internal organs, especially when longer scan times from either one modality are required, can be an issue. Thus, the use of advanced nonrigid image fusion algorithms or the simultaneous acquisition using a multimodality scanner can be essential when the situation includes fast internal organ movement or demands high registration accuracy.

2 PET/CT

2.1 Technical Aspects of PET/CT

Positron emission tomography (PET) has evolved to be one of the most meaningful functional imaging technologies due to the high sensitivity in the picomolar range as well as the ability to observe metabolic processes over time and track radiolabeled bio markers, so called tracers, in vivo (Czernin and Phelps 2002). Although PET data are very quantitative, they do, however, lack good spatial resolution and do not provide sufficient anatomical information, especially if very specific tracers are used. This limitation often requires the need to have morphological data *underlayed* in order to be more accurate in oncological diagnosis, tumor staging, or radiation therapy planning (Beyer et al. 2000; Townsend et al. 2004).

The first choice modality used to add anatomical information to the PET data is X-ray computed tomography (CT), since it is well established in clinical oncological imaging and provides a very good spatial resolution. In general, the realization of a hybrid PET/CT device is basically the two individual devices mounted next to each other with a patient bed able to transfer the patient from one device to the other (Fig. 1). Both devices are controlled from one computer console. A very fast obtainable CT projection scan (topogram or scout scan) is generally used for anatomical orientation and to plan the examination regions for the PET and CT scan (Fig. 1a). After planning, low-dose or diagnostic CT scans are performed. Following the CT scans, the PET images are acquired in a multibed position mode to cover the whole body of the patient (Fig. 1c). Special fusion software implemented into the console is used to overlay both acquired image data sets (Fig. 1d).

When gamma rays penetrate through tissue there is certain likelihood that they will get absorbed. In PET, this absorption is called *attenuation* which leads to a subsequent quantification error (Ostertag et al. 1989). Conventional stand-alone PET scanners measure this gamma-ray attenuation by using an external positron emitting source, such as Ge-68, which has the same emission energy (511 keV) as the isotopes used for PET tracer (Huesman et al. 1988). Thus, the measured attenuation maps can be directly applied to correct the PET emission data.

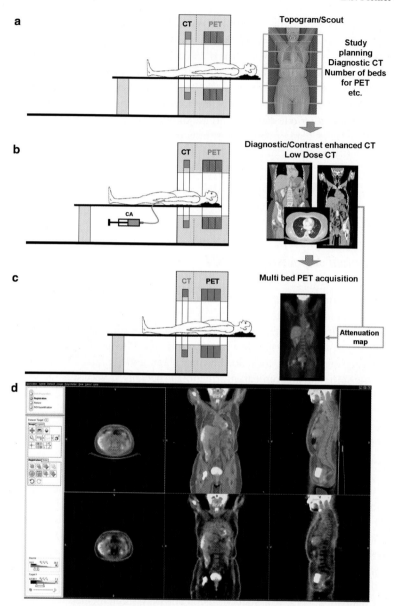

Fig. 1 a–d Schematic workflow of the PET/CT examination. **a** A fast scout scan is used to determine examination regions for PET and diagnostic CT. **b** The second step in a PET/CT workflow is the acquisition of either a low-dose or diagnostic CT scan. **c** PET data are acquired at multiple bed positions, reconstructed and corrected for attenuation using the previously acquired CT data. **d** PET and CT images are registered and displayed as fused images. The analysis software allows dynamic and individual adjustment of image contrast and fusion intensity

In a PET/CT system, the CT scan can be used for attenuation correction, although these data are acquired at a lower energy, typically at 80–120 keV, and need to be up-scaled to the tissue absorption factors for 511 keV (Fig. 1b). The CT scan can be performed much faster than the conventional transmission scans, resulting in a drastic reduction of the overall examination time. This, combined with the additional anatomical information provided from the CT, is a major advantage of combined PET/CT over conventional PET (Beyer et al. 2002; Mohnike 2006; Townsend and Beyer 2002; Townsend et al. 2003).

2.2 Impact for Clinical Diagnosis

Since the installation of the first combined PET scanner in 2001, it has been shown that nearly 80% of the performed PET/CT acquisitions are carried out in the field of oncology (Juweid and Cheson 2006; Weber 2005). The use of a combined PET/CT system allows for tumor detection and staging as well as therapy monitoring and planning in a single device (Antoch et al. 2004; Francis et al. 2005). Several studies show the clear advantage of combined PET/CT over PET or CT alone or when carried out side by side. A study by Antoch et al. (2004) performed on 260 patients having different kinds of tumor diseases revealed that the staging accuracy was 84% when combined PET/CT was used, compared with an accuracy of only 76% when images where evaluated side-by-side. The staging accuracy was only 63% or 64 % respectively, when only CT or PET information was used alone. A study of Bar-Shalom et al. (2003) showed that in 204 tumor patients, 49% of the examinations revealed additional information obtained from a PET/CT scan compared with information obtained from either using PET or CT alone. This led to an alternation in treatment in 14% of the cases. Pfannenberg et al. (2007) could show that whole-body PET in combination with a protocol, including an arterial and portal-venous contrast enhanced scan, compared with PET/CT with a low-dose nonenhanced CT scan, revealed additional diagnostic value in 52 out of 100 patients with different malignant tumors. An example of a 60-year-old melanoma patient is shown in Fig. 2, where the FDG-PET image shows an increased tracer uptake in the right lower abdomen (Fig. 2a) corresponding to the colon ascendes in the CT scan (Fig. 2b). However, the low-dose CT shows minimal pericolic streaking but no mass (Fig. 2c). In sharp contrast to Fig. 2c, the diagnostic CT performed with intravenous and oral contrast agent clearly shows enhanced intraluminal boarders of a lesion (Fig. 2d).

PET/CT has also great potential in the planning of radiation therapy, especially when tumor regions are difficult to define. Having both PET and CT information available, a more accurate definition of the irradiation regions is possible. Areas showing high tumor activity in PET images may not necessarily be detected by CT and might thus be overseen by conventional therapy planning based on CT alone. Furthermore, tissue appearing as lesion expansion in a CT may be indicated as benign in a PET scan and thus not be unnecessarily irradiated (Herrmann 2005; Scarfone et al. 2004).

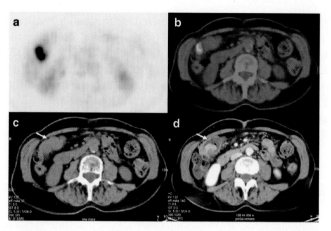

Fig. 2 a–d An example of how the use of a contrast agent can improve the localization of pathological FDG uptake in a 60-year-old patient with melanoma (Pfannenberg et al. 2007). **a** The
transaxial PET image and **b** the fusion with the low-dose CT show a focal spot of FDG uptake in
the lower right abdomen, which corresponds to the colon ascendes. **c** The transaxial low dose CT
shows only discrete pericolic compression but no mass. **d** The diagnostic CT using intravenous and
oral contrast agent clearly shows an intraluminal contrast enhanced lesion (*arrow*)

2.3 Potential and Limitations of Combined PET/CT

PET/CT offers significant shorter scan times compared with stand-alone PET scanners, where the attenuation correction is not based on an ultrafast CT scan. The
linear scaling of attenuation coefficients, measured at an energy of up to 140 kVp,
to 511 kV PET values is a valid method for soft tissue and bones (Kinahan et al.
1998, 2003). Beside the advantage of the shorter scan time, the CT-based attenuation
map also has higher statistics and, therefore, a lower noise contribution than conventional attenuation measured with 511 keV gamma sources. However, in regions with
high-density materials, such as inlays or obese patients, CT causes beam-hardening
artifacts by attenuating the lower X-ray energy more than the high energies, resulting in a shift of the polychromatic X-ray spectra to higher energies. This effect can
cause significant artifacts in the CT images and lead to false attenuation values for
the PET images (Fig. 3). Beam hardening artifacts are also the reason why whole-
body PET/CT examinations are performed with the patient's arms raised above the
head rather than at the side of the body as usually performed in PET. This also
avoids truncation artifacts caused by exceeding the CT field of view, which would
subsequently lead to an incorrect quantification in the PET images (Ohnesorge et al.
2000).

2.3.1 Co-registration Errors

The latest generations of PET/CT scanners implement 3D PET data acquisition
technology and fast scintillator materials, such as lutetium oxy-orthosilicate (LSO)

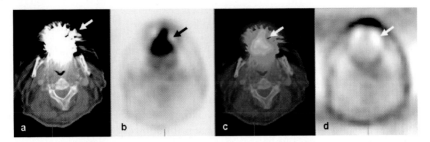

Fig. 3 a Metal artifact in a CT image, and **b** its impact on the attenuation correction of the PET data. **c** The hyper-dense implants in the jaw lead to a misinterpretation of the attenuation data, which cause an artificially increased uptake in the PET data. **d** However, the PET image without attenuation correction does not show this increased uptake and can thus be used to verify that the increased uptake in the PET image is related to wrong attenuation

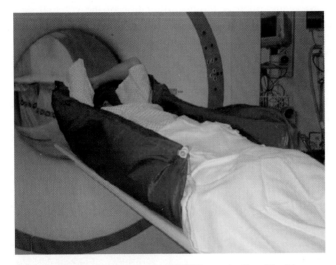

Fig. 4 Immobilization of the patient during a PET/CT examination. The blue vacuum mattress supports the patient to hold the "arms up" position during the 20–30 min scan time, without having major movement

or gadolinium oxy-orthosilicate (GSO), allowing short scan times of only 3–4 min per bed position. Shorter scan times result in more comfort for the patient and reduced probability for a misalignment of PET and CT data caused by patient-induced motion artifacts. Nevertheless, a 4-min scan time per bed position still results in a 20–30 min PET scan for a whole body examination with five to eight bed positions and a 16-cm axial field of view of the PET scanner. This is still a significant time-window between the CT scan and the last PET bed position. Thus, to avoid patient motion during the acquisition, comfortable and secured patient bedding is mandatory (Fig. 4).

2.3.2 Breathing Artifacts

Another source of misaligned PET and CT data are breathing artifacts. CT scans are usually very fast and acquired in inspiration phase according to standard diagnostic CT scan protocols. The PET scan is acquired over several minutes while the patient breathes normally. This can lead to a mismatch of PET and CT data, especially in areas of the diaphragm, thorax, and abdomen. To avoid such artifacts, adapted examination protocols with instructed respiration cycles — mid expiration, breath hold — (Beyer et al. 2003) or CT scans in normal respiration are performed (Brechtel et al. 2006; Goerres et al. 2002, 2003).

2.3.3 Contrast Agents

Diagnostic CT usually requires the application of contrast media, intravenously and orally. Contrast agents improve the discrimination of the vascular system and digestive tract from other soft tissue. However, the effects of CT contrast agents are not included in the linear scaling model to calculate PET attenuation correction data from X-ray absorption factors. CT contrast agents contain iodine and cover a range approximately from 100 up to a 1,000 Hounsfield units (Mohnike 2006). Thus, contrast-enhanced structures are considered as bone in the attenuation map and might lead to a false PET attenuation correction if the PET/CT examination protocols are not adjusted accordingly. However, a careful comparison of CT image and the contrast-enhanced regions with the PET images as well as the review of the uncorrected PET data generally help to avoid misinterpretation in clinical diagnosis (Fig. 5).

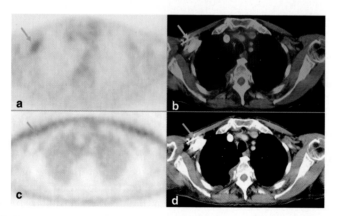

Fig. 5 a–d Contrast-media-related artifact. The attenuation corrected PET image **a** shows increased uptake in the right supraclavicular region due to increased contrast agent concentration in the right vena subclavia **d**. The fused PET/CT image **b** shows that the high uptake region corresponds to the vessel. The PET image not attenuation corrected **c** does not show the increased uptake and can thus prove that this is related due to the high contrast agent uptake from the CT and the resulting erroneous attenuation correction data

2.3.4 Advanced PET/CT Applications

The ultimate goal of combined PET/CT is to replace separate PET and CT examinations by a combined PET/CT scan, where both examinations operate at their full diagnostic value. Since the introduction of the first combined PET/CT scanner in 2000, which utilized a single-slice CT, the latest PET/CT generation is based on a 64-slice spiral CT, allowing the full range of diagnostics, equal to a state-of-the-art stand-alone CT. These advanced machines are especially of interest for cardiology (Di Carli and Dorbala 2007; Namdar et al. 2005). Dedicated respiratory and cardiac gating options (Nehmeh et al. 2003) allow for a fast acquisition of perfectly matched PET and CT data of the heart with excellent image quality.

2.4 PET/CT in Preclinical Research

The realm of preclinical imaging using small laboratory animals to investigate pathological processes in vivo or accelerate the development of drugs and biomarkers is an emerging field in biomedicine. However, dedicated imaging systems with much enhanced performance, compared with clinical scanners, in terms of resolution and sensitivity, are necessary to accommodate the much smaller anatomy of mice and rats. Industry has replied to this need by introducing commercial animal scanners in the early 2000s. While the first generation of animal imaging systems were stand-alone PET or CT systems, General Electric, Gamma Medica, and Siemens have recently introduced combined PET/CT machines for small-animal imaging (Fig. 6). Dedicated small-animal state-of-the-art PET scanners offer a resolution in the range 1–1.5 mm with a sensitivity of up to 11% (Tai et al. 2005; Wang et al. 2006) The excellent image resolution allows for quantitative assessment of tiny structures, such as the ribs or vertebral bodies of a mouse (Fig. 7). Small-animal CT systems can achieve an image resolution of less than 20 μm, which allows the quantitative assessment of the trabecular bone density in a mouse femur (Fig. 8). Subsequently, the combined PET/CT modality provides synergy of the best features of the individual scanners, allowing the fusion of morphology and functional information with the highest possible accuracy for noninvasive small animal imaging.

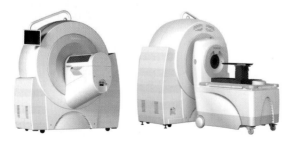

Fig. 6 State-of-the-art preclinical PET/CT and dockable PET and CT device

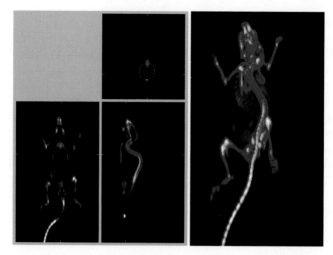

Fig. 7 ^{18}F–flouride PET scan of a mouse. The large axial FOV of 12 cm can cover the whole animal. In comparison with a clinical system, the much higher resolution enables resolving small bones such as the ribs of a mouse. *Right*: 3D maximum intensity projection (MIP). *Left*: typical 3D card display (transversal, coronal and, sagittal view)

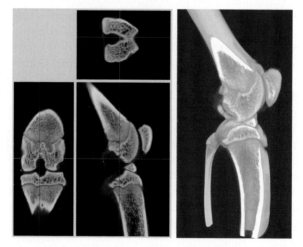

Fig. 8 CT bone scan of a mouse knee joint using a dedicated small-animal CT scanner, which provides an image resolution of 40 μm. *Right*: 3D rendering display of the knee. *Left*: typical 3D card display (transversal, coronal and, sagittal view). The tiny trabecular bone structures in the bone can be resolved

3 PET/MR – A New Tool for Science and Clinic?

The combination of PET and CT has already shown great value in clinical and preclinical applications. The advantage of having quantitative functional information underlayed with the anatomy can lead, in many situations, to more accurate diagnosis and optimized therapy protocols. A limitation of CT is that adequate soft-tissue contrast can not be achieved. Despite the use of contrast agents, sufficient morphology is not revealed in many cases. Furthermore, the CT radiation dose which is necessary to achieve a good image quality is significant (Brix et al. 2005). Although the strength of CT lies in bone and lung imaging, supplementing the PET with magnetic resonance imaging (MRI) would be an advantage over PET/CT for many applications due to the excellent soft-tissue contrast of MRI in regions such as the brain or abdomen. In addition, MRI examinations do not require the use of ionizing radiation and therefore do not engender an additional radiation dose for the patient. Studies with high-field magnets (9.4 Tesla) confirmed that MRI can be performed without risk for the patient (Vaughan et al. 2006). A PET/MRI system can probably not replace PET/CT since both MRI and CT have their own individual strength, but the combination of PET and MRI would definitely stimulate the emerging field of molecular imaging.

3.1 Technical Challenges

The combination of two imaging modalities is always a challenge. One reason for this is the question of whether the two modalities can operate together without performance compromise and without mutual interference.

The main challenge in merging the hardware of PET and MRI into a one single device is that conventional PET detector designs use photomultiplier tubes (PMT) for the light detection. Due to their functional principle — accelerating electrons in a high electric field inside a vacuum tube — PMTs are very sensitive to magnetic fields, and hence, are not suitable for use near or inside a high magnetic field. Also, if the PET and MRI are combined to be used simultaneously, both fields of view have to be physically aligned. This means that the PET detectors have to be built within the MRI bore, resulting in very limited space for the PET detectors.

3.1.1 PET Light Detectors

An alternative light detector for PET, which is capable of detecting the very small amounts of scintillation light, is the avalanche photodiode (APD) (Grazioso et al. 2005; Pichler et al. 2001). This solid-state detector has already been used for small-animal PET scanner approaches (Lecomte et al. 2001; Pichler et al. 2004; Ziegler et al. 2001). Although the internal gain of APDs is only in the order of 10^2–10^3 and they furthermore require a charge sensitive preamplifier for readout, APDs provide sufficiently fast and low-noise electrical signals. APDs are proven to be insensitive to magnetic fields and are very small in size, with only a few millimeters' thickness. Thus, APDs are ideal candidates to be used as PET detectors inside a high-magnetic field. However, for combined PET/MRI the charge sensitive preamplifiers require very careful design in order to avoid potential interference with MRI radiofrequencies or gradients.

3.1.2 PET Detector Materials in the MR Field

MRI requires a homogeneous static magnetic field. Whenever this magnetic field is distorted or inhomogeneous the acquired MR images will show artifacts. The tendency of material to interact with the magnetic field and cause distortions is quantified by the material's susceptibility.

Integrating a PET detector inside a magnet requires the insertion of different materials, such as scintillator crystals, light detector, electronics and electronic shielding materials. All these different components need to be magnetically compatible with susceptibilities close to human tissue in order to maintain the MRI performance. Nonmagnetic materials are not necessarily MRI compatible. Metals have certain conductivity where MRI gradients, which are varying magnetic fields during MRI, can induce eddy currents. These eddy currents distort the MR images and lead to chemical-shift artifacts. In addition, electro-conductive materials can interact with the radiofrequency (RF) probe and alter the B_1-field, which subsequently excites the protons in the object being measured.

While scintillating materials such as LSO, BGO or GSO cause only mild artifacts when located very close to the object inside a MR scanner (Marsden et al. 2002; Shao et al. 1997; Yamamoto et al. 2002), the electronic circuit boards and light detectors, which essentially contain metallic and even ferro-magnetic parts, are more likely to cause distortions of the homogeneous MR field or interact with the gradient or RF system.

Most of the material-related MRI artifacts can be avoided if the PET detector is located outside the RF probe and preserves a certain distance to the object (Fig. 9). A PET detector which is used inside a magnetic field has to be carefully selected to be "transparent" to the MRI scanner. Subsequently, this means that all electronic components, such as capacitors, amplifiers, and resistors, need to be nonmagnetic and large solid areas of metal need to be avoided.

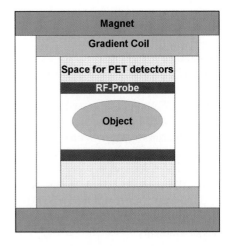

Fig. 9 Schematic (side) view of the setup of a PET/MRI system. The PET detectors are usually located between the gradient set and the RF probe to avoid interference during MRI

3.2 History of PET/MR Development

While PET/CT could be relatively easily realized by combining two existing, more-or-less standard imaging systems, linked together by one patient bed and one operating console, PET/MRI involves major modifications, especially in the PET detector technology.

Figure 10 shows three basic concepts to combine PET and MRI. Although the easiest realization is to mount the PET and MRI side by side (Fig. 10a), this design does result in limited latitude for the data acquisition. The major drawback of this PET/CT-like solution for a PET/MRI is that the scans can not be performed simultaneously. This not only adds significant examination time, since the MRI is much slower than CT imaging, it also rules out the possibility of acquiring two different sets of information simultaneously by PET and MRI. Such a synchronous data acquisition could be of high interest in preclinical research and clinical diagnosis if, for example, the perfusion needs to be temporally correlated with receptor expression. Such an isochronal acquisition of PET and MRI data could also be of great

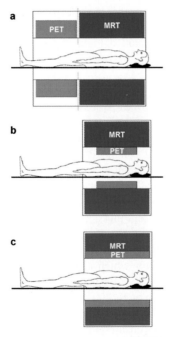

Fig. 10 a–c Potential realizations of PET/MRI scanners. **a** PET/MRI side by side. Two individual devices are mounted back-to-back to each other and have a common control unit, similar to a PET/CT. **b** PET insert within an MRI. The MRI system remains untouched and can also be operated without the PET insert; however, the bore size is drastically reduced and the PET detectors have to be compact. **c** PET detector embedded into an MRI system. Both devices are merged together into one multimodality scanner. This approach requires major modifications of both the PET and MRI technologies

interest in brain as well as in tumor imaging. In sharp contrast to PET/CT, where an integration of PET detectors inside the CT seems impossible due to the high X-ray flux of the CT, the PET/MRI is set apart and paves the way for many interesting applications in biomedical and clinical research. Furthermore, for cardiac imaging, the acquisition of temporally matched information on perfusion and metabolic viability of the myocardium might be of importance.

To achieve a simultaneous PET/MRI data acquisition, a PET detector fully integrated inside the MRI scanner is mandatory. In general, there are two different ways to construct an integrated PET/MRI scanner, first by inserting a PET in a standard MRI (Fig. 10b), which will reduce the bore size drastically but still allows for use of the MRI scanner without the PET, and secondly, by fully embedding the PET detectors into the MRI scanner hardware, maintaining a larger clear MRI bore (Fig. 10c).

Although the latter is definitely the solution of choice, it is, however, the most expensive and most challenging realization of a PET/MRI system. Currently, at least one major medical imaging company decided for the PET insert solution and constructs a dedicated PET/MRI scanner for brain examination in research and clinic (Fig. 10b). The first encouraging results of this approach were presented at the 2006 Radiology Society of North America (RSNA) conference in Chicago.

The integration of the PET scanner in the MRI scanner bore means that the PET detectors need to operate at the maximum magnetic field strength. Thus, the use of PMTs in this environment is excluded. Figure 11 shows schematically four different approaches for "MR compatible" PET detector designs.

3.2.1 Light-fiber-based PET/MRI Systems

Using long light fibers to transport the scintillation light to the PMTs residing outside the high-magnetic field in a shielded environment (Figs. 11a, 12) has been investigated for many years (Marsden et al. 2002; Shao et al. 1997). However, this method impacts the PET signal quality by a light loss caused in the fibers (Catana et al. 2005; Marsden et al. 2002; Raylman et al. 2006). Both the energy and timing resolution of the PET suffer from this approach. With the introduction of reliably working APDs (Lecomte et al. 1990; Pichler et al. 1998), which can be operated inside magnetic fields, the group at the University of California, Davis, USA, has designed a hybrid PET detector which can be operated inside a 7-Tesla magnet (Catana et al. 2006) (Figs. 11, 13). Basically, scintillation crystals are coupled to position-sensitive APDs (Shah et al. 2002) via short light fibers; this avoids materials other than the nonmetallic scintillator and light fibers being located inside the MRI field of view (FOV). This ensures a minimized probability that either the PET interferes with the MRI or the MRI affects the PET signals. The short light fibers, having only a length of 10 cm, still maintain a good PET signal quality. The crystal blocks are assembled to a ring which is located between the limited space (3 cm) between gradient and RF coil of a small-animal 7-Tesla MRI system. This approach has a limited axial field of view (14 mm) and does not allow for an easy axial extension since all the space is already occupied by the light fibers. Nevertheless, the

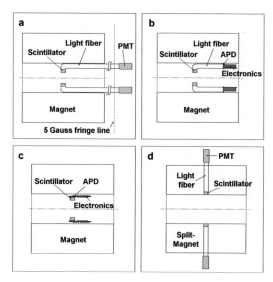

Fig. 11 a–d Schematics of four different approaches to design a PET/MRI system. **a** Long optical fibers coupled to PMTs. The long fibers lead the scintillation light away from the magnetic file so that PMTs can be operated. **b** Hybrid approach with fibers and APDs. Very short fibers are used to couple the scintillators to the APDs, which reside outside the MR FOV. **c** APDs directly coupled to the scintillator block. This approach requires careful design to have no interference of the PET detectors with the MRI. However it offers a very compact design. **d** Split magnet approach. This approach uses well-established PMT technology with a modified split magnet, where the PET detector is built in between the two magnet halves

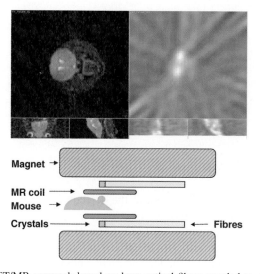

Fig. 12 *Bottom*: PET/MR approach based on long optical fibers coupled to outside PMTs. The PET ring consists of a ring of scintillation crystals coupled to long light fibers, whose read-out is analyzed outside the magnet. *Top*: images show simultaneously acquired PET/MR images of a rat head injected with FDG. The 3D PET volume image was acquired by stepping the mouse through the PET scanner in 2-mm steps (10 min per step) (Marsden et al. 2002)

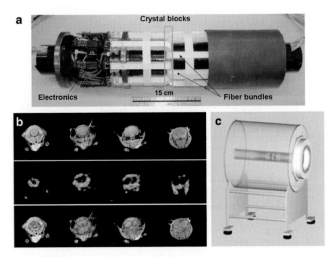

Fig. 13 a–c PET/MRI system built at the University of Davis, California, USA (Catana et al. 2006). **a** Photograph of the PET insert with cover taken off. **b** Acquired PET/MR images of a dead mouse injected with ^{18}F-fluoride. **c** Schematic of the PET insert when it is located inside the MRI scanner

losses in energy and timing resolution inherent to the use of long light fibers are minimized and the system can take full advantage of having an MRI FOV free of metallic objects, since only the crystal blocks and the light fibers reside at the center of the MRI. The first encouraging results and mouse images have been shown by using this approach (Fig. 13) (Catana et al. 2006).

The manufacturing of light-fiber-based PET systems can be very delicate. Even though short light fibers have already been successfully used in existing state-of-the-art small-animal PET scanners (Tai et al. 2005), they bear limitations for a PET/MRI application since the radially available space for the PET detectors in such a combined system is very limited. The more axial PET detector layers are added to the system, the more fibers are needed to read out the individual crystals, thus limiting the axial FOV.

3.2.2 Integrated PET/MRI Systems

The use of fibers to transfer the light to the detector is always associated with a loss of energy and timing resolution, even if very short light fibers are used. To avoid these losses, the light detector needs to be directly coupled to the scintillator. This implies that the presence of metallic material inside the MRI FOV can not be avoided. In the approach of the University of Tübingen, Germany, a 3×3 APD array is directly coupled to the crystal block (Judenhofer et al. 2007; Pichler et al. 2006). To avoid long signal tracks, which would provide a large contact surface for distortions and noise to interact with the detector, the preamplifier is mounted as close as possible to the APD array and implemented as an integrated circuit. The

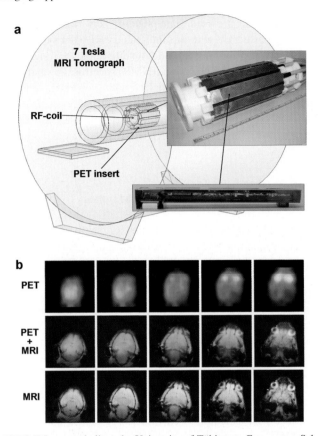

Fig. 14 a, b PET/MRI system built at the University of Tübingen, Germany. **a** Schematic of the PET when inserted in the 7-Tesla MRI system. Small images show the assembled integrated PET insert and one detector cassette with LSO crystal, and attached electronics. **b** Acquired PET/MR images of a mouse head injected with ^{18}F-FDG. The high PET uptake matches the location of the harderian glands when overlayed with the MRI data (Judenhofer et al. 2007)

arrangement of crystal block, APD array, and preamplifier electronics is all located at the centre of the MRI FOV between the gradient and RF coil of a 7-Tesla small-animal MRI system (Fig. 14). The presence of the RF-coil and the switching of the gradients require good RF shielding for the PET detector. The best shielding would be achieved by encapsulating the complete detector assembly in a solid metal box made of copper, yet the use of large solid metal surfaces is problematic as eddy currents can be induced. Thus, for the PET detector shielding, 10-µm, thin, double-sided, copper-coated plastic was used, which is sufficient enough for shielding but does not interfere with the MRI. In addition, each detector is encapsulated by itself, which reduces the overall continuous surfaces and thus the area for eddy currents to be created. This approach provides the potential to design a PET scanner with a large axial FOV if highly integrated electronics, which only occupy the space behind the crystal block and APD, are used. First phantom performance measurements and animal studies were performed with this integrated PET/MRI system. The initial results indicate a nearly uncompromised functionality of the PET and MRI, and might even allow for nuclear magnetic resonance (NMR) spectroscopy and functional MRI (fMRI). Figure 14 shows a mouse head injected with [^{18}F]FDG, simultaneously imaged with a prototype fully integrated PET/MRI (Judenhofer et al. 2007). A similar approach of directly coupling the scintillator to the APD is already used for investigation and construction of a first clinical head PET/MRI system by Siemens Medical Solutions.

3.2.3 PET/MRI Approaches using Modified Magnets

So far, all the described PET/MRI approaches require a significant modification of the PET detector technology in order to avoid mutual interference between the two imaging systems and to make the PET scanner basically invisible for the MRI. However, the MRI system remains more or less untouched.

Two groups, at the University of Cambridge, UK, and the University of Western Ontario, Canada, are working on a PET/MRI system using advanced MRI technology and, more or less, state-of-the-art PET detector technology. This is either done by using a split magnet, where PET detectors are built in between the two halves of the magnet, or by using a field-cycled MRI scanner where the magnetic field is close to 0 Tesla when the PET signals are read out by PMTs (Gilbert et al. 2006; Lucas et al. 2006). Both approaches are currently under investigation, since the split magnet needs a special gradient coil design to bridge the axial gaps between the two magnet halves. The PET detectors used in between are based on a commercially available animal PET scanner detector technology using 12×12 LSO crystal arrays with an individual crystal size of $1.5 \times 1.5 \times 10\,\text{mm}^3$ coupled to position-sensitive PMTs via a short light-fiber bundle (Tai et al. 2005). The fiber bundles are elongated to 1.2 m in order to lead out the scintillation light in radial direction to the PMT. However, the split magnet allows a radial guidance of the fibers which does not require bending, subsequently having only little light loss and space constraints (Fig. 15). Nevertheless, the MRI system is based on a 1-Tesla magnet, which will limit the signal-to-noise ratio of the MR images (Lucas et al. 2006).

Both, PET/MRI systems, the one based on the split magnet and the one based on the field-cycled MRI need to prove their feasibility, in order to allow the construction of a high-quality PET/MRI scanner at reasonable cost.

3.3 PET Attenuation Correction based on MRI Data

As already discussed for PET/CT, for an accurate PET quantification, correction for the 511-keV photon attenuation caused by the tissue is mandatory. In sharp contrast to PET/CT, where the CT image data provide an attenuation map for PET images,

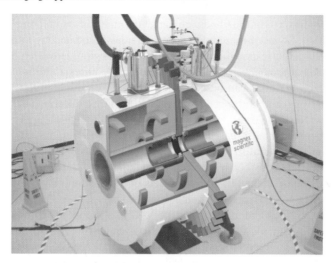

Fig. 15 Split magnet PET/MR approach of the University of Cambridge. A 1-Tesla magnet with a schematic of PET system superimposed. The cut-away shows a ring of scintillating crystal blocks (at the center), fiber optic bundles, and screened PMTs (outside magnet cryostat) (Lucas et al. 2006)

MR image data contain the information about tissue proton density. The proton density does not necessarily reflect the photon attenuation probability. For example: bone, which is a very dense tissue, has a high attenuation factor in CT images, but only low proton density. Hence, bones provide no signal in MR images and are similar to the MRI signal of air. Thus, a simple re-mapping of MR signal intensities would not provide an accurate PET attenuation correction.

The use of a measured attenuation correction with an external source, such as carried out on stand alone PET scanner, does not seem adequate for PET/MRI since the space within the MRI scanner is already limited and a mechanical implementation of the rotation mechanism is challenging. In addition, the transmission measurement would increase the total examination time and contribute to the radiation exposition.

This problem calls for new approaches so as to derive PET attenuation data for a combined PET/MRI scanner from the MR image data.

First approaches, based on regional segmentation of the image into body regions and organs have already been successfully implemented. Usually, they only provide sophisticated data when applied to rigid body parts such as the head (Zaidi and Hasegawa 2003; Zaidi et al. 2003). Here, the circular shape and also the distribution of the tissue, such as skull, brain, liquor, etc., have only small variations from examination to examination. Thus, algorithms can segment regions based on a set of a-priori information. While these algorithms perform well on rigid and well defined structures such as the head, they tend to fail or require manual user assistance if applied on other body regions; for example, the thorax or abdomen. Furthermore, a simple segmentation of MR images to reveal an attenuation map for PET will not include MR image truncation artifacts caused by the limited MR FOV. For these cases, new algorithms and methods are currently under investigation (Montandon and Zaidi 2005). Some of these approaches are atlas based and try to use more a-priori information corresponding to the investigated region. However, the creation of sophisticated atlases is very time-consuming and requires a multiplicity of data sets from which the atlas can be derived. Furthermore, different body regions as well as gender, age, and body size or weight will require a different atlas to achieve proper results. Nevertheless, it remains unclear how pathologies (e.g., large tumors) can be implemented in atlas-based attenuation correction.

A new approach is to utilize so-called support vector machines (Zien et al. 2000), which are algorithms that can learn from given templates. The aim is to apply such algorithms on well-matched training data sets of attenuation maps derived from a transmission or a CT scan and MRI data from the same subject. The algorithms try to find certain textures and attributes of the MRI image data matching to a certain attenuation value from the attenuation data. However, to have a sophisticated trained algorithm, several hundred ideally matched training data sets are necessary.

Overall, it is up to now unclear which attenuation correction approach for PET/MRI data is the best to be used. All listed algorithms have their strength and weaknesses, and probably a combination of all will lead to an adequate and automated MRI-based attenuation correction.

3.4 Preclinical Research Gains from PET/MRI

PET is a powerful molecular imaging tool with a number of demonstrated applications in the study of experimental animal models. Through the use of highly specific radiolabeled molecular probes, PET provides exceptionally sensitive assays of a wide range of biological processes and is therefore a novel method to study animal models of diseases. However, the principal drawback of PET is its relatively poor spatial resolution, thus making an accurate localization of high uptake extremely difficult in many cases. This is particularly true when using highly specific radiolabeled probes that do not produce images with significant anatomical information for reference. On the other hand, MRI provides exquisite high resolution and anatomical information as well as access to volume-specific chemical and physical information (e.g., metabolite concentrations and water diffusion characteristics). However, the sensitivity of MRI is much lower compared with nuclear imaging approaches. Absolute quantification in MRI is also challenging due to the nonlinear relationship between probe concentration and its effect on image intensity. Each modality has its advantages as well as its limitations. Merging these two modalities in the study of experimental animal models will allow the strengths of both techniques to be exploited in a synergistic fashion. Accurate morphological information can also improve the quantification accuracy by correcting for partial volume effects (Meltzer et al. 1990; Rousset et al. 1998). Besides the better soft tissue contrast, MRI has the big advantage compared with CT that it does not use ionizing radiation. For whole-body mouse CT scan with a spatial resolution of about 50 µm, the dose per scan is about 0.6 Gy, which is approximately 5% of the LD 50 (lethal dose for 50%) value for mice (Weissleder 2002). Several studies indicate that even X-ray doses below 0.1 Gy can influence the expression of cytokines such as IL-10 or IL-12 in animal models (Liu et al. 2003). Thus, radiation exposure is definitely a substantial problem in preclinical research using small animals. In sharp contrast to PET, the radiation dose of CT is usually by factors higher than the radiation dose from the positron emitters. Therefore, small-animal imaging might profit immensely from a combined PET/MRI system. In addition, the flexibility of MRI scans by using different sequences to investigate different soft-tissue types presents a large choice of imaging protocols for preclinical studies. The simultaneous acquisition of PET and MRI data is an advantage not only because it reduces the total scan time but also because it allows a temporal coregistration of PET and MRI data.

3.5 Roadmap for Clinical PET/MRI

The described approaches to combining PET and MRI into one device are mostly based on preclinical research systems. For a clinical multimodality PET/MRI scanner investigations are pursued to develop a PET insert which can be used in combination with a standard 3-Tesla clinical patient scanner. Due to limited available space inside the MRI machine, the PET insert can be used exclusively for imaging of the head and neck regions. It uses a standard MR head-coil, which will be located in the PET insert. While such a system will provide an ideal platform for studies in the fields of neurology, neuro-oncology and psychiatry, the ultimate goal would definitely be a whole-body PET/MRI system. Such a system would not only be valuable for whole-body oncological examinations but also allow for advanced motion correction by simultaneous PET and MRI data acquisition. This option of improved motion correction is another benefit of PET/MRI over PET/CT.

3.6 PET/MRI: Goes the Potential beyond Dual-Modality Imaging?

The original aim of combining PET and MRI as a dual modality imaging system was to cover weaknesses of the existing PET/CT systems, which are lack of soft-tissue contrast and the relatively high radiation dose applied from the CT. However, MR imaging goes far beyond acquiring anatomical images with high- quality and high soft-tissue contrast; MRI offers also functional information such as fMRI and proton spectroscopy. Thus, complementary functional information from PET and MRI can be correlated, providing additional information for kinetic modeling. The potential of simultaneous PET/MRI, therefore, goes beyond revealing tracer uptake and morphology towards multifunctional imaging.

References

Antoch G, Saoudi N, Kuehl H, Dahmen G, Mueller SP et al (2004) Accuracy of whole-body dual-modality fluorine-18-2-fluoro-2-deoxy-D-glucose positron emission tomography and computed tomography (FDG-PET/CT) for tumor staging in solid tumors: comparison with CT and PET. J Clin Oncol 22:4357–4368

Bar-Shalom R, Yefremov N, Guralnik L, Gaitini D, Frenkel A et al (2003) Clinical performance of PET/CT in evaluation of cancer: additional value for diagnostic imaging and patient management. J Nucl Med 44:1200–1209

Beyer T, Antoch G, Blodgett T, Freudenberg LF, Akhurst T, Mueller S (2003) Dual-modality PET/CT imaging: the effect of respiratory motion on combined image quality in clinical oncology. Eur J Nucl Med Mol Imaging 30:588–596

Beyer T, Townsend DW, Blodgett TM (2002) Dual-modality PET/CT tomography for clinical oncology. Q J Nucl Med 46:24–34

Beyer T, Townsend DW, Brun T, Kinahan PE, Charron M et al (2000) A combined PET/CT scanner for clinical oncology. J Nucl Med 41:1369–1379

Brechtel K, Klein M, Vogel M, Mueller M, Aschoff P et al (2006) Optimized contrast-enhanced CT protocols for diagnostic whole-body 18F-FDG PET/CT: technical aspects of single-phase versus multiphase CT imaging. J Nucl Med 47:470–476

Brix G, Lechel U, Glatting G, Ziegler SI, Munzing W et al (2005) Radiation exposure of patients undergoing whole-body dual-modality 18F-FDG PET/CT examinations. J Nucl Med 46: 608–613

Catana C, Stickel J, Judenhofer M, Pichler B, Cherry S (2005) Simultaneous PET-MRI- from Detector Modules to Imaging System. Society for Molecular Imaging, Fourth Annual Meeting in Cologne, Germany, September 7–10, 2005, p. 4

Catana C, Wu Y, Judenhofer MS, Qi J, Pichler BJ, Cherry SR (2006) Simultaneous acquisition of multislice PET and MR images: initial results with a MR-compatible PET scanner. J Nucl Med 47:1968–1976

Czernin J, Phelps ME (2002) Positron emission tomography scanning: current and future applications. Annu Rev Med 53:89–112

Di Carli MF, Dorbala S (2007) Cardiac PET-CT. J Thorac Imaging 22:101–106

Francis IR, Brown RK, Avram AM (2005) The clinical role of CT/PET in oncology: an update. Cancer Imaging 5(Spec No A):S68–S75

Gilbert KM, Handler WB, Scholl TJ, Odegaard JW, Chronik BA (2006) Design of field-cycled magnetic resonance systems for small animal imaging. Phys Med Biol 51:2825–2841

Goerres GW, Burger C, Schwitter MR, Heidelberg TN, Seifert B, von Schulthess GK (2003) PET/CT of the abdomen: optimizing the patient breathing pattern. Eur Radiol 13:734–739

Goerres GW, Kamel E, Heidelberg TN, Schwitter MR, Burger C, von Schulthess GK (2002) PET-CT image co-registration in the thorax: influence of respiration. Eur J Nucl Med Mol Imaging 29:351–360

Grazioso R, Aykac M, Casey ME, GG, Schmand M (2005) APD Performance in Light Sharing PET Applications. IEEE Trans Nucl Sci 52:1413–1416

Herrmann T (2005) Radiation oncology and functional imaging. Nuklearmedizin 44(Suppl 1): S38–S40

Huesman R, Derenzo SE, Cahoon JL, Geyer AB, Moses WW et al (1988) Orbiting transmission source for positron tomography. IEEE Trans Nucl Sci:735

Judenhofer MS, Catana C, Swann BK, Siegel S, Jung W-I et al (2007) PET/MR images acquired with a compact MRI compatible PET detector in a 7 Tesla magnet. Radiology 244:807–814

Juweid ME, Cheson BD (2006) Positron-emission tomography and assessment of cancer therapy. N Engl J Med 354:496–507

Kinahan PE, Hasegawa BH, Beyer T (2003) X-ray-based attenuation correction for positron emission tomography/computed tomography scanners. Semin Nucl Med 33:166–179

Kinahan PE, Townsend DW, Beyer T, Sashin D (1998) Attenuation correction for a combined 3D PET/CT scanner. Med Phys 25:2046–2053

Lecomte R, Cadorette J, Jouan A, Heon M, Rouleau D, Gauthier G (1990) High resolution positron emission tomography with a prototype camera based on solid state scintillation detectors. IEEE Trans Nucl Sci 37:805–811

Lecomte R, Pepin CM, Lepage MD, Pratte J-F, Dautet H, Binkley DM (2001) Performance analysis of phoswich/APD detectors and low-noise CMOS preamplifiers for high-resolution PET systems. IEEE Trans Nucl Sci 48:650–655

Liu XD, Ma SM, Liu SZ (2003) Effects of 0.075 Gy x-ray irradiation on the expression of IL-10 and IL-12 in mice. Phys Med Biol 48:2041–2049

Lucas AJ, Hawkes RC, Ansorge RE, Williams GB, Nutt RE et al (2006) Development of a combined microPET-MR system. Technol Cancer Res Treat 5:337–341

Marsden PK, Strul D, Keevil SF, Williams SC, Cash D (2002) Simultaneous PET and NMR. Br J Radiol 75(Spec No):S53–S59

Meltzer CC, Leal JP, Mayberg HS, Wagner HN Jr, Frost JJ (1990) Correction of PET data for partial volume effects in human cerebral cortex by MR imaging. J Comput Assist Tomogr 14:561–570

Mohnike WHG (2006) PET/CT Atlas. Springer, Berlin Heidelberg New York

Montandon ML, Zaidi H (2005) Atlas-guided non-uniform attenuation correction in cerebral 3D PET imaging. Neuroimage 25:278–286

Namdar M, Hany TF, Koepfli P, Siegrist PT, Burger C et al (2005) Integrated PET/CT for the assessment of coronary artery disease: a feasibility study. J Nucl Med 46:930–935

Nehmeh SA, Erdi YE, Rosenzweig KE, Schoder H, Larson SM et al (2003) Reduction of respiratory motion artifacts in PET imaging of lung cancer by respiratory correlated dynamic PET: methodology and comparison with respiratory gated PET. J Nucl Med 44:1644–1648

Ohnesorge B, Flohr T, Schwarz K, Heiken JP, Bae KT (2000) Efficient correction for CT image artifacts caused by objects extending outside the scan field of view. Med Phys 27:39–46

Ostertag H, Kubler WK, Doll J, Lorenz WJ (1989) Measured attenuation correction methods. Eur J Nucl Med 15:722–726

Pfannenberg AC, Aschoff P, Brechtel K, Muller M, Klein M et al (2007) Value of contrast-enhanced multi-phase CT in combined PET/CT protocols for oncological imaging. Br J Radiol 80:437–445

Pichler B, Böning G, Lorenz E, Mirzoyan R, Pimpl W et al (1998) Studies with a prototype high resolution PET scanner based on LSO-APD modules. IEEE Trans Nucl Sci 45:1298–1302

Pichler BJ, Bernecker F, Böning G, Rafecas M, Pimpl W et al (2001) A 4 × 8 APD array, consisting of two monolithic silicon wafers, coupled to a 32-channel LSO matrix for high-resolution PET. IEEE Trans Nucl Sci 48:1391–1396

Pichler BJ, Judenhofer MS, Catana C, Walton JH, Kneilling M et al (2006) Performance test of an LSO-APD detector in a 7-T MRI scanner for simultaneous PET/MRI. J Nucl Med 47:639–647

Pichler BJ, Swann BK, Rochelle J, Nutt RE, Cherry SR, Siegel SB (2004) Lutetium oxyorthosilicate block detector readout by avalanche photodiode arrays for high resolution animal PET. Phys Med Biol 49:4305–4319

Raylman RR, Majewski S, Lemieux SK, Velan SS, Kross B et al (2006) Simultaneous MRI and PET imaging of a rat brain. Phys Med Biol 51:6371–6379

Rousset OG, Ma Y, Evans AC (1998) Correction for partial volume effects in PET: principle and validation. J Nucl Med 39:904–911

Scarfone C, Lavely WC, Cmelak AJ, Delbeke D, Martin WH et al (2004) Prospective feasibility trial of radiotherapy target definition for head and neck cancer using 3-dimensional PET and CT imaging. J Nucl Med 45:543–552

Shah KS, Farrell R, Grazioso R, Harmon ES, Karplus E (2002) Position-sensitive avalanche photodiodes for gamma-ray imaging. IEEE Trans Nucl Sci 49:1687

Shao Y, Cherry SR, Farahani K, Slates R, Silverman RW et al (1997) Development of a PET detector system compatible with MRI/NMR systems. IEEE Trans Nuclear Sci 44:1167–1171

Shekhar R, Walimbe V, Raja S, Zagrodsky V, Kanvinde M et al (2005) Automated 3-dimensional elastic registration of whole-body PET and CT from separate or combined scanners. J Nucl Med 46:1488–1496

Slomka PJ (2004) Software approach to merging molecular with anatomic information. J Nucl Med 45(Suppl 1):36S–45S

Tai YC, Ruangma A, Rowland D, Siegel S, Newport DF et al (2005) Performance evaluation of the microPET focus: a third-generation microPET scanner dedicated to animal imaging. J Nucl Med 46:455–463

Townsend DW, Beyer T (2002) A combined PET/CT scanner: the path to true image fusion. Br J Radiol 75(Spec No):S24–S30

Townsend DW, Beyer T, Blodgett TM (2003) PET/CT scanners: a hardware approach to image fusion. Semin Nucl Med 33:193–204

Townsend DW, Carney JP, Yap JT, Hall NC (2004) PET/CT today and tomorrow. J Nucl Med 45(Suppl 1):4S–14S

Vaughan T, DelaBarre L, Snyder C, Tian J, Akgun C et al (2006) 9.4T human MRI: preliminary results. Magn Reson Med 56:1274–1282

Wang Y, Seidel J, Tsui BM, Vaquero JJ, Pomper MG (2006) Performance evaluation of the GE healthcare eXplore VISTA dual-ring small-animal PET scanner. J Nucl Med 47:1891–900

Weber WA (2005) Use of PET for monitoring cancer therapy and for predicting outcome. J Nucl Med 46:983–995

Weissleder R (2002) Scaling down imaging: molecular mapping of cancer in mice. Nat Rev Cancer 2:11–18

Yamamoto S, Kuroda K, Senda M (2002) Scintillator selection for MR compatible gamma detectors. Presented at the Nuclear Science Symposium Conference Record, 2002 IEEE, vol 3, pp 1632–1635

Zaidi H, Hasegawa B (2003) Determination of the attenuation map in emission tomography. J Nucl Med 44:291–315

Zaidi H, Montandon ML, Slosman DO (2003) Magnetic resonance imaging-guided attenuation and scatter corrections in three-dimensional brain positron emission tomography. Med Phys 30:937–948

Ziegler SI, Pichler BJ, Boening G, Rafecas M, Pimpl W et al (2001) A prototype high-resolution animal positron tomograph with avalanche photodiode arrays and LSO crystals. Eur J Nucl Med 28:136–143

Zien A, Ratsch G, Mika S, Scholkopf B, Lengauer T, Muller KR (2000) Engineering support vector machine kernels that recognize translation initiation sites. Bioinformatics 16:799–807

Part II
Imaging Probes

Contrast Agents: Magnetic Resonance

Carmen Burtea, Sophie Laurent, Luce Vander Elst, and Robert N. Muller(✉)

Abstract Even though the intrinsic magnetic resonance imaging (MRI) contrast is much more flexible than in other clinical imaging techniques, the diagnosis of several pathologies requires the involvement of contrast agents (CAs) that can enhance the difference between normal and diseased tissues by modifying their intrinsic parameters. MR CAs are *indirect* agents because they do not become visible by themselves as opposed to other imaging modalities. The signal enhancement produced by MRI CAs (i.e., the efficiency of the CAs) depends on their *longitudinal* (r_1) and *transverse* (r_2) *relaxivity* (expressed in s^{-1} $mmol^{-1}$ l), which is defined as the increase of the nuclear relaxation rate (the reciprocal of the relaxation time) of water protons produced by 1 mmol per liter of CA.

Paramagnetic CAs (most of them complexes of gadolinium) are frequently used in clinics as extracellular, hepatobiliary or blood pool agents. Low molecular weight paramagnetic CAs have similar effects on R_1 and R_2, but the predominant effect at

Robert N. Muller

Department of General, Organic and Biomedical Chemistry, NMR and Molecular Imaging Laboratory, University of Mons-Hainaut, 24, Avenue du Champ de Mars, 7000 Mons, Belgium
robert.muller@umh.ac.be

W. Semmler and M. Schwaiger (eds.), *Molecular Imaging I.*
Handbook of Experimental Pharmacology 185/I.
© Springer-Verlag Berlin Heidelberg 2008

low doses is that of T_1 shortening (and R_1 enhancement). Thus, organs taking up such agents will become bright in a T_1-weighted MRI sequence; these CAs are thus called *positive contrast media*.

The CAs known as *negative agents* influence signal intensity mainly by shortening T_2^* and T_2, which produces the darkening of the contrast-enhanced tissue. These CAs are generally composed of superparamagnetic nanoparticles, consisting of iron oxides (magnetite, Fe_3O_4, maghemite, γFe_2O_3, or other ferrites). Iron oxide nanoparticles are taken up by the monocyte-macrophage system, which explains their potential application as MRI markers of inflammatory and degenerative disorders.

Most of the contemporary MRI CAs approved for clinical applications are non-specific for a particular pathology and report exclusively on the anatomy and the physiological status of various organs. A new generation of MRI CAs is progressively emerging in the current context of *molecular imaging*, agents that are designed to detect with a high specificity the cellular and molecular hallmarks of various pathologies.

1 Introduction

Clinical magnetic resonance imaging (MRI) relies on the magnetic properties of ^1H, as one of the most abundant naturally occurring nuclei in the human body. Particularly detailed anatomical images are obtained by exposing ^1H nuclei to an external magnetic field and to excitation pulses in the form of radio waves (oscillating electromagnetic field). Spatial information about the distribution of magnetic nuclei in the body is achieved by exposing them to an inhomogeneous magnetic field that varies linearly over the body, forming a so-called *magnetic field gradient*. The magnetic field gradient causes identical nuclei to precess at different Larmor frequencies, which are proportional to the field strength. The larger the gradient strength the larger the frequency range, and thereby the characteristically outstanding contrast between various anatomic structures in the human body is obtained by MRI (Lauterbur 1973; Petersen et al. 1985; Rinck 1993; Muller 1996).

The term *contrast* defines the relative difference in intensities between two adjacent regions within an examined object on a gray (or color) scale. The numerical difference between the intensities of pixels or voxels creates the contrast. The contrast of an MR image is the result of various contributing *intrinsic* [proton longitudinal and transverse relaxation times, T_1 and T_2, respectively, the T_2-star (T_2^*), proton density, flow, diffusion, and perfusion] and *extrinsic* (type of pulse sequence, timing parameters of the pulse sequence, strength of magnetic field) parameters.

Even though the intrinsic MRI contrast is much more flexible than in other clinical imaging techniques, the diagnosis of several pathologies requires the involvement of contrast agents (CAs) that can enhance the difference between normal and diseased tissues by modifying their intrinsic parameters. This is the result of increasing (*positive agents* like paramagnetic CAs) or of decreasing (*negative agents* like superparamagnetic CAs) the signal intensity by shortening the proton relaxation times of the imaged organs and tissues. Accordingly, MR CAs are *indirect* agents because they do not become visible by themselves as opposed to other imaging modalities.

The signal enhancement produced by MRI CAs (i.e. the CAs' efficiency) depends on their *relaxivity* (r_1 and r_2), which is defined as the increase of relaxation rate ($R_1 = 1/T_1$; $R_2 = 1/T_2$) produced by 1 mmol per liter of CA (expressed in s^{-1} $mmol^{-1}$ l) (1). The r_1 and r_2 are the main physicochemical parameters that are considered in the development of an effective magnetic label, and they depend essentially on the size and chemical structure of a CA molecule and on the accessibility of water molecules to the magnetic center (1).

$$R_{i(obs)} = \frac{1}{T_{i(obs)}} = \frac{1}{T_{i(diam)}} + r_i C; \quad i = 1 \; or \; 2 \tag{1}$$

where:

$R_{i(obs)}$ and $1/T_{i(obs)}$ = global relaxation rate of the aqueous system (s^{-1})
$T_{i(diam)}$ = relaxation time of the system before addition of the CA(s)
C = the concentration of the paramagnetic center ($mmol\,l^{-1}$)
r_i = the relaxivity ($s^{-1}\,mmol^{-1}$ l)

It should be emphasized that tissue concentration of CA is not the only parameter that contributes to its efficiency. The CA distribution within the image voxel, the proton density and the diffusion as well as the chemical environment are not negligible contributors to the efficiency of signal enhancement.

The CAs for MRI should fulfill several requirements for clinical applications: adequate relaxivity and susceptibility effects, tolerance, safety, low toxicity, stability, optimal biodistribution, elimination and metabolism. Most of the MRI CAs do not highlight specific pathologies, but rather unspecific pathological alterations. Those with a wide clinical application can be classified as extracellular, blood pool, and hepatobiliary agents, as well as pharmaceuticals enhancing the lymph nodes, liver and tumors.

2 Relaxation Mechanisms

2.1 Paramagnetic Relaxation

Quantitative theoretical models have been developed to express the relaxivity of paramagnetic centers. The efficiency of CAs is linked to molecular motions and to intrinsic properties of the nuclei (magnetic moment, gyromagnetic ratio, spin). The paramagnetic relaxation is classically explained by two mechanisms: the "inner sphere" (IS) and "outer sphere" (OS) contributions (Muller 1996). The principle of "inner sphere" relaxation (Fig. 1) relies on a chemical exchange during which one (or several) water molecule(s) in contact with the electronic spins leaves the first coordination sphere of the paramagnetic center and is (are) replaced by other

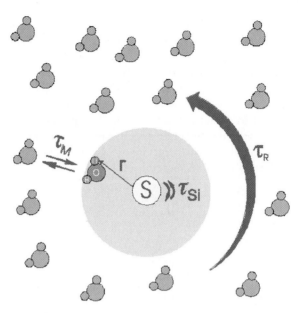

Fig. 1 Schematic representation of the inner sphere relaxation mechanism

molecules (residence time τ_M). This mechanism allows the propagation of the paramagnetic effect to the totality of the solvent since the water molecule exchanges between two sites (bound to the paramagnetic center and bulk water). The IS model has been described by the Solomon-Bloembergen-Morgan theory (SBM) (Solomon 1955; Bloembergen 1957).

The relaxation time of water protons located in the first coordination sphere of the metal is T_{1M}. The contribution of the inner sphere mechanism is given by:

$$R_1{}^{IS} = fq \frac{1}{T_{1M} + \tau_M} \tag{2}$$

where:

f = the relative concentration of the paramagnetic complex and of the water molecules

q = the number of water molecules in the first coordination sphere

τ_M = the water residence time

Calculation of T_{1M} is based on a model which includes the amplitude of the magnetic interaction, its temporal modulation and the effect of the strength of the external magnetic field (3).

$$\frac{1}{T_{1M}} = \frac{2}{15} \left(\frac{\mu_0}{4\pi} \right)^2 \gamma_H^2 \gamma_S^2 \hbar^2 S(S+1) \frac{1}{r^6} \left[\frac{7\tau_{c2}}{1 + (\omega_S \tau_{c2})^2} + \frac{3\tau_{c1}}{1 + (\omega_H \tau_{c1})^2} \right] \tag{3}$$

$$\text{where } \frac{1}{\tau_{ci}} = \frac{1}{\tau_R} + \frac{1}{\tau_M} + \frac{1}{\tau_{si}} \tag{4}$$

$$\frac{1}{\tau_{S1}} = \frac{1}{5\tau_{SO}} \left[\frac{1}{1 + \omega_S^2 \tau_V^2} + \frac{4}{1 + 4\omega_S^2 \tau_V^2} \right] \tag{5}$$

$$\frac{1}{\tau_{S2}} = \frac{1}{10\tau_{SO}} \left[3 + \frac{5}{1 + \omega_S^2 \tau_V^2} + \frac{2}{1 + 4\omega_S^2 \tau_V^2} \right] \tag{6}$$

where:

γ_S and γ_H = the gyromagnetic ratios of the electron (S) and of the proton (H), respectively

$\omega_{S,H}$ = the angular frequencies of the electron and of the proton

r = the distance between coordinated water protons and unpaired electron spins

$\tau_{c1,2}$ = the correlation times modulating the interaction; they are defined by (4)

Where:

τ_R = the rotational correlation time of the hydrated complex

$\tau_{s1,2}$ = the longitudinal and transverse relaxation times of the electron

These latter parameters are field dependent (5 and 6).

τ_{SO} = the value of $\tau_{s1,2}$ at zero field

τ_v = the correlation time characteristic of the electronic relaxation times

The second contribution to the paramagnetic relaxation is the "outer sphere" relaxation (Fig. 2). It is explained by the dipolar interaction at long-distance between the spin of the paramagnetic substance and the nuclear spin. This mechanism is modulated by the translational correlation time (τ_D) that takes into account the relative diffusion (D) of the paramagnetic center and the solvent molecule, as well as their distance of closest approach (d) (7). The OS model has been described by Freed (1978).

$$\tau_D = d^2 / D \tag{7}$$

The complexity of equations describing the relaxation rate explains the important number of parameters describing the IS and OS relaxation (eight parameters: τ_M, q, τ_R, D, r, d, τ_V, τ_{S0}). Considering this high number of parameters, the estimation of all of them by the technique of field cycling is often ambiguous. Thus, the determination of some parameters by independent methods facilitates the theoretical adjustment of the proton nuclear magnetic relaxation dispersion (NMRD) profiles (Fig. 3). This curve characterizes the efficiency of CA at different magnetic fields (Vander Elst et al. 1997; Muller et al. 1999; Laurent et al. 2000, 2004a, 2004b).

Rotational correlation time (τ_R)

The rotational correlation time characterizes the reorientation of the vector between Gd^{3+} and the protons of the water molecule. Generally, for a low molecular weight complex, τ_R limits the relaxivity of the complex at imaging field. The rotational correlation time can be obtained by various methods, such as: (1) analysis of ^{17}O longitudinal relaxation on Gd complexes (Micskei et al. 1993a, 1993b),

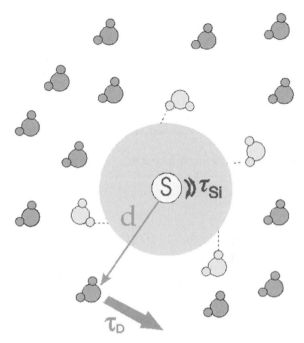

Fig. 2 Schematic representation of the outer sphere relaxation mechanism

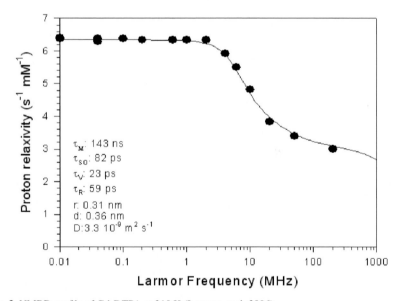

Fig. 3 NMRD profile of Gd-DTPA at 310 K (Laurent et al. 2006)

(2) measurement of the longitudinal relaxation rate in ^{13}C-NMR (Shukla et al. 1991), (3) fluorescence polarization spectroscopy (Helms et al. 1997), and (4) ^{2}H-NMR on deuterated lanthanum complexes (Vander Elst et al. 1997).

Electronic relaxation times (τ_{S1} and τ_{S2})

Longitudinal and transverse electronic relaxation times (τ_{S1} and τ_{S2}, respectively) describe the process of return to equilibrium of the magnetization associated to electrons during transitions between electronic levels of paramagnetic center. These transitions produce fluctuations that allow the relaxation of protons.

Number of coordinated water molecules (q)

The number of coordinated water molecules strongly influences the IS contribution. For complexes like Gd-DTPA, if the number of coordinated water molecules increases from 1 to 2, the relaxivity increases by approximately 30%, but nearly all Gd-DTPA derivatives have a q value equal to 1. The value of q can be estimated either in solid phase (X-rays or neutron diffraction) or in solution [fluorescence of Eu or Yb complexes, LIS (lanthanide-induced shift) method in ^{17}O-NMR].

Proton-metal distance (r)

In the presence of paramagnetic centers, the IS contribution relies on dipolar interactions. The efficiency of dipolar mechanism is proportional to $1/r^6$, where r is the metal-proton distance. So, even a weak modification of this distance has an important impact on the complex relaxivity.

Coordinated water residence time (τ_M)

The mechanism of IS relaxation is based on an exchange between water molecules surrounding the complex and the water molecule(s) coordinated to the lanthanide. Consequently, the exchange rate ($k_{ex} = 1/\tau_M$) is an essential parameter for transmission of the "relaxing" effect to the solvent. This parameter has been studied in many complexes to understand the influence of various factors, like the charge, the presence of amide bonds, etc. (Micskei et al. 1993a, 1993b; Gonzalez et al. 1994; Aime et al. 1999; Zhang et al. 2001; Toth et al. 1996, 1998, 1999).

2.2 Superparamagnetic Relaxation

The proton relaxation in superparamagnetic colloids like iron oxide particles occurs because of the fluctuations of the dipolar magnetic coupling between the nanocrystal magnetization and the proton spin. These superparamagnetic crystals of iron oxide exhibit extremely high magnetic moments due to a cooperative alignment of the electronic spins of the individual paramagnetic ions.

The relaxation is described by an outer sphere model where the dipolar interaction fluctuates because of both the translational diffusion process and the Néel relaxation process (Roch et al. 1992, 1999a, 1999b, 2001; Muller et al. 2001; Ouakssim et al. 2004).

The analysis of the proton NMRD profiles (Fig. 4) of superparamagnetic particles gives thus:

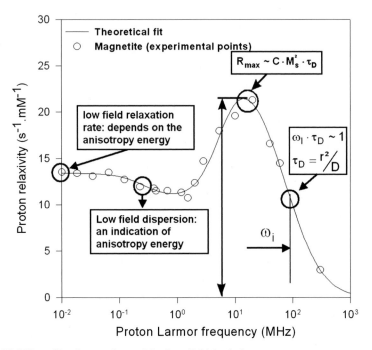

Fig. 4 NMRD profile of magnetite particles in colloidal solution

1. *The average radius (r)*: at high magnetic fields, the relaxation rate depends only on τ_D and the inflection point corresponds to the condition $\omega_I \cdot \tau_D \sim 1$. As shown in (8), the determination of τ_D gives the crystal size r; r, D and ω_I are the average radius of the superparamagnetic crystals, the relative diffusion coefficient, and the proton Larmor frequency, respectively.

$$\tau_D = r^2/D \qquad (8)$$

2. *The specific magnetization (M_s)*: at high magnetic fields, M_s can be obtained from the equation $M_s \approx (R_{max}/C \cdot \tau_D)^{1/2}$, where C is a constant and R_{max} the maximal relaxation rate.
3. *The crystal anisotropy energy (Ea)*: the absence or the presence of an inflection point at low fields informs about the magnitude of the anisotropy energy. For crystals characterized by a high Ea value as compared to the thermal agitation, the low field dispersion disappears. This was confirmed in a previous work with cobalt ferrites (Roch et al. 1999b), which are known to have high anisotropy energy.
4. *The Néel relaxation time (τ_N)*: this characterizes the spatial fluctuations of the global magnetization of the superparamagnetic particle. The relaxation rate at very low field R_0 is governed by a "zero magnetic field" correlation time τ_{C0}, which is equal to τ_N if $\tau_N \ll \tau_D$. However, this situation is often not met, so that τ_N is often reported as a qualitative value in addition to the crystal size and the specific magnetization.

3 Clinical Contrast Agents

3.1 Positive Contrast Agents

Paramagnetic CAs are actually the most frequently used in clinical applications after the first introduction of paramagnetic ions (Mn^{2+}) by Lauterbur et al. (1978). These compounds enhance the image contrast by lowering the T_1 of water protons in the adjacent tissues. Most of them are complexes of the lanthanide gadolinium(III) (Gd), which is chelated with hydrophilic poly(aminocarboxylate) ligands to reduce the toxicity of the heavy metal. The favorable magnetic properties of Gd(III) (seven unpaired electrons and slow electronic relaxation time) make of it the preferred paramagnetic ion for MRI applications (in addition to Mn^{2+}, Dy^{3+} and Fe^{3+}), while the number of water molecules coordinated directly to the paramagnetic center depends on the denticity of the chelate molecule. Low molecular weight paramagnetic CAs have similar effects on R_1 and R_2, but since the intrinsic R_1 of tissues is much lower than R_2, the predominant effect at low doses is that of T_1 shortening (and R_1 enhancement). Thus, organs taking up such agents will become bright in a T_1-weighted MRI sequence; these CAs are thus called *positive contrast media*.

Gd-DTPA and Gd-DOTA were the first ionic compounds of a new generation of imaging agents. These complexes are characterized by low toxicity, high thermodynamic and kinetic stability. Although well tolerated, these two compounds are high osmolar CAs (Weinmann et al. 1984; Magerstadt et al. 1986). Thus, two neutral non-ionic gadolinium chelates, Gd-DTPA-BMA (Bousquet et al. 1988) and Gd-HP-DO3A (Cacheris et al. 1990) have been developed. More recently, another neutral paramagnetic complex has been used as an extracellular CA, Gd-DO3A-butrol (Vogler et al. 1995; Platzek et al. 1997; Tombach et al. 2002). Since the detection of metastatic focal liver disease is a key health strategy, efforts have been focused to obtain hepatobiliary CAs for MRI, like Gd-BOPTA (Uggeri et al. 1995) or Gd-EOB-DTPA (Weinmann et al. 1991; Vander Elst et al. 1997) (Fig. 5).

3.1.1 Extracellular Agents

The most commonly used MRI contrast media in radiology are extracellular agents (Table 1). They are typically small molecular weight compounds that distribute nonspecifically in the blood plasma and extracellular space of the body after administration. Due to the hydrophilicity of their chelating agent, most of them have a rapid excretion through the kidneys with an elimination half-life of about 15–90 min. Accordingly, they are efficient agents for imaging the leakage through the blood-brain barrier, and their typical use concerns the detection of brain tumors (Fig. 6). The first CA approved for clinical MRI applications in human beings was the anionic gadolinium diethylenetriaminepentaacetate complex, Gd-DTPA, which is nowadays routinely used for contrast enhancement under the name of Magnevist (Schering, Berlin, Germany) (Lauffer 1988; Harpur et al. 1993; Tweedle et al. 1995; Vogler et al. 1995; Caravan et al. 1999; Rohrer et al. 2005; Herborn et al. 2007).

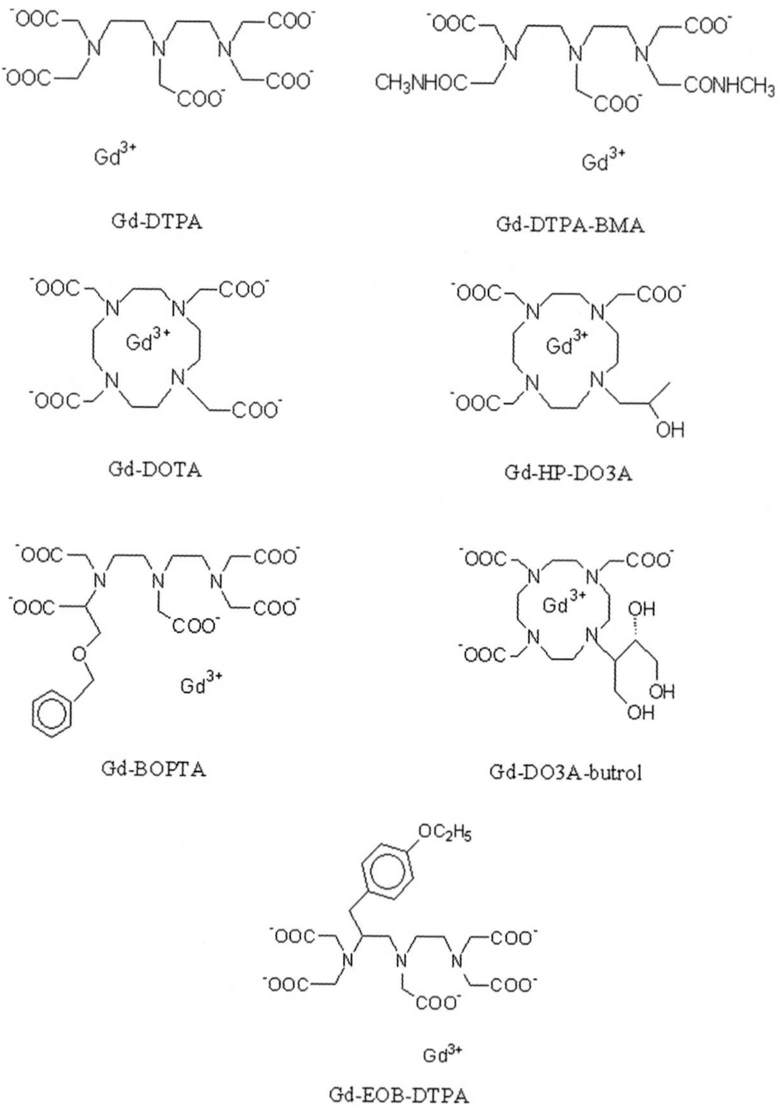

Fig. 5 Structure of paramagnetic contrast agents

This class of MRI contrast media has limited adverse effects (i.e., headache, nausea, "metallic" taste), mainly because of their efficient and rapid excretion from the body, which minimizes exposure to drug and possible cell internalization by endocytosis. They are largely excreted unaltered by oxidation or conjugation (Caravan et al. 1999). Though, the possible in-vivo decomplexation and transmetallation by endogenous ions represents a matter of great concern in the development of new contrast media because both metal ions and free organic ligands are highly toxic (Tweedle et al. 1991).

Table 1 Extracellular MRI contrast agents currently used in clinical practice

Name of the compound/ Generic name	Trade name	Relaxivity[a] $(s^{-1}\,mM^{-1})$ (1.5T, 37°C, water)	Distribution/ excretion	Indication/dosage LD_{50}
Gd-DTPA Gadopentetate dimeglumine	Magnevist	$r_1 = 3.3$ $r_2 = 3.9$	Intravascular, extracellular Renal excretion	Neuro/whole body 0.1–0.3 mmol/kg $LD_{50} = 6.4$ mmol/kg
	Magnevist enteral		Bowel marking	Gastrointestinal 100 ml oral (0.001 mol/l)
Gd-DOTA Gadoterate meglumine	Dotarem	$r_1 = 2.9$ $r_2 = 3.2$	Intravascular, extracellular Renal excretion	Neuro/whole body 0.1 mmol/kg $LD_{50} =$ 10.6 mmol/kg
Gd-DTPA-BMA Gadodiamide	Omniscan	$r_1 = 3.3$ $r_2 = 3.6$	Intravascular, extracellular Renal excretion	Neuro/whole body 0.1–0.2 mmol/kg $LD_{50} = 34$ mmol/kg
Gd-HP-DO3A Gadoteridol	ProHance	$r_1 = 2.9$ $r_2 = 3.2$	Intravascular, extracellular Renal excretion	Neuro/whole body 0.1 mmol/kg $LD_{50} = 12$ mmol/kg
Gd-DTPA-BMEA Gadoversetamide	Optimark	$r_1 = 3.8$ $r_2 = 4.2$	Intravascular, extracellular Renal excretion	Neuro/whole body 0.1 mmol/kg $LD_{50} = 26$ mmol/kg
Gd-DO3A-butrol Gadobutrol	Gadovist	$r_1 = 3.3$ $r_2 = 3.9$	Intravascular, extracellular Renal excretion	Neuro/whole body 0.1 mmol/kg $LD_{50} = 23$ mmol/kg
Gd-BOPTA Gadobenate dimeglumine	MultiHance	$r_1 = 4.0$ $r_2 = 4.3$	Extracellular, hepatobiliary Renal and biliary excretion	Central nervous system (CNS), liver 0.1 mmol/kg (CNS) 0.05 mmol/kg (liver) $LD_{50} = 7.9$ mmol/kg

[a]For more information see Rohrer et al. (2005)
LD_{50} median lethal dose

Commonly, linear chelates of gadolinium (e.g., Gd-DTPA) and bisamide derivatives (e.g., Gd-DTPA-BMA) are less stable than macrocyclic systems (e.g., Gd-DOTA) and C4-substituted compounds like Gd-ethoxybenzyl (EOB)-DTPA (hepatobiliary agent). In-vivo dissociation may result from the chelate interaction with endogenous entities or by spontaneous processes. The biological interaction may be related to the size, shape, charge, and lipophilicity of the chelate, while the thermodynamics and kinetics of metal-ligand binding govern the spontaneous processes (Wedeking et al. 1992; Laurent et al. 2001; Cabella et al. 2006; Idée J-M et al. 2006). Thomsen (2006) has reported recently that Omniscan, an extracellular nonionic low osmolar CA, may produce a serious adverse reaction called nephrogenic systemic fibrosis (NSF), which in some cases can lead to serious physical disability.

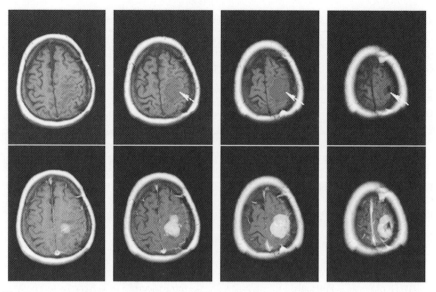

Fig. 6 Patient with a brain tumor before (*top row*: precontrast) and after the injection of Magnevist (*bottom row*: contrast enhanced). The slightly opaque mass in the patient's left hemisphere observed in precontrast images (*arrows*) is clearly delineated only in contrast-enhanced images. Extracellular agents enhance the absence or breakdown of the blood-brain barrier and the high vascular lesions. Serial axial slices of the brain were acquired at 1.5 T on a Siemens Symphony MRI system with a T_1-weighted spin-echo sequence (repetition time, TR = 552 ms; echo time, TE = 17 ms; matrix = 192×256; field of view, FOV = 173×230; slice thickness 5 mm). [Images courtesy of Dr. Divano L, Chambor Clinic of Medical Imaging, Mons, Belgium]

3.1.2 Blood Pool Agents

Magnetic resonance angiography (MRA), one of the clinical imaging techniques used to image blood vessels, is of paramount importance for the diagnosis of pathologies that are characterized by vascular injuries and flow reduction, i.e., traumatic injuries, ulcers, infectious diseases, tumors, embolism, atherosclerosis. The vascular system can be visualized by MRA in the absence of any exogenous CA, unlike X-ray angiography and other angiographic techniques, but diagnosis is sometimes challenging because the contrast is flow-dependent and sensitive to artifacts at locations of turbulent flow, such as behind a stenosis. Faster MRA protocols and the development of CAs dedicated to this application have greatly improved the clinical value of this technique, known nowadays as contrast enhanced MRA (CE-MRA) (Den Boer and Hoogeveen 2001). CE-MRA (Fig. 7) has, moreover, the advantage of not being invasive, since no exposure to ionizing radiation or nephrotoxic iodinated CA is involved as opposed to X-ray angiography and CT angiography (Schneider et al. 2005).

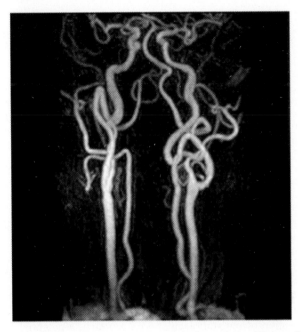

Fig. 7 Three-dimensional CE-MRA of the neck vessels (normal carotid artery bifurcations are well represented) in a healthy individual obtained after the first pass of a bolus of Dotarem. Coronal images were acquired at 1.5 T on a Siemens Symphony MR imaging system with a 3D time-of-flight (TOF) sequence (TR = 3.7 ms; TE = 1.5 ms; matrix = 180×384; FOV = 188×300; slice thickness 0.8 mm). [Images courtesy of Dr. Divano L, Chambor Clinic of Medical Imaging, Mons, Belgium]

For a proper evaluation of the vascular system by CE-MRA, angiographic CAs must have an enhanced T_1 relaxivity, a prolonged vascular residence time and a limited extravasation to allow repeated image acquisitions after a single administration. Other prerequisite attributes are the low toxicity, biological inertness, excretability from the blood stream, low accumulation in the reticulo-endothelial system (RES), absence of metabolic conversion and low immunogenicity (Bogdanov et al. 1999). Several strategies were developed for the prolongation of the vascular residence time and for the enhancement of T_1 relaxivity (increased rotational correlation time, τ_R, and decreased water residence time, τ_M). Thus, some of the MRA CAs mimic the circulating blood cells (liposomes or micelles) (Anelli et al. 2001; Parac-Vogt et al. 2006), while others mimic plasma proteins (macromolecules and colloids) (Corot et al. 1997; Kobayashi et al. 2001; Gaillard et al. 2002; Wang et al. 2003) or reversibly bind to plasma proteins (Parmelee et al. 1997; Bremerich et al. 2001; Sharafuddin et al. 2002; Hovland et al. 2003; Parac-Vogt et al. 2005).

However, different disadvantages limit the clinical application of these approaches for CE-MRA. The concerns regarding patient safety and manufacturing costs restrict their utilization for the development as blood-pool CAs and only a limited

Table 2 Blood pool contrast agents approved for phase III clinical trials

Name of the compound/ Trade name	Relaxivity $(s^{-1}\,mM^{-1})$ $(37\,^{\circ}C)$	Mechanism of blood enhancement	Excretion, Plasma half-life, LD_{50}	Indication/dosage
MS-325 Vasovist (formerly AngioMARK)	$r_1 = 5.1$ in water and 25 in 4% HSA at 0.47 T, and ~5 in water at 1.41 T[a]	Transient binding to albumin	Biliary and partly renal excretion Half-life = 23 min in rats, 1.97 h in rabbits, and 3.52 h in primates $LD_{50} = 5$–6 mmol/kg	Peripheral vascular disease and coronary artery disease 0.05 mmol/kg
P792 Gadomelitol Vistarem	$r_1 = 38.5$ in water and 40 in 4% HSA at 0.47 T, and 24.9 in water at 1.41 T[b]	Macro-molecular Gd-DOTA derivative	Renal excretion Half-life = 20 min in rats and 41 min in rabbits $LD_{50} > 1.88$ mmol/kg	Myocardial perfusion, vascular imaging and tumor characterization 0.015 mmol/kg

[a] Muller et al. (1999)
[b] Vander Elst et al. (2005)

number has progressed to clinical trials to date (Table 2). For example, liposomes leave the circulation rapidly and accumulate in liver and spleen. The prolonged blood pool retention of macromolecular CAs represent a potential risk to the patient, while the relaxivity gain obtained by increasing the molecule size is often less than expected (Aime et al. 1998). The main drawback of plasma protein mimetics is their opsonization and recognition by the reticulo-endothelial system, which leads to fast plasma depletion and decrease of the blood pool signal. Cardiac toxicity, immunogenicity, and prolonged retention in liver and bone characterize albumin-chelate conjugates, whereas poly(L-lysine) chelate conjugate is retained in kidneys and adrenal glands. The foremost disadvantage of dextran-based conjugates is their polydispersity, which is responsible for the fast elimination from the blood.

Low molecular weight CAs that bind noncovalently to plasma albumin produce an efficacious alternative to macromolecule-based MR blood pool agents, which solve the clearance problems. For instance, MS-325 is a small-molecule chelate with a molecular weight of 957 Da that binds strongly and reversibly to human serum albumin (HSA) after injection and thus becomes a macromolecular complex (68 KDa in the bound form) with blood-pool distribution. At a clinical dose of 0.05 mmol/kg, one or two MS-325 molecules will be bound per molecule of HSA. The equilibrium between free and protein-bound MS-325 allows that a small amount of MS-325 be excreted through the kidneys (Kroft et al. 1999; Muller et al. 1999; Caravan et al. 2002; McMurry et al. 2002; Farooki et al. 2004).

Another molecular approach with potential clinical benefits is represented by the intermediate size (MW = 6.47 kDa) blood-pool agents like P792, which is a macro-cyclic gadolinium complex having a Gd-DOTA core on which hydrophilic bulky groups are linked to ensure biocompatibility. The agent is rapidly eliminated mainly via the urinary route, does not bind to albumin and does not cross the healthy blood-brain barrier. Combining intravascular retention with no extravascular diffusion, the rapid body clearance and the marked T_1 effect, P792 presents optimal attributes for angiographic applications, allowing a favorable contrast between vessels and adjacent tissue (Turetschek et al. 2001; Gaillard et al. 2002; Corot et al. 2003; Mandry et al. 2005).

3.1.3 Hepatobiliary Agents

The CAs used for MRI of the liver were designed to improve the discrimination and diagnosis of focal hepatic lesions. Paramagnetic extracellular CAs may improve the differential diagnosis, but they rapidly distribute in the interstitial space, do not pass plasma membranes, while their hepatocellular uptake and biliary excretion are negligible. More accurate depiction of all types of hepatic lesions has raised the necessity to develop liver-specific agents, despite the progress in liver-dedicated T_1- or T_2-weighted MRI protocols. Two main classes of liver CAs were designed to overcome the limitations of unspecific tissue uptake of extracellular low molecular weight gadolinium chelates. These are hepatobiliary CAs, with uptake into hepatocytes followed by variable biliary excretion, and superparamagnetic iron oxide (SPIO), with uptake by the macrophages of RES mainly into the liver and spleen (Semelka and Helmberger 2001; Weinmann et al. 2003; Reimer et al. 2004a; Karabulut and Elmas 2006). Considering that these latter agents belong to the class of negative contrast media and they are not specific to hepatocytes, they will be covered subsequently in the sub-chapter 3.2.

The only hepatobiliary CAs that are approved for clinical use are mangafodipir trisodium (Mn-DPDP, Teslascan) and gadobenate dimeglumine (Gd-BOPTA, MultiHance). Gadoxetic acid (Gd-EOB-DTPA, Eovist, Primovist) is in phase III clinical trials in USA and Europe, has finished phase III studies in Japan, and has been approved for clinical use in Sweden (Table 3). The enhancement produced by these agents during the distribution phase depends mainly on tumor vascularity and its blood supply, while late enhancement relies on cell specificity. In the case of mangafodipir, its active uptake by differentiated carcinoma cells allows diagnosis of primary hepatocellular liver tumors (Rofsky et al. 1993). Experimental studies with gadobenate dimeglumine did not show any intracellular uptake within hepatocellular carcinomas (Marchal et al. 1993).

The chemical similitude of Mn-DPDP [manganese (II)-N, N'-dipiridoxylethylenediamine-N, N'-diacetate-5, 5'-bis(phosphate) sodium salt] with vitamin B_6 (DPDP is a vitamin B_6 analog) contributes to its hepatocyte uptake, but some of the liver accumulation is related to the metabolism of the parent compound with release of free Mn^{2+} ions. Mn-DPDP is metabolized in-vivo by dephosphorylation and transmetallation by Zn^{2+}, while free Mn^{2+} ions are probably bound by α_2-macroglobulin and transported to the liver (Elizondo et al. 1991; Toft et al. 1997a, 1997b). After intravenous administration $(5\,\mu mol/kg)$, the manganese ion accumulates in liver, bile, pancreas, kidneys, and cardiac muscle. The physiological status of liver parenchyma influences the degree of liver enhancement, which starts within 1–2 min post injection, attains a steady-state level within 5–10 min and persists for several hours. Compared with Gd chelates, this pattern of liver

Table 3 Properties of hepatobiliary contrast agents approved for clinical use or in phase III clinical trials

Name of the compound/ Trade name	Relaxivity $(s^{-1}mM^{-1})$ $(0.47\,T,\ 37\,°C)$	Transport	Excretion, Plasma half-life, LD$_{50}$	Indication/dosage
Mangafodipir trisodium Mn-DPDP Teslascan	$r_1 = 2.8$ in water solution and 21.7 in liver tissue[a]	Vitamin B$_6$ transporter and α_2- macroglobulin	15% renal, 59% biliary Half-life = 120 min, LD$_{50}$ = 5.4 mmol/kg	Metastases, additional pancreatic enhancement 0.005 mmol/kg
Gadobenate dimeglumine Gd-BOPTA MultiHance	$r_1 = 4.2$ in water solution[b] and 30 in liver tissue[c]	Organic anion	75–90% renal, 10–25% biliary Half-life = 15 min LD$_{50}$ = 5.7–7.9 mmol/kg	Metastases Biliary obstruction limits liver uptake 0.05 mmol/kg
Gadoxetic acid Gd-EOB- DTPA Eovist, Primovist	$r_1 = 4.9$ in water solution[d] and 10.7 in liver tissue[e]	Organic anion	41% renal, 57% biliary Half-life = 60 min, LD$_{50}$ > 10 mmol/kg	Metastases Biliary obstruction limits liver uptake 0.0125–0.025 mmol/kg

[a]Elizondo et al. (1991); [b]Laurent et al. (2006); [c]Reimer et al. (2004a); [d]Vander Elst et al. (1997); [e]Shuter et al. (1996)

enhancement allows greater flexibility in scanning protocols and patient scheduling (Bellin et al. 2005). The lesion-liver contrast is significantly improved by Mn-DPDP because, generally, the compound is not taken up by nonhepatocellular liver lesions. Thus, Mn-DPDP-enhanced MRI was comparable or superior to CT in detecting small metastases and improved the tumor-liver contrast up to 218% on T$_1$-weighted gradient-echo images. However, the benefits of Mn-DPDP in the detection of hepatocellular carcinomas (HCCs) are rather conflicting because HCCs may contain variable amounts of functioning hepatocytes. Furthermore, a considerable variability of Mn-DPDP uptake was also found in the case of adenomas, which does not allow a reliable differentiation between them and HCC (Reimer et al. 2004a).

The adverse events produced by Mn-DPDP are probably related to the in-vivo dechelation of the CA. Among them, the most frequently reported by patients were flushing, warmth, nausea, increase of the blood pressure and heart rate, and dizziness.

Gd-BOPTA (gadolinium benzyloxypropionictetraacetate) (Uggeri et al. 1995; Morisetti 1999; Schima et al. 1999) and Gd-EOB-DTPA (gadolinium ethoxybenzyl diethylenetriaminepentaacetic acid) (Weinmann et al. 1991; Schuhmann-Giampieri 1992; Hamm et al. 1995; Shuter B et al. 1996) are water-soluble gadolinium complexes with a lipophilic moiety that intermediates hepatocellular uptake through the anionic-transporter protein (van Montfoort et al. 1999; Reimer et al. 2004a). The transporter is a membrane protein located in the sinusoidal and canalicular side of hepatocytes. The intracellular transport of gadolinium chelates is partly energy-dependent and they accumulate in bile with no metabolic alteration. Although the two compounds exhibit similar chemical structure, the bile sequestration of Gd-BOPTA is minimal and its diffusion back into the plasma is possible. Thus,

Gd-BOPTA has a less important biliary elimination in comparison with Gd-EOB-DTPA (Table 3).

The hepatic uptake of Gd-BOPTA represents only 2–4% of the injected dose, and its transient albumin binding makes this CA potentially suitable for MR angiography. During the first minutes after administration, Gd-BOPTA acts as a conventional extracellular CA. A marked and long-lasting enhancement of normal liver parenchyma is produced 40–120 min after administration. Gd-BOPTA is indicated for the detection of focal liver lesions in patients with known or suspected primary liver cancer (e.g., hepatocellular carcinoma) or metastatic disease, which appear hypointense on MR images (Reimer et al. 2004a; Bellin et al. 2005). Gd-BOPTA was particularly efficient in the detection of hypervascular lesions on delayed post-contrast images (i.e., 40–120 min post injection). The most common adverse events reported by patients (1–2.6%) were headache, flushing, nausea, abnormal taste, and reaction at the injection site.

Similar to Gd-BOPTA, Gd-EOB-DTPA is able to bind to plasma proteins, which results in an increase of T_1 relaxivity ($8.7 s^{-1}$ mM^{-1}, bovine plasma, $0.47 T$) (Rohrer et al. 2005). Gd-EOB-DTPA has a short phase of extracellular behavior, while the delayed phase starts 15–20 min after administration, when 30% of the compound is taken-up by hepatocytes. This increases the signal intensity of normal liver parenchyma with an improved lesion-to-liver contrast because most of the malignant tumors do not contain functioning hepatocytes. Compared with CT, Gd-EOB-DTPA-enhanced MRI was able to detect small lesions at a higher rate, with a lower frequency of false positive results. Due to excretion through the biliary system, Gd-EOB-DTPA has a potential application for contrast-enhanced MR cholangiography. The adverse events currently reported as being definitely, possibly or probably related to Gd-EOB-DTPA administration were nausea, vasodilation, headache, taste perversion and pain at the injection site.

3.2 Negative Contrast Agents

The CAs known as *negative agents* influence signal intensity mainly by shortening T_2^* and T_2, which at a given echo time produces darkening of the contrast-enhanced tissue. Conversely, they can act as positive agents (T_1 shortening and image brightening) when appropriate imaging sequences are involved. These CAs are composed of superparamagnetic nanoparticles, consisting of iron oxides (magnetite, Fe_3O_4, maghemite, γFe_2O_3, or other ferrites), which have a net magnetic dipole that is large compared with the sum of its individual unpaired electrons. This large magnetic moment alters the magnetic field in tissues and creates a large magnetic-field heterogeneity, through which water molecules diffuse. Diffusion induces dephasing of the proton magnetic moments, resulting in T_2 shortening. Such CAs are also called *susceptibility agents* because of their effect on the magnetic field, which increases with the crystal size and is a long-distance effect, as opposed to the paramagnetic IS process of relaxation, which requires a close interaction with water protons (Rinck 1993; Okuhata 1999).

The superparamagnetic nanoparticles are composed of an iron oxide nucleus of several nanometers diameter. To increase their stability in aqueous medium, particles are coated with small molecules (citrate, oleate, silane, etc.) or polymers (dextran, synthetic polymers, starch, etc.) and form colloidal suspensions. Iron oxides are divided into two classes according to their global size: if the diameter is >50 nm, they are called SPIO, while USPIO (ultra small particles of iron oxide) have a diameter of <50 nm. The most common method for the synthesis of superparamagnetic nanoparticles involves coprecipitation of ferrous and ferric salts in an alkaline medium. Although coprecipitation methods are used for their simplicity, the nanoparticles are fairly polydisperse. Thus, several other techniques are currently being developed to obtain nanoparticles with more uniform dimensions (Willard et al. 2004; Thorek et al. 2006).

Various kinds of nanoparticles have been developed and are used for clinical applications: Sinerem (Guerbet, France) (Jung and Jacobs 1995), Clariscan (Nycomed, Norway) (Kellar et al. 2000), Endorem (Guerbet, France) (Groman et al. 1989) and Resovist (Schering, Germany) (Bremer et al. 1999; Reimer et al. 1999) (Table 4).

Superparamagnetic nanoparticles have currently become very popular because of their strong magnetic efficacy and because they are composed of biodegradable iron, which is biocompatible and can thus be reused/recycled by cells using normal biochemical pathways for iron metabolism (Bulte and Kraitchman 2004). In addition, their surface coating allows chemical linkage of functional groups and vectorizing molecules that render them able to target a certain organ or disease (Corot et al. 2006; Thorek et al. 2006).

Conversely, their main disadvantage for MRI applications is represented by the fast opsonization after intravenous administration, which leads to a massive uptake by macrophages and mainly by the Kupffer cells in liver. Sometimes, these agents can produce on MR images a strong effect of magnetic susceptibility called "blooming", which manifests by a pronounced decrease of signal intensity that causes the distortion or obliteration of organ boundaries (Wang et al. 2001).

3.2.1 Passive Targeting

Iron oxide nanoparticles are taken up by the monocyte-macrophage system, which explains their capture by liver, spleen and bone marrow and their potential application as MRI markers of inflammatory and degenerative disorders characterized by an enhanced phagocytic activity of the macrophages. Their capture by phagocytes, which is expressed in terms of stability, biodistribution, opsonization, metabolism and clearance from the vascular system, is modulated by the same properties that influence the MRI efficacy, i.e., the size of iron oxide crystals, the hydrodynamic size of the coated particle, the charge, the nature of coating, etc. (Corot et al. 2006). As a general rule, larger-sized particles such as SPIOs are taken-up faster than USPIO, but the charge of the coating material plays a decisive role. Hence, the blood half-life is shorter for ionic dextran (carboxy and carboxy-methyl) than for nonionic dextran, while very small USPIO (VSOP) that are coated with citrate have the shortest blood

Table 4 Properties of superparamagnetic nanoparticles approved for clinical use or under clinical investigations[a]

Names of the compound Company	Hydrodynamic Size (nm)[b] Coating agent	Relaxivity $(s^{-1}\,mM^{-1})$ $(1.5\,T, 37\,^{\circ}C,$ water or plasma)	Half-life in humans (hours) Dosage (μmol Fe/kg)	Applications
Ferumoxides, AMI-25 Endorem/Feridex Guerbet, Advanced Magnetics	120–180 Dextran T10	$r_1 = 10.1$ $r_2 = 120$	2 30	Liver imaging Cellular labeling
Ferumoxtran-10, AMI-227 BMS-180549 Sinerem/Combridex Guerbet, Advanced Magnetics	15–30 Dextran T10, T1	$r_1 = 9.9$ $r_2 = 65$	24–36 45	Metastatic lymph node imaging Macrophage imaging Blood pool agent Cellular labeling
Ferumoxytol Code 7228 Advanced Magnetics	30 Carboxylmethyl-dextran T10	$r_1 = 15$ $r_2 = 89$	10–14 18–74	Macrophage imaging Blood pool agent Cellular labeling
Ferumoxsil AMI-121 Lumirem/ Gastromark Guerbet, Advanced Magnetics	300 Silicon	n.a.	Oral	Gastrointestinal imaging
Ferucarbotran SHU-555A Resovist Schering	60 Carboxydextran	$r_1 = 9.7$ $r_2 = 189$	2.4–3.6 8–12	Liver imaging Cellular labeling
SHU-555C Supravist Schering	21 Carboxydextran	$r_1 = 10.7$ $r_2 = 38$	6 40	Blood pool agent Cellular labeling
Feruglucose NC100150 Clariscan (abandoned) Ferristene Abdoscan GE-Healthcare	20, Pegylated starch (Clariscan) 3,500, Sulphonated styrene-divinylbenzene copolymer (Ferristene Abdoscan®)	n.a. n.a.	6 36 Oral	Blood pool agent Gastrointestinal imaging
VSOP-C184 Ferropharm	7 Citrate	$r_1 = 14$ $r_2 = 33.4$	0.6–1.3 15–75	Blood pool agent Cellular labeling

[a]For more information see Corot et al. (2006)
[b]Determined by laser light scattering

half-life in humans due to their anionic surface. However, the blood half-life is dose-dependent due to the progressive saturation of macrophage uptake and is generally longer in humans than in animals. It is worthy to mention that the total amount of iron oxide (50–200 mg Fe) injected for clinical MRI has a satisfactory safety profile and chronic iron toxicity can develop only if liver iron concentration exceeds 4 mg/gram of tissue (Bonnemain 1998).

Clinical applications of iron oxide nanoparticles depend on their biodistribution. Thus, SPIO is well adapted for imaging of liver tumors and metastases because of the intense macrophage (Kupffer cells) uptake. In these conditions, the contrast of liver tumors is possible because only healthy liver tissue has a dark signal on T_2 or T_2^*-weighted images, while the signal intensity of tumors is not changed. Liver tumors or metastases as small as 2–3 mm can thus be detected (Stark et al. 1988; Tanimoto and Kuribayashi 2005; Yoshikawa et al. 2006).

USPIO with prolonged half-life and minor macrophage uptake are useful for imaging metastatic lymph nodes because these iron particles are progressively taken up by macrophages in healthy lymph nodes (they appear dark on MR images) but no modification of contrast is observed in metastatic tissue. Comparatively, USPIO are useful for macrophage imaging in inflammatory and/or degenerative diseases (Weissleder et al. 1990; Hudgins et al. 2002; Mack et al. 2002). For instance, USPIO were used to detect inflammation associated with ischaemic stroke (Saleh et al. 2004) or to image macrophage-rich areas in unstable atherosclerotic plaques (Ruehm et al. 2001; Trivedi et al. 2004). They were also useful for in-vivo imaging of macrophage activity in experimental autoimmune encephalomyelitis (EAE) (Xu et al. 1998) or in patients with multiple sclerosis (Dousset et al. 2006).

Iron oxide particles coated by inert silicon (ferumoxsil) or polystyrene (ferristene) were developed for oral administration and improvement of differentiation between the gastrointestinal tract and surrounding tissues (Johnson et al. 1996; Jacobsen et al. 1996).

3.2.2 Blood-pool Imaging

Small sized (7–30 nm) iron oxide nanoparticles like Sinerem/Combidex, Ferumoxytol-7228, SHU-555C, VSOP-C184, and MION (monocrystalline iron oxide nanocompounds) have optimal physicochemical and biological properties for blood-pool imaging (Table 4). Their low levels of macrophage uptake and prolonged half-lives, as well as T_1-shortening effect with certain MRI protocols and when injected at low doses (15–50 µmol Fe/kg) were exploited for MRA applications, e.g., angiography, evaluation of cerebral, myocardial or renal perfusion, detection of hepatic vascular lesions (Ahlstrom et al. 1999; Corot et al. 2003; Reimer et al. 2004b). These compounds, known as slow-clearance blood pool agents, provide a larger time window for image acquisition of the vascular system, both for the first-pass and for the equilibrium-phase MRA. Unfortunately, major drawbacks of these applications were observed due to the superparamagnetic nature of iron oxide nanoparticles, which was responsible for the loss of blood signal mainly when higher doses of CA were injected. In these conditions, the T_2^* effects prevail over the T_1 effects, even when using MRI sequences with very short echo times. In addition, images acquired during the equilibrium-phase show both arterial and venous contrast enhancement, which complicates the interpretation of the vascular tree (Schneider et al. 2005; Corot et al. 2006).

4 Perspectives

Among the modern methods of clinical imaging, MRI has prevailed as the foremost diagnostic technique because it is able to furnish, noninvasively and with a high spatial resolution, both anatomical and physiological information. Most of the contemporary MRI CAs approved for clinical applications are nonspecific for a particular pathology and report exclusively on the anatomy and the physiological status of various organs. Nevertheless, a new generation of MRI CAs is progressively emerging in the current context of *molecular imaging*. These new agents are designed to detect with a high specificity the cellular and molecular hallmarks of various pathologies. It is, however, generally accepted that conventional gadolinium chelates have a quite low efficiency in the detection of molecular events because of their sensitivity in the order of micromolar concentrations. Thus, the development of MRI CAs with improved efficiency represents a challenge with respect to the choice of the most adequate method of chemical synthesis and to the development of MRI protocols adapted for their detection.

As a new and rapidly expanding discipline, molecular imaging integrates cell and molecular biology with the final purpose to develop new diagnostic technologies able to identify, in-vivo, biochemical processes involved in pathological mechanisms which are often produced a long time before the morphological ones. Their early detection may represent a decisive advantage for the choice of adequate therapeutic strategies (Gupta and Weissleder 1996; Nunn et al. 1997; Weissleder and Mahmood 2001; Massoud and Gambhir 2003; Meade et al. 2003; Rollo 2003; Rudin et al. 2003; Sosnovik and Weissleder 2006).

The new generation of MRI CAs under development in biomedical research is represented by complex assemblies made of a magnetic reporter, the *contrastophore*, conjugated via a linker to a *vectorizing moiety* (ligand) specific to the structure to be targeted. Various vector and carrier molecules have been developed to deliver magnetic labels to specific target sites, such as antibodies, peptides, polysaccharides, aptamers, and synthetic compounds (e.g., peptide mimetics). The high specific affinity for the target of these ligand molecules and its preservation after conjugation to the magnetic reporter are prerequisite requirements for success in molecular targeting.

Another constraint is related to the minimal concentration of the magnetic reporter able to exert a significant effect on the relaxation rate of tissue water and therefore on the MRI signal. Since cellular receptors are present in nano- or even picomolar concentrations, the CA bound to these targets should bring an effective magnetic payload in order to defeat the signal dilution in the image voxel.

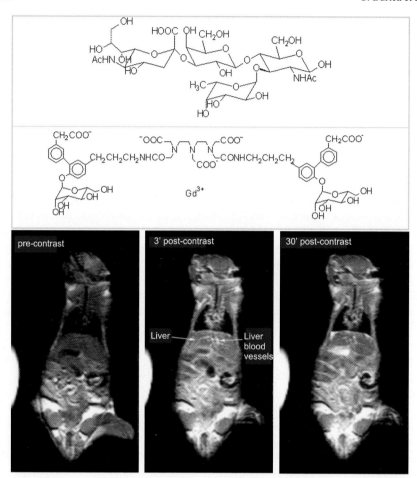

Fig. 8 Molecular imaging of inflammation with Gd-DTPA-B(sLe^x)A, an E-selectin-targeted CA (Boutry et al. 2005). Chemical structure of sialyl-Lewis^x, the natural ligand of E-selectin (adhesion molecule expressed in inflammation) (*top row*), and of Gd-DTPA-B(sLe^x)A which is vectorized to E-selectin with a mimetic of sialyl-Lewis^x conjugated to Gd-DTPA (*middle row*). MR coronal images of a mouse with hepatitis (induced by the co-administration of D-galactosamine and lipopolysaccharide) before (pre-contrast) and several time intervals (3 min and 30 min post-contrast) after i.v. administration of Gd-DTPA-(middle row)(sLe^x)A are presented in the bottom row. The liver blood vessels appear bright in the postcontrast images due to the binding of Gd-DTPA-B(sLe^x)A to E-selectin. The images were acquired at 1.0 T with a Siemens Magnetom Impact System by using a T1-weighted spin-echo sequence (TR/TE $=$ 600/20 ms; FOV $=$ 5 $\times$ 10 cm; matrix $=$ 90 $\times$ 256; slice thickness $=$ 3 mm; spatial resolution $=$ 0.555 $\times$ 0.390 mm)

These limitations can be solved by increasing the efficiency of CAs either by a greater intrinsic relaxivity (modulation of physical properties like q, τ_M and τ_R) or by the attachment of many magnetic centers to the ligand. Among the magnetic materials able to be detected at low tissue concentrations, one can point out the superparamagnetic particles (Corot et al. 2006), the paramagnetic dendrimers

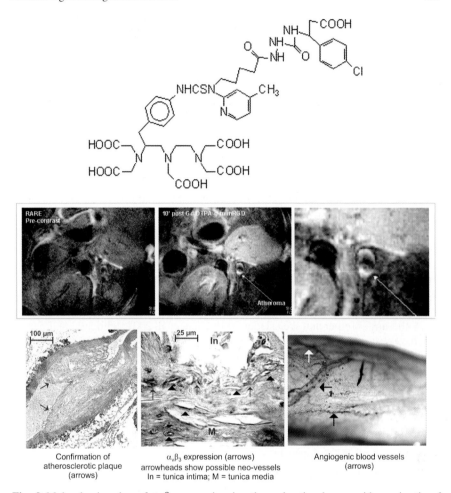

Fig. 9 Molecular imaging of $\alpha_v\beta_3$ expression in atherosclerotic plaques with a mimetic of RGD peptide conjugated to Gd-DTPA (Burtea et al. 2008). Chemical structure of $\alpha_v\beta_3$-targeted contrast agent, Gd-DTPA-g-mimRGD is shown in top row. Axial slices at the level of abdominal aorta of a transgenic mouse model of atherosclerosis (ApoE$^{-/-}$ mouse) before and 10 min after the administration of Gd-DTPA-g-mimRGD are presented in the middle row. The images were acquired at 4.7 T with a Bruker AVANCE-200 imaging system (RARE imaging protocol, TR/TE = 1,048.5/4 ms, RARE factor = 4, NEX = 4, matrix = 256, FOV = 2.3 cm, slice thickness 0.8 mm, spatial resolution = 90 μm). The external structures of the aortic wall (probably adventitia and partly tunica media) are strongly enhanced, while in the enlarged image the more profound layers (toward the aortic lumen) of the aortic wall (possibly tunica media and intima) can be distinguished. The presence of atherosclerotic plaques (bottom row) was confirmed on histologic sections (stained with hemalun and Luxol fast blue), which were validated by immunohistochemistry for $\alpha_v\beta_3$ expression (anti-α_v antibody; color developed with diaminobenzidine) and for the presence of angiogenic blood vessels (anti-PECAM antibody on whole-mount aorta)

(Wiener et al. 1994), and the perfluorocarbon nanoparticles (Lanza et al. 2003). It should, however, be noticed that specific binding of low molecular-weight CAs to cell membrane receptors could by itself increase the relaxation rate by slowing down the rotational motion of the magnetic reporter, which results in the enhancement of MRI signal.

The success of molecular imaging with MRI CAs furthermore depends on issues like a long half-life of elimination (to allow an optimal contact with binding sites), low toxicity, a significant enhancement of the signal/noise ratio and an optimal and economic industrial and clinical implementation. Nevertheless, the necessity to deliver magnetic payloads in sufficient quantity at binding sites and the long elimination half-lives could result in a high background noise and the consequent diminution of the signal/noise ratio. In addition, the saturation of cell receptors is possible. This last biochemical limitation was tentatively solved by targeting receptors involved in cellular transport (e.g., receptor mediated endocytosis) or readily accessible to the vascular system.

Despite various drawbacks, the current developments in MR molecular imaging have a wide diversity of potential applications, which range from the diagnosis of a particular pathology (Figs. 8, 9) (Barber et al. 2004; Sibson et al. 2004; Boutry et al. 2005, 2006; Burtea et al. 2008) to the monitoring of gene therapy or chemotherapy (Bremer and Weissleder 2001; Zhao et al. 2001; Ichikawa et al. 2002; Schellenberger et al. 2002). Cellular imaging is another growing field of interest for medical research and clinical applications which uses superparamagnetic CAs to image cell migration and trafficking after transplantation (Bulte and Kraitchman 2004; Corot et al. 2006; George et al. 2006).

Finally, in-vitro MR techniques were proposed for diagnostic applications (Burtea et al. 2005) in which CAs are exploited as magnetic relaxation switches capable of sensing biochemical interactions (De León-Rodriguez et al. 2002; Högemann et al. 2002; Perez et al. 2002; Meade et al. 2003). In fact, the molecular interactions result in a 30–40% change in the relaxation rate, which can be evaluated by MR relaxometry or MRI.

References

Ahlstrom KH, Johansson LO, Rodenburg JB, Ragnarsson AS, Akeson P, Borseth A (1999) Pulmonary MR angiography with ultrasmall superparamagnetic iron oxide particles as a blood pool agent and a navigator echo for respiratory gating: pilot study. Radiology 211:865–869

Aime S, Botta M, Fasano M, Terreno E (1998) Lanthanide(III) chelates for NMR biomedical applications. Chem Soc Rev 27:19–29

Aime S, Botta M, Fasano M, Terreno E (1999) Prototropic and water-exchange processes in aqueous solutions of Gd(III) chelates. Acc Chem Res 32:941–949

Anelli PL, Lattuada L, Lorusso V, Schneider M, Tourner H, Uggeri F (2001) Mixed micelles containing lipophilic gadolinium complexes as MRA contrast agents. MAGMA 12:114–120

Barber PA, Foniok T, Kirk D, Buchan AM, Laurent S, Boutry S, Muller RN, Hoyte L, Tomanek B, Tuor UI (2004) Magnetic resonance molecular imaging (MRMI) of early endothelial activation in focal ischemia in mice. Ann Neurol 56:116–120

Bellin M-F, Webb JAW, Van Der Molen AJ, Thomsen HS, Morcos SK (2005) Safety of MR liver specific contrast media. Eur Radiol 15:1607–1614

Bloembergen NJ (1957) Proton relaxation times in paramagnetic solutions. Chem Phys 27: 572–573

Bogdanov AA Jr, Lewin M, Weissleder R (1999) Approaches and agents for imaging the vascular system. Adv Drug Delivery Rev 37:279–293

Bonnemain B (1998) Superparamagnetic agents in magnetic resonance imaging, physicochemical characteristics and clinical applications. A review. J Drug Target 6:167–174

Bousquet JC, Saini S, Stark DD, Hahn PF, Nigam M, Wittenberg J, Ferrucci JT (1988) Gd-DOTA: characterization of a new paramagnetic complex. Radiology 166:693–698

Boutry S, Burtea C, Laurent S, Vander Elst L, Muller RN (2005) Magnetic resonance imaging of inflammation with a specific selectin-targeted contrast agent. Magn Reson Med 53:800–807

Boutry S, Laurent S, Vander Elst L, Muller RN (2006) Specific E-selectin targeting with a superparamagnetic MRI contrast agent. Contrast Med Mol Imaging 1:15–22

Bremer C, Allkemper T, Bärmig J, Reimer P (1999) RES-specific imaging of the liver and spleen with iron oxide particles designed for blood pool MR-angiography. J Magn Reson Imaging 10:461–467

Bremer C, Weissleder R (2001) In vivo imaging of gene expression: MR and optical technologies. Acad Radiol 8:15–23

Bremerich J, Colet J-M, Giovenzana GB, Aime S, Scheffler K, Laurent S, Bongartz G, Muller RN (2001) Slow clearance gadolinium-based extracellular and intravascular contrast media for three-dimensional MR angiography. J Magn Reson Imaging 13:588–593

Bulte JWM, Kraitchman DL (2004) Iron oxide MR contrast agents for molecular and cellular imaging. NMR Biomed 17:484–499

Burtea C, Laurent S, Roch A, Vander Elst L, Muller RN (2005) C-MALISA (cellular magnetic-linked immunosorbent assay), a new application of cellular ELISA for MRI. J Inorg Biochem 99:1135–1144

Burtea C, Laurent S, Murariu O, Rattat D, Toubeau G, Verbruggen A, Vansthertem D, Vander Elst L, Muller RN (2008) Molecular imaging of alpha-v beta-3 integrin expression in atherosclerotic plaques with a mimetic of RGD peptide grafted to Gd-DTPA, Cardiovasc Res, doi: 10.1093/cvr/cvm115.

Cabella C, Geninatti Crich S, Corpillo D, Barge A, Ghirelli C, Bruno E, Lorusso V, Uggeri F, Aime S (2006) Cellular labeling with Gd(III) chelates: only high thermodynamic stabilities prevent the cells acting as 'sponges' of Gd^{3+} ions. Contrast Med Mol Imaging 1:23–29

Cacheris WP, Quay SC, Rocklage SM (1990) The relationship between thermodynamics and toxicity of gadolinium complexes. Magn Reson Imaging 8:467–481

Caravan P, Ellison JJ, McMurry TJ, Lauffer R (1999) Gadolinium (III) chelates as MRI contrast agents: structure, dynamics, and applications. Chem Rev 99:2293–2352

Caravan P, Cloutier NJ, Greenfield MT, McDermid SA, Dunham SU, Bulte JWM, Amedio JC, Looby RJ, Supkowski RM, Horrocks WD, McMurry TJ, Lauffer RB (2002) The interaction of MS-325 with human serum albumin and its effect on proton relaxation rates. J Am Chem Soc 124:3152–3162

Corot C, Schaefer M, Beauté S, Bourrinet P, Zehaf S (1997) Physical, chemical and biological evaluations of CMD-A2-Gd-DOTA - A new paramagnetic dextran polymer. Acta Radiol 38: 91–99

Corot C, Violas X, Robert P, Gagneur G, Port M (2003) Comparison of different types of blood pool agents (P792, MS325, USPIO) in a rabbit MR angiography-like protocol. Invest Radiol 38:311–319

Corot C, Robert P, Idée J-M, Port M (2006) Recent advances in iron oxide nanocrystal technology for medical imaging. Adv Drug Deliv Rev 58:1471–1504

De León-Rodriguez LM, Ortiz A, Weiner AL, Zhang S, Kovacs Z, Kodadek T, Sherry AD (2002) Magnetic resonance imaging detects a specific peptide-protein binding event. J Am Chem Soc 124:3514–3515

Den Boer JA, Hoogeveen R (2001) Contrast enhanced MR angiography. Medica Mundi 45:10–22

Dousset V, Brochet B, Deloire MSA, Lagoarde L, Barroso B, Caille JM, Petry KJ (2006) MR imaging of relapsing multiple sclerosis patients using ultra-small-particle iron oxide and compared with gadolinium. Am J Neuroradiol 27:1000–1005

Elizondo G, Fnetz CJ, Stank DD, Scott M. Rocklage SM, Quay SC, Wonah D, Tsang YM, Chia-Mei Chen M, Ferrucci JT (1991) Preclinical evaluation of MnDPDP: New paramagnetic hepatobiliary contrast agent for MR imaging. Radiology 178:73–78

Farooki A, Narra V, Brown J, Gadofosveset EPIX/Schering (2004) Curr Opin Investig Drugs 5: 967–976

Freed JH (1978) Dynamic effects of pair correlation functions on spin relaxation by translational diffusion in liquids. II. Finite jumps and independent T_1 processes. J Chem Phys 68:4034–4037

Gaillard S, Kubiak C, Stolz C, Bonnemain B, Chassard D (2002) Safety and pharmacokinetics of P792, a new blood-pool agent: results of clinical testing in nonpatient volunteers. Invest Radiol 37:161–166

George AJT, Bhakoo KK, Haskard DO, Larkman DJ, Reynolds PR (2006) Imaging molecular and cellular events in transplantation. Transplantation 82:1124–1129

Gonzalez G, Powell DH, Tissières V, Merbach AE (1994) Water-exchange, electronic relaxation and rotational dynamics of the MRI contrast agent [Gd(DTPA-BMA)(H$_2$O)] I aqueous solution: a variable pressure, temperature, and magnetic field ^{17}O NMR study. J Phys Chem. 98:53–59

Groman EV, Josephson L. Lewis JM (1989) US Patent, 4827945

Gupta H, Weissleder R (1996) Targeted contrast agents in MR imaging. Magn Reson Imaging Clin N Am 4:171–184

Hamm B, Staks T, Mühler A, Bolbow M, Taupitz M, Frenzel T, Wolf K-J, Weinmann H-J, Lange L (1995) Phase I clinical evaluation of Gd-EOB-DTPA as a hepatobiliary MR contrast agent: safety, pharmacokinetics, and MR imaging. Radiology 195:785–792

Harpur ES, Worah D, Hals P-A, Holtz E, Furuhama K, Nomura H (1993) Preclinical safety assessment and pharmacokinetics of gadodiamide injection, a new magnetic resonance imaging contrast agent. Invest Radiol 28:S28–S432

Helms MK, Petersen CE, Bhagavan NV, Jameson DM (1997) Time-resolved fluorescence studies on site-directed mutants of human serum albumin FEBS Letters, 408:67–70

Herborn CU, Honold E, Wolf M, Kemper J, Kinner S, Adam G, Barkhausen J (2007) Clinical safety and diagnostic value of the gadolinium chelate gadoterate meglumine (Gd-DOTA). Invest Radiol 42:58–62

Högemann D, Ntziachristos V, Josephson L, Weissleder R (2002) High throughput magnetic resonance imaging for evaluating targeted nanoparticle probes. Bioconjugate Chem 13:116–121

Hovland R, Aasen AJ, Klaveness J (2003) Preparation and in vitro evaluation of GdDOTA-(BOM)$_4$; a novel angiographic MRI contrast agent. Org Biomol Chem 1:1707–1710

Hudgins PA, Anzai Y, Morris MR, Lucas MA (2002) Ferumoxtran-10, a superparamagnetic iron oxide as a magnetic resonance enhancement agent for imaging lymph nodes: A phase 2 dose study. Am J Neuroradiol 23:649–656

Ichikawa T, Högemann D, Saeki Y, Tyminski E, Terada K, Weissleder R, Chiocca EA, Basilion JP (2002) MRI of transgene expression: correlation to therapeutic gene expression. Neoplasia. 4:523–530

Idée J-M, Port M, Raynal I, Schaefer M, Le Greneur S, Corot C (2006) Clinical and biological consequences of transmetallation induced by contrast agents for magnetic resonance imaging: a review. Fundam Clin Pharmacol 20:563–576

Jacobsen TF, Laniado M, Van Beers BE, Dupas B, Boudghene FP, Rummeny E, Falk TH, Rinck PA, MacVicar D, Lundby B (1996) Oral magnetic particles (ferristene) as a contrast medium in abdominal magnetic resonance imaging. Acad Radiol 3:571–580

Johnson WK, Stoupis C, Torres GM, Rosenberg EB, Ros RR (1996) Superparamagnetic iron oxide (SPIO) as an oral contrast agent in gastrointestinal (GI) magnetic resonance imaging (MRI): comparison with state-of-the-art computed tomography (CT). Magn Reson Imaging 14:43–49

Jung, CW, Jacobs P (1995) Physical and chemical properties of superparamagnetic iron oxide MR contrast agents: ferumoxides, ferumoxtran, ferumoxsil. Magn Reson Imaging 13:661–674

Karabulut N, Elmas N (2006) Contrast agents used in MR imaging of the liver. Diagn Interv Radiol 12:22–30

Kellar KE, Fujii DK, Guther WHH, Briley-Saebo K, Spiller M, Bjornerud A, Koenig SH (2000) NC100150 Injection, a preparation of optimized iron oxide nanoparticles for positive-contrast MR angiography. J Magn Reson Imaging 11:488–494

Kobayashi H, Kawamoto S, Saga T, Sato N, Hiraga A, Ishimori T, Konishi J, Togashi K, Brechbiel MW (2001) Positive effects of polyethylene glycol conjugation to generation-4 polyamidoamine dendrimers as macromolecular MR contrast agents. Magn Reson Med 46:781–788

Kroft LJM, de Roos A (1999) Blood pool contrast agents for cardiovascular MR imaging. J Magn Reson Imaging 10:395–403

Lanza GM, Lamerichs R, Caruthers S, Wickline SA (2003) Molecular imaging in MR with targeted paramagnetic nanoparticles. Medica Mundi 47:34–39

Lauffer R (1988) Paramagnetic metal complexes as water proton relaxation agents for MRI: theory and design. Chem Rev 187:901–927

Laurent S, Vander Elst L, Houzé S, Guérit N, Muller RN (2000) Synthesis and characterization of various benzyl diethylenetriaminepentaacetic acids (DTPA) and their paramagnetic complexes: potential organ specific contrast agents for MRI. Helv Chim Acta 83:394–406

Laurent S, Vander Elst L, Copoix F, Muller RN (2001) Stability of MRI paramagnetic contrast media. A proton relaxometric protocol for transmetallation assessment. Invest Radiol 36:115–122

Laurent S, Botteman F, Vander Elst L, Muller RN, (2004a) Optimising the design of paramagnetic MRI contrast agents: influence of backbone substitution on the water exchange rate of Gd-DTPA derivatives. Magn Reson Mater Phys Biol Med 16:235–245

Laurent S, Botteman F, Vander Elst L, Muller RN (2004b) Relaxivity and transmetallation stability of new benzyl-substituted derivatives of gadolinium-DTPA complexes. Helv Chim Acta 87:1077–1089

Laurent S, Vander Elst L, Muller RN (2006) Comparative study of the physicochemical properties of six clinical low molecular weight gadolinium contrast agents. Contrast Med Mol Imaging 1:128–137

Lauterbur PC (1973) Image formation by induced local interactions – examples employing nuclear magnetic resonance. Nature 242:190–191

Lauterbur PC, Mendonça-Dias MH, Rudin AM (1978) Augmentation of tissue water proton spin-lattce relaxation rates by in-vivo addition of paramagnetic ions. In: Dutton PO, Leigh J, Scarpa A (eds) Frontiers of Biological Energetics. Academic Press, New York, pp 752–759

Mack MG, Balzer JO, Straub R, Eichler K, Vogl TJ (2002) Superparamagnetic iron oxide-enhanced MR imaging of head and neck lymph nodes. Radiology 222:239–244

Magerstadt M, Gansow OA, Brechbiel MW, Colcher D, Balzer L, Knop RH, Girton ME, Naegele M (1986) Gadolinium-(DOTA): an alternative to gadolinium – (DTPA) as a T1, 2 relaxation agent for NMR imaging or spectroscopy. Magn Reson Med 3:808–812

Mandry D, Pedersen M, Odile F, Robert P, Corot C, Felblinger J, Grenier N, Claudon M (2005) Renal functional contrast-enhanced magnetic resonance imaging; Evaluation of a new rapid-clearance blood pool agent (P792) in Sprague-Dawley rats. Invest Radiol 40:295–305

Marchal G, Zhang X, Ni Y, Van Hecke P, Yu J, Baert AL (1993) Comparison between Gd-DTPA, Gd-EOB-DTPA, and Mn-DPDP in induced HCC in rats: a correlation study of MR imaging, microangiography, and histology. Magn Reson Imaging 11:665–674

Massoud TF, Gambhir SS (2003) Molecular Imaging in living subjects: seeing fundamental biological processes in new light. Genes Dev 17:545–580

McMurry TJ, Parmelee DJ, Sajiki H, Scott DM, Ouellet HS, Walovitch RC, Tyeklàr Z, Dumas S, Bernard P, Nadler S, Midelfort K, Greenfield M, Throughton J, Lauffer RB (2002) The effect of a phosphodiester linking group on albumin binding. Blood half-life, and relaxivity of intravascular diethylentriaminepentaacetato aquo gadolinium(III) MRI contrast agents. J Med Chem 45:3465–3474

Meade TJ, Taylor AK, Bull SR (2003) New magnetic resonance contrast agents as biochemical reporters. Curr Opin Biotechnol 13:597–602

Micskei K, Helm L, Brucher E, Merbach AE (1993a) ^{17}O NMR study of water exchange on $[Gd(DTPA)H2O]^{2-}$ and $[Gd(DOTA)H2O]^{-}$ related to NMR imaging. Inorg Chem 32: 3844–3850

Micskei K, Powell DH, Helm L, Brücher E, Merbach AE (1993b) Water exchange on $[Gd(H_2O)_8]^{3+}$ and $[Gd(PDTA)(H_2O)_2]^{-}$ in aqueous solution: a variable-pressure, -temperature and -magnetic field ^{17}O NMR study. Magn Reson Chem 31:1011–1020

Morisetti A, Bussi S, Tirone P, de Haën C (1999) Toxicological safety evaluation of gadobenate dimeglumine 0.5 M solution for injection (MultiHance), a new magnetic resonance imaging contrast medium. J Comput Assist Tomogr 23:S207–S217

Muller RN (1996) Contrast agents in whole body magnetic resonance: operating mechanisms. In: Grant DM, Harris RK (eds) Encyclopedia of nuclear magnetic resonance. Wiley, New York, pp 1438–1444

Muller RN, Raduchel B, Laurent S, Platzek J, Piérart C, Mareski P, Vander Elst L (1999) Physico-chemical characterization of MS-325, a new gadolinium complex, by multinuclear relaxometry. Eur J Inorg Chem 1949–1955

Muller RN, Roch A, Colet JM, Ouakssim A, Gillis P (2001) Particulate magnetic contrast agents. In: Merbach AE, Toth E (eds) The chemistry of contrast agents in medical magnetic resonance imaging. Wiley, New York, pp 417–435

Nunn AD, Linder KE, Tweedle MF (1997) Can receptors be imaged with MRI agents? Q J Nucl Med 41:155–162

Okuhata Y (1999) Delivery of diagnostic agents for magnetic resonance imaging. Adv Drug Deliv Rev 37:121–137

Ouakssim A, Fastrez S, Roch A, Laurent S, Gossuin Y, Pierart C, Vander Elst L, Muller RN (2004) Control of the synthesis of magnetic fluids by relaxometry and magnetometry. J Magn Magn Mater 272–276:e1711–e1713

Parac-Vogt TN, Kimpe K, Laurent S, Vander Elst L, Burtea C, Chen F, Muller RN, Ni Y, Verbruggen A, Binnemans K (2005) Synthesis, characterization and pharmacokinetic evaluation of a potential MRI contrast agent containing two paramagnetic centers with albumin binding affinity. Chem Eur J 11:3077–3086

Parac-Vogt TN, Kimpe K, Laurent S, Piérart C, Vander Elst L, Muller RN, Binnemans K (2006) Paramagnetic liposomes containing amphiphilic bisamide derivatives of Gd-DTPA with aromatic side chain groups as possible contrast agents for magnetic resonance imaging. Eur Biophys J 35:136–144

Parmelee DJ, Walovitch RC, Ouellet HS, Lauffer RB (1997) Preclinical evaluation of the pharmacokinetics, biodistribution, and elimination of MS-325, a blood pool agent for magnetic resonance imaging. Invest Radiol 32:741–747

Perez JM, Josephson L, O'Loughlin T, Högemann D, Weissleder R (2002) Magnetic relaxation switches capable of sensing molecular interactions. Nat Biotechnol 20:816–820

Petersen SB, Muller RN, Rinck PA (eds) (1985) An introduction to biomedical nuclear magnetic resonance. Thieme, Stuttgart New York

Platzek J, Blaszkiewicz P, Gries H, Luger P, Mishl G, Muller-Fahrnow A, Raduchel B, Sulzle D (1997) Synthesis and structure of a new macrocyclic polyhydroxylated gadolunium chelate used as a contrast agent for magnetic resonance imaging. Inorg Chem 36:6086–6093

Reimer P, Muller M, Marx C, Wiedermann D, Muller RN, Rummeny EJ, Ebert W, Shamsi K, Peters PE (1998) T1 effects of a bolus-injectable superparamagnetic iron oxide, SH U 555 A: dependence on field strength and plasma concentration–preliminary clinical experience with dynamic T1-weighted MR imaging. Radiology 209:831–836

Reimer P, Schneider G, Schima W (2004a) Hepatobiliary contrast agents for contrast-enhanced MRI of the liver: properties, clinical development and applications. Eur Radiol 14:559–578

Reimer P, Bremer C, Allkemper T, Engelhardt M, Mahler M, Ebert W, Tombach B (2004b) Myocardial perfusion and MR angiography of chest with SH U 555 C: Results of placebo-controlled clinical phase I study. Radiology 231:474–481

Rinck PA (ed) (1993) Magnetic resonance in medicine. The basic textbook of the European Magnetic Resonance Forum, 3rd edn. Blackwell, Oxford London Edinburgh Boston Melbourne Paris Berlin Vienna

Roch A, Muller RN (1992) Longitudinal relaxation of water protons in colloidal suspensions of superparamagnetic crystals. Proc11th Annual Meeting of the Society of Magnetic Resonance in Medicine. 11:1447

Roch A, Muller RN, Gillis P (1999a) Theory of proton relaxation induced by superparamagnetic particles. J Chem Phys 110:5403–5411

Roch A, Gillis P, Ouakssim A, Muller RN (1999b) Proton magnetic relaxation in superparamagnetic aqueous colloids: a new tool for the investigation of ferrite crystal anisotropy. J Magn Magn Mater 201:77–79

Roch A, Muller RN, Gillis P (2001) Water relaxation by SPM particles: Neglecting the magnetic anisotropy? A caveat. J Magn Reson Imaging 14:94–96

Roch A, Moiny F, Muller RN, Gillis P (2002) Water magnetic relaxation in superparamagnetic colloid suspensions: the effect of agglomeration. In: Fraissard J, Lapina O (eds) Magnetic resonance in colloid and interface science. Kluwer, Dordrecht, pp 383–392

Rofsky NM, Weinreb JC, Bernardino ME, Young SW, Lee JK, Noz ME (1993) Hepatocellular tumors: characterization with Mn-DPDP-enhanced MR imaging. Radiology 188:53–59

Rohrer M, Bauer H, Mintorovitch J, Requardt M, Weinmann H-J (2005) Comparison of magnetic properties of MRI contrast media solutions at different magnetic field strengths. Invest Radiol, 40:715–724

Rollo FD (2003) Molecular imaging: an overview and clinical applications. Radiol Manage 25:28–32

Rudin M, Weissleder R (2003) Molecular imaging in drug discovery and development. Nat Rev Drug Discov 2:123–131

Ruehm SG, Corot C, Vogt P, Kolb S, Debatin JF (2001) Magnetic resonance imaging of atherosclerotic plaque with ultrasmall superparamagnetic particles of iron oxide in hyperlipidemic rabbits. Circulation 103:415–422

Saleh A, Wiedermann D, Schroeter M, Jonkmanns C, Jander S, Hoehn M (2004) Central nervous system inflammatory response after cerebral infarction as detected by magnetic resonance imaging. NMR Biomed 17:163–169

Schellenberger EA, Hogemann D, Josephson L, Weissleder R (2002) Annexin V-CLIO: a nanoparticle for detecting apoptosis by MRI. Acad Radiol 9:S310–S311

Schima W, Saini S, Petersein J, Weissleder R, Harisinghani M, Mayo-Smith W, Hahn PF (1999) MR imaging of the liver with Gd-BOPTA: quantitative analysis of T1-weighted images at two different doses. J Magn Reson Imaging 10:80–83

Schneider G, Prince MR, Meaney JFM, Ho VB (eds) (2005) Magnetic resonance angiography – Techniques, indications and practical applications. Springer, Milan Berlin Heidelberg New York.

Schuhmann-Giampieri G, Schmitt-Willich H, Press WR, Negishi C, Weinmann HJ, Speck U (1992) Preclinical evaluation of Gd-EOB-DTPA as a contrast agent in MR imaging of the hepatobiliary system. Radiology 183:59–64

Semelka RC, Helmberger TKG (2001) Contrast agents for MR imaging of the liver. Radiology 218:27–38

Sharafuddin MJ, Stolpen AH, Dang YM, Andresen KJ, Roh B-S (2002) Comparison of MS-325- and gadodiamide enhanced MR venography of iliocaval veins. J Vasc Interv Radiol 13:1021–1027

Shukla R. Zhang X, Tweedle M. (1991) In vitro determination of correlation times independent of nuclear magnetic resonance dispersion. Inverst Radiol 26:S224–S225

Shuter B, Tofts PS, Wanga S-C, Pope JM (1996) The relaxivity of Gd-EOB-DTPA and Gd-DTPA in liver and kidney of the Wistar rat. Magn Reson Imaging 14:243–253

Sibson NR, Blamire AM, Bernades-Silva M, Laurent S, Boutry S, Muller RN, Styles P, Anthony DC (2004) MRI detection of early endothelial activation in CNS inflammation. Magn Reson Med 51:248–252

Solomon I (1955) Relaxation processes in a system of two spins. Phys Rev 99:559–565

Sosnovik DE, Weissleder R (2006) Emerging concepts in molecular MRI. Curr Opin Biotechnol 17:1–7

Stark DD, Weissleder R, Elizondo G, Hahn PF, Saini S, Todd LE, Wittenberg J, Ferrucci JT (1988) Superparamagnetic iron oxide: Clinical application as a contrast agent for MR imaging of the liver. Radiology 168:297–301

Tanimoto A, Kuribayashi S (2005) Hepatocyte-targeted MR contrast agents: Contrast enhanced detection of liver cancer in diffusely damaged liver. Magn Reson Med Sci 4:53–60

Thomsen HS (2006) Nephrogenic systemic fibrosis: a serious late adverse reaction to gadodiamide. Eur Radiol 16:2619–2621

Thorek DLJ, Chen AK, Czupryna J, Tsourkas A (2006) Superparamagnetic iron oxide nanoparticle probes for molecular imaging. Ann Biomed Eng 34:23–38

Toft KG, Hustvedt SO, Grant D, Friisk GA, Skotland T (1997a) Metabolism of mangafodipir trisodium (MnDPDP), a new contrast medium for magnetic resonance imaging, in beagle dogs. Eur J Drug Metab Pharmacokinet 22:65–72

Toft KG, Hustvedt SO, Grant D, Martinsen I, Gordon PB, Friisk GA, Korsmo AJ, Skotland T (1997b) Metabolism and pharmacokinetics of MnDPDP in man. Acta Radiol 38:677–689

Tombach B, Heindel W (2002) Value of 1.0-M gadolinium chelates: review of preclinical and clinical data on gadobutrol. Eur Radiol 12:1550–1556

Toth E, Pubanz D, Vauthey S, Helm L, Merbach AE (1996) High-pressure NMR kinetics. 72. The role of water exchange in attaining maximum relaxivities for dendrimeric MRI contrast agents. Chem Eur J 2:1607–1615

Toth E, Van Uffelen I, Helm L, Merbach AE, Ladd D, Briley-Saebo K, Kellar KE (1998) Gadolinium-based linear polymer with temperature-independent proton relaxivities: a unique interplay between the water exchange and rotational contributions. Magn Reson Chem 36:S125–S134

Toth E, Helm L, Kellar KE, Merbach AE (1999) Gd(DTPA-bisamide)alkyl copolymers: A hint for the formation of MRI contrast agents with very high relaxivity. Chem Eur J 5:1202–1211

Trivedi RA, U-King-Im JM, Graves MJ, Kirkpattrick PJ, Gillard JH (2004) Noninvasive imaging of carotid plaque inflammation. Neurology 63:187–188

Turetschek K, Floyd E, Shames DM, Roberts TPL, Preda A, Novikov V, Corot C, Carter WO, Brasch RC (2001) Assessment of a rapid clearance blood pool MR contrast medium (P792) for assays of microvascular characteristics in experimental breast tumors with correlations to histopathology. Magn Reson Med 45:880–886

Tweedle MF, Hagan JJ, Kumar K, Mantha S, Chang CA (1991) Reaction of gadolinium chelates with endogenously available ions. Magn Reson Imaging 9:409–415

Tweedle MF, Wedeking P, Kumar K (1995) Biodistribution of radiolabeled, formulated gadopentetate, gadoteridol, gadoterate, and gadodiamide in mice and rats. Invest Radiol 30:372–380

Uggeri F, Aime S, Anelli PL, Botta M, Brocchetta M, de Haen C, Ermondi G, Grandi G, Paoli P (1995) Novel contrast agents for magnetic resonance imaging. Synthesis and characterization of the ligand BOPTA and its Ln(III) complexes (Ln = Gd, La, Ln). X-ray structure of disodium (TPS-9-145337286-C-S)-[4-carboxy-5,8,11-tris(carboxymethyl)-1-phenyl-2-oxa-5,8,11-triazatridecan-13-oato(5-)]gadolinite (2-) in a mixture with its enantiomer. Inorg Chem 34:633–642

Vander Elst L, Maton F, Laurent S, Seghi F, Chapelle F, Muller RN (1997) A multinuclear MR study of Gd-EOB-DTPA: comprehensive preclinical characterization of an organ specific MRI contrast agent. Magn Reson Med 38:604–614

Vander Elst L, Raynal I, Port M, Tisnès P, Muller RN (2005) In vitro relaxometric and luminiscence characterization of P792 (Gadomelitol, Vistarem) an efficient and rapid clearance blood pool MRI contrast agent. Eur J Inorg Chem 1142–1148

van Montfoort JE, Stieger B, Meijer DKF, Weinmann H-J, Meier PJ, Fattinger KE (1999) Hepatic uptake of the magnetic resonance imaging contrast agent gadoxetate by the organic anion transporting polypeptide Oatp1. J Pharmacol Exp Ther 290:153–157

Vogler H, Platzek J, Schuhmann-Giampieri G, Frenzel T, Weimann H-J, Radüchel B, Press W-R (1995) Pre-clinical evaluation of gadobutrol: a new neutral, extracellular contrast agent for magnetic resonance imaging. Eur J Radiol 21:1–10

Wang SJ, Brechbiel M, Wiener EC (2003) Characteristics of a new MRI contrast agent prepared from polypropyleneimine dendrimers, generation 2. Invest Radiol 38:662–668

Wang Y-XJ, Hussain SM, Krestin GP (2001) Superparamagnetic iron oxide contrast agents: physicochemical characteristics and applications in MR imaging. Eur Radiol 11:2319–2331

Wedeking P, Kumar K, Tweedle MF (1992) Dissociation of gadolinium chelates in mice: relationship to chemical characteristics. Magn Reson Imaging 10:641–648

Weinmann H-J, Brasch RC, Press W-R, Wesbey GE (1984) Characteristics of gadolinium -DTPA complex, apotential NMR contrast agent. Am J Roentgenol 142:619–624

Weinmann HJ, Schuhmann-Giampiepi G, Schmitt-Willich H, Vogler H, Frenzei, Gries H (1991) A new lipophilic gadolinium chelate as a tissue-specific contrast medium for MRI. Magn Reson Med 22:233–237

Weinmann H-J, Ebert W, Misselwitz B, Schmitt-Willich H (2003) Tissue-specific MR contrast agents. Eur J Radiol 46:33–44

Weissleder R, Elizondo G, Wittenberg J, Rabito CA, Bengele HH, Josephson L (1990) Ultrasmall superparamagnetic iron oxide: Characterization of a new class of contrast agents for MR imaging. Radiology 175:489–493

Weissleder R, Mahmood U (2001) Molecular imaging. Radiology 219:316–333

Wiener EC, Brechbiel MW, Brothers H, Magin RL, Gansow OA, Tomalia DA, Lauterbur PC (1994) Dendrimer-based metal chelates: a new class of magnetic resonance imaging contrast agents. Magn Reson Med 31:1–8

Willard MA, Kurihara LK, Carpenter EE, Calvin S, Harris VG (2004) Chemically prepared magnetic nanoparticles. In: Nalwa HS (ed) Encyclopedia of science and nanotechnology, vol 1, pp 815–848

Xu S, Jordan E, Brocke S, Bulte JW, Quigley L, Tresser N, Ostuni JL, Yang Y, mcFarland HF, Frank JA (1998) Study of relapsing remitting experimental allergic encephalomyelitis SJL mouse model using MION-46L enhanced in-vivo MRI: early histopathological correlation. J Neurosci Res 52:549–558

Yoshikawa T, Mitchell DG, Hirota S, Ohno Y, Oda K, Maeda T, Fuji M, Sugimura K (2006) Gradient- and spin-echo T2-weighted imaging for SPIO-enhanced detection and characterization of focal liver lesions. J Magn Reson Imaging 23:712–719

Zhang S, Wu K, Sherry AD (2001) Gd3+ complexes with slowly exchanging bound-water molecules may offer advantages in the design of responsive MR agents. Invest Radiol 36:82–86

Zhao M, Beauregard DA, Loizou L, Davletov B, Brindle M (2001) Non-invasive detection of apoptosis using magnetic resonance imaging and a targeted contrast agent. Nature Med 7: 1241–1244

Contrast Agents: X-ray Contrast Agents and Molecular Imaging – A Contradiction?

Ulrich Speck

Abstract It is the purpose of this article to discuss whether and how X-ray contrast media may contribute to molecular imaging. X-ray contrast media are small molecules containing heavy elements, preferentially iodine. Modern CT allows precise, fast and reliable quantification of contrast media concentrations in large volumes with excellent spatial resolution throughout the body. The main disadvantage is the low contrast sensitivity requiring iodine concentrations of ≥ 0.5 mg/ml. Various approaches of the past and the present to specific contrast agents reflecting physiological, cellular or molecular processes are presented and options for the future are discussed.

1 Introduction

The term 'molecular imaging' reflects the desire for earlier detection of abnormalities developing into diseases, earlier detection of responses to therapy and more precise and specific information on the quality and site of disease processes. According to a consensus of a group of experts, *molecular imaging* shall mean to 'directly or indirectly monitor and record the spatiotemporal distribution of molecular or cellular

Ulrich Speck
Institut für Radiologie, Universitätsklinikum Charité - Humboldt-Universität Schumannstraße 20/21, 10098 Berlin-Mitte, Gremany
ulrich.speck@charite.de

W. Semmler and M. Schwaiger (eds.), *Molecular Imaging I.*   167
Handbook of Experimental Pharmacology 185/I.
© Springer-Verlag Berlin Heidelberg 2008

processes' (Thakur and Lentle 2005). Although MR spectroscopy detects and quantifies endogenous biomolecules, reflecting molecular and cellular processes, the basic idea is to achieve the goal via visible pharmaceuticals distributing in the living organism and either accumulating in specific areas and/or generating or changing a signal which can be detected by imaging equipment.

It is the purpose of this article to discuss the question if and in which way X-ray contrast media may contribute to molecular imaging.

2 Basic Properties of X-ray Contrast Agents

X-ray contrast agents absorb X-rays either more or less than the usual body constituents, primarily water. Due to low density, gas does not absorb X-rays to an extent which is relevant to medical imaging. It is still used to outline body cavities but in most cases is replaced by dense compounds containing heavy elements. The most commonly used X-ray contrast agents are water-soluble tri-iodinated derivatives of benzoic acid (Fig. 1). This class of compounds has been developed during a selection process which began with the discovery of X-rays. For more than 50 years all new X-ray contrast molecules belonged to this class of compounds. Only after the introduction of metal chelates (Fig. 2) as contrast agents for MRI have other elements besides iodine been considered. Up to now, however, none of the chelates has been approved for X-ray imaging.

Whereas imaging agents devoted to detecting molecular and cellular processes must in some way directly or indirectly participate in these processes or interact with components participating in the processes, the development of X-ray contrast agents led in the opposite direction: molecules displaying the least possible interaction with body constituents and processes were preferred because of advantages in tolerability (Dawson et al. 1999).

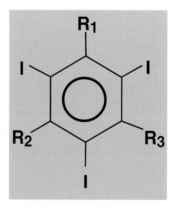

Fig. 1 Basic chemical structure of water-soluble iodinated X-ray contrast agents

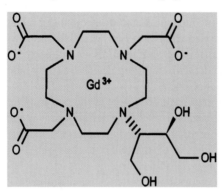

Fig. 2 Gadobutrol, a metal chelate used in magnetic resonance imaging. Metal content: 26% of weight

X-ray contrast media are usually highly concentrated aqueous solutions. A typical product contains 300–370 mg iodine/ml, which means about 600–800 mg of the iodinated organic molecule per ml. The high concentration of the contrast substance leaves limited room for water (about 0.7 ml per ml of contrast agent) and restricts the design of the molecules because limitations regarding osmolality and viscosity of the final preparation must be observed, in addition to solubility, chemical stability and cost. One of the important restrictions is the requirement of an extremely high content of iodine or another heavy element in the molecules. The iodine content of molecules in currently available X-ray contrast media is in the range of 44–49%. It is a drawback of metal chelates that their metal content reaches only half this value. The larger the proportion of the organic constituents contributing very little to X-ray absorption, the less room remains for water, which results in a further increase in viscosity and osmolality. Due to the very high content of iodine, the specific weight of X-ray contrast agents reaches up to 1.4 g/ml, which is much higher than the specific weight of any tissue.

3 Sensitivity

X-ray imaging is applicable to the whole body. X-rays penetrate all body constituents with modest scattering, which allows precise localisation of objects deep in the tissue.

X-ray absorption is a well understood process. It provides precise quantification of, e.g. contrast agent concentration in the tissue or body cavities, and excellent spatial and temporal resolution. Diagnostic applications do not require advancing the X-ray source or detector in body cavities by endoscopic methods as used in optical imaging or as in case of special coils improving the image quality in MRI.

Most disease-specific molecular and cellular processes involve low concentrations and display low capacities. Therefore, molecular imaging requires high sensitivity of the imaging modalities in the detection and quantification of the imaging probes as it is obtained with short lived radioisotopes. Optical imaging and ultrasound are next in sensitivity. MRI requires a contrast agent concentration that is too high to enable the detection of biomolecules, e.g. by labelled antibodies, or to trace intracellular metabolism.

The most relevant drawback of X-rays is the low contrast sensitivity. Even in CT, a minimum concentration of 0.5 mg iodine/ml is required to achieve a detectable change of about 10–15 Hounsfield units (HU) and ten times this concentration would be desirable. At 0.5 mg iodine/ml, there is a 1–4 mM concentration of a molecule labelled with 1–3 iodine atoms.

Examples of X-ray contrast agents which reach sufficient concentrations by active transport mechanisms are compiled in Table 1. The least dose is about 3 g iodine in case of cholegraphic agents and about 3 g gadolinium in case of liver parenchyma enhancing Gd-EOB-DTPA (Fig. 3a). Targeting smaller volumes of tissue than liver parenchyma may require less contrast material. Small lesions will, however, receive

Table 1 Examples of X-ray contrast agents monitoring molecular and cellular processes

Target	Contrast material	Commercial product or experimental	Biological mechanism	Reference
Liver, spleen, lymph nodes	Thorium oxide	Thorotrast	Uptake by macrophages, RES	Urich 1995
Liver, spleen	Liposomes, lipiodol emulsions, iodipamide particles	Experimental, phase I, II clinical trials	Uptake by macrophages, RES	Weichert et al. 2000; Leander et al. 1998; Violante et al. 1981
Gall bladder	Various oral cystographic agents, e.g. iopanoic acid	Telepaque, etc.	Anion transport	Urich and Speck 1991
Bile ducts	Various intravenous cholegraphic agents, e.g. iodipamide	Biligrafin	Anion transport	Lin et al. 1977
Urinary tract	Early ionic urographic agents including iodamide	Uromiro	Tubular secretion	Difazio et al. 1978
Pancreas	Oral cholecystographic agent iopanoat (?)	Experimental	Unknown; excretion into pancreatic duct	Schmiedl et al. 1994
Liver	Gadolinium EOB DTPA	Primovist; MRI product, not approved for CT; phase I, II clinical trials	Uptake into hepatocytes	Schmitz et al. 1997
Liver	Selected hepatobiliary agents	Experimental, phase I clinical trial	Uptake into hepatocytes	Mützel et al. 1982; Leander et al. 1998

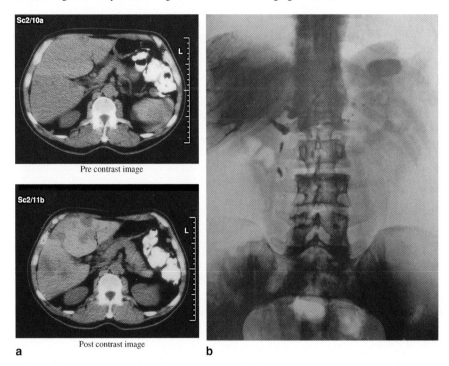

Fig. 3 a, b Examples of X-ray contrast agents which display contrast due to intracellular uptake. **a** Liver enhancement following intravenous administration of a lanthanide chelate. **b** Visualisation of e.g., lymph nodes following intravenous injection of colloidal thorium oxide. Although severely toxic, it indicates that specific uptake of radio-opaque compounds can be sufficient to opacify small structures in conventional radiographs (Börner et al. 1960)

only a small proportion of cardiac output. If perfusion is in the same range as in best perfused normal tissue, i.e. 1 ml/g/min, it will take almost 10 h until the blood volume of 5 l passes a 10-ml lesion. Meanwhile, competing processes will have diminished blood concentration. If the extraction is 100% during one passage of the blood and a contrast enhancement of 50 HU in the 10 ml of tissue is desired, this would mean a dose of 100 mg iodine or 500 mg contrast agent under optimistic assumptions (Table 2).

Improvements in contrast sensitivity require higher radiation doses or the application of lower energy X-rays; both are not acceptable in most patients and indications. The use of monoenergetic X-rays or X-rays with narrow energy distribution allows better use to be made of the sudden rise in absorption occurring at the k-edge of iodine and other heavy elements, but none of these measures would result in dramatic improvements regarding sensitivity. Consequently, molecular imaging applying X-ray imaging is restricted to the detection of high capacity molecular or cellular processes, the detection of molecules which occur in high concentration, or those processes which result in physicochemical states leading to the accumulation of contrast agent molecules independently of an active transport or specific binding.

Table 2 Estimation of minimum dose necessary to achieve a 50-HU contrast enhancement by a specifically binding or transported iodinated contrast agent

- 50 HU means 2 mg iodine/ml tissue
- 10 g tissue requires 20 mg iodine
- 20 mg iodine is contained in 5 l blood if a dose of 100 mg iodine is injected and the mean blood level for the next 10 h is 20% of the theoretical initial concentration (80% loss due to biodegradation, diffusion into tissues, excretion; most likely losses will be higher)
- 100% extraction of the contrast agent during first pass, 10-h perfusion
- If the specific contrast agent molecule contains 20% (weight) iodine the total dose required is 500 mg

4 Specificity of Extracellular X-ray Contrast Agents

Although frequently called 'non-specific' the currently dominating extracellular X-ray and MR contrast agents display very useful specificities for a large variety of diseases. The contrast media are distributed throughout the body by the blood flow and diffusion according to the permeability of capillaries and the size of the interstitial space (Krause and Schuhmann-Gampieri 1998). Perfusion, capillary permeability and the proportion of extracellular space differ in ischemic state, inflammation and tumours (Vaupel et al. 1989). The faster the imaging becomes and the larger the volumes simultaneously scanned are, the better the early distribution phase of rapidly injected contrast media can be displayed. This early distribution allows the best differentiation between perfusion and diffusion, depending on differences in contrast. As scanners were much slower in the past, the potential benefits of the extracellular contrast media were not fully recognised.

Limitations are obvious if the diseased tissue does not differ from normal tissue in respect of the above-mentioned criteria, or if treatment, although efficacious, does not change these parameters, or if the contrast enhancement changes dramatically after treatment even though treatment is not effective. Another drawback is the short-lasting contrast, which requires repeated injections if the diagnosis is missed during the first scan or if persistent visualisation of a lesion is required during an interventional procedure.

5 Monitoring of Molecular and Cellular Processes by X-ray Contrast Agents

Molecular and cellular processes have been visualised by X-ray contrast agents long before the term 'molecular imaging' became popular and even before the advent of early CT (Table 1). Because of the above-mentioned limitations in the sensitivity of contrast detection by X-ray radiography, this applies to high capacity transport mechanisms and the non-specific uptake of particles by cells specialised in this process.

None of the products or experimental preparations is currently in clinical use or under development. Thorium oxide was not excreted at all; furthermore, it proved to be toxic because of long-lived α-radiation (Martling et al. 1999). Also, other agents displayed various types of toxicity, or at least did not reach the same level of tolerance as the extracellular contrast agents. With the exception of thorium dioxide (Fig. 3b), none of them resulted in a reliable and satisfactory degree of contrast, nor did they provide important diagnostic information which could not been obtained by more recently established imaging methods with at least a similar quality. In spite of an everlasting interest in specific contrast agents, one after the other of these specific contrast agents has disappeared from the market.

Admittedly, previous 'specific' X-ray contrast agents did not address currently important diagnostic problems such as early tumour detection, non-obstructive inflammatory arterial disease or degenerative cerebral disease.

6 Directions of Future Research

The application of X-ray contrast agents to molecular imaging is not very likely. The minimal concentration required is probably far too high to be reached by specific binding, even if small molecules are used to direct iodine or other radio-opaque elements to diseased tissue. Nevertheless, some metabolic or transport processes operate with high capacity. If the metabolized or transferred contrast agents accumulate in the cells, tissues or cavities where the process takes place, the required concentration may be reached. Such accumulation may happen if the contrast agent is caught in the cells or cavity because of unidirectional transport, the biotransformation towards charged or more hydrophilic, non-diffusible metabolites, or the concentration exceeds solubility resulting in precipitation.

Other mechanisms more indirectly depending on molecular or cellular processes indicating abnormalities may be used to achieve sufficient accumulation of X-ray contrast agents: several disease processes result in changes of, for example, the extracellular pH, the accumulation of calcium, extracellular matrix materials (Orford et al. 2000; Vaupel et al. 1989). It is conceivable that specifically designed contrast agent molecules accumulate at acidic pH by precipitation or formation of large aggregates, bind to calcium deposits, thus enhancing the weak X-ray absorption of calcium, or bind to matrix molecules. The process may be enhanced if the contrast agent molecules tend to bind to each other either in aqueous solution or after they change their shape or ionicity following any kind of reaction or binding at the target location.

Although a variety of concepts seem to offer opportunities for the development of X-ray contrast media with specificities which differ from the currently used inert small molecules with extracellular distribution, one has to consider the following obstacles:

- In the past 100 years many approaches have been tried, intentionally or unintentionally, which failed. They may be repeated because these experiments have never been reported or the knowledge has been lost.
- Most likely mechanisms resulting in sufficient specificity and contrast medium concentration will be complicated multi-step reactions.
- The toxicity of accumulating X-ray contrast agents requires specific attention.
- Cost caused by expensive development and production must be balanced against the medical benefit.

Nevertheless, increasing spatial and to some extent also contrast resolution of X-ray equipment, advances in the understanding of disease processes and chemistry are in favour of improved X-ray contrast agents which provide important additional information.

7 Conclusions

Molecular imaging and X-ray contrast agents sound like an unresolvable contradiction. Extracellular, well tolerated and cheap non-ionic contrast media displaying perfusion, permeability and the proportion of interstitial space set a standard which is very hard to overcome. Yet, X-ray contrast media meeting a broad definition of molecular imaging have been used in the past. They failed because the processes displayed were of too little medical significance and/or tolerance was not satisfactory. An X-ray contrast agent indicating a universal process such as pH lowering or extracellular matrix accumulation may find a place within the broad range of diagnostic imaging methods.

References

Börner W, Moll E, Schneider P, Stucke K (1960) Zur Problematik der Thorotrastschäden. Klinische und radiologische Untersuchungen zum Verhalten von Thorium und seiner Zerfallsprodukte im Organismus. Rofo 93:287–297

Dawson P, Cosgrove DO, Grainger RG (eds) (1999) Textbook of contrast media. Isis Medical Media, Oxford

Difazio LT, Singhvi SM, Heald AF, McKinstry DN, Brosman SA, Gillenwater JY, Willard DA (1978) Pharmacokinetics of iodamide in normal subjects and in patients with renal impairment. J Clin Pharmacol 18:35–41

Krause W, Schuhmann-Gampieri G (1998) Pharmacokinetics of contrast media. In: Dawson P, Clauss W (eds) Contrast media in practice. Springer, Berlin Heidelberg New York, pp 31–39

Leander P, Höglund P, Kloster Y (1998) New liposomal liver-specific contrast agent for CT: first human phase I clinical trial assessing efficacy and safety. Acad Radiol 5(Suppl 1):S6–S8

Lin SK, Moss AA, Riegelman S (1977) Iodipamide kinetics: Capacity-limited biliary excretion with simultaneous pseudo-first-order renal excretion. J Pharm Sci 66:1670–1674

Martling U, Mattsson A, Travis LB, Holm LE, Hall P (1999) Mortality after long-term exposure to radioactive Thorotrast: a forty-year follow-up survey in Sweden. Radiat Res 151:293–299

Mitsutomo O (1930) Klinische Anwendung der "Lienographie", einer neuen Methode zur röntgenologischen Darstellung von Milz und Leber. Rofo 41:892–898

Mützel W, Wegener OH, Souchon R, Weinmann H-J (1982) Water-soluble contrast agents for computed tomography of the liver: experimental studies in dog. In: Amiel M, Moreau JF (eds) Contrast media in radiology Appraisal and prospects. Springer, Berlin Heidelberg New York, pp 320–323

Orford JL, Selwyn AP, Ganz P, Popma JJ, Rogers C (2000) The comparative pathobiology of atherosclerosis and restenosis. Am J Cardiol 86(Suppl):6H–11H

Schmiedl U, Schmoll K, Horn J, Speck U, Freeny P (1994) Imaging of exocrine pancreatic function investigation of the biovailability of weak organic acids as potential pancreatic contrast agents for computed tomography. Invest Radiol 29:689–694

Schmitz SA, Häberle JH, Balzer T, Shamsi K, Boese-Landgraf J, Wolf K-J (1997) Detection of focal liver lesions: CT of the hepatobiliary system with gadoxetic acid disodium, or Gd-EOB-DTPA. Radiology 2002:399–405

Thakur M, Lentle BC (2005) Report of a summit on molecular imaging. Radiology 236:753–755

Urich K, Speck U (1991) Biliary excretion of contrast media. Progr Pharmacol Clin Pharmacol 8:307–322

Urich K (1995) Successes and failures in the development of contrast media. Blackwell, Berlin

Vaupel P, Kallinowski F, Okunieff P (1989) Blood flow, oxygen and nutrient supply, and metabolic microenvironment of human tumors: a review. Cancer Research 49:6449–6465

Violante MR, Mare K, Fischer HW (1981) Biodistribution of a particulate hepatolienographic CT contrast agent: A study of iodipamide ethyl ester in the rat. Invest Radiol 16:40–45

Weichert JP, Lee FT, Chosy SG, Longino MA, Kuhlman JE, Helsey DE, Leverson GE (2000) Combined hepatocyte-selective and blood-pool contrast agents for the CT detection of experimental liver tumors in rabbits. Radiology 216:865–871

Radiopharmaceuticals: Molecular Imaging using Positron Emission Tomography

Gunnar Antoni and Bengt Långström(✉)

Abstract We describe the use of molecules labeled with short-lived emitting radionuclides for molecular imaging in combination with the positron emission tomography technique. How to use molecular probes to visualize and quantitatively determine rates of specific biochemical events such as synaptic transmission, enzymatic processes and binding to specific receptor proteins is highlighted. The sensitivity of the PET technique and the ability to measure and validate relationships between molecular events and biological functions is a key factor for the successful application of PET in biomedical research. In specific applications, the opportunity of using molecules labeled in specific positions may be critical. Molecular imaging using PET is also gaining increasing interest as a tool in drug development, especially when applied to early proof of concept studies in man.

In this chapter, the concept of molecular imaging is exemplified and the use of position-specific labeling of tracer molecules as a tool to gain understanding of complex biological processes will be discussed.

Bengt Långström

Department of Biochemistry and Organic Chemistry BMC, Uppsala University, Box 576, 751 23 Uppsala, Sweden

bengt.langstrom@biorg.uu.se

W. Semmler and M. Schwaiger (eds.), *Molecular Imaging I.*
Handbook of Experimental Pharmacology 185/I.

177

1 Introduction

The era of diagnostic imaging using radiation started with the discovery of X-rays by Roentgen in 1895. Other milestones in utilizing radiation for diagnostic purpose were when Lawrence and Livingstone used a particle accelerator to produce radioactivity followed by the discovery of nuclear fission. Since then nuclear medicine has developed into a medical specialty all over the world. At the end of the 1970s, positron emission tomography (PET) was developed, but not until the 1990s was the full potential of the technique acknowledged outside the scientific community.

Modern high-resolution computerized tomography (CT) and nuclear magnetic resonance imaging (MRI) equipment give exquisite detailed anatomical information, including soft tissue, and a variation of the latter, nuclear magnetic resonance spectroscopy (MRS), can be used to obtain information related to specific molecules and may be classified as a molecular imaging tool (Sonnewald et al. 1994). In this context, the sensitivity is important and PET using tracers with high specific radioactivity allows detection of radioactivity that corresponds to picomolar concentrations. This is significantly lower than the detection limit using MRS, which is in the millimolar range. Molecular imaging is thus mainly performed using PET and single photon emission computed tomography (SPECT) (Jazczak and Tsui 1995), which are based on tracers designed to interact with a certain molecular target or measure a physiological process. All these modalities, except for MRI and MRS, involve the use of ionizing radiation, and PET and SPECT also involve the administration of a radioactive substance, a radiopharmaceutical or a tracer.

PET and SPECT not only provide time-resolved three-dimensional images but also dynamic information. The main difference between these two is the opportunity with PET to obtain highly accurate and quantitative measurements of radioactivity (Hoffman et al. 1986). With knowledge of the specific radioactivity of the administered tracer, the regional uptake of radioactivity can be used to assess the concentration of a certain compound, assuming that all radioactivity is associated with the administered tracer molecule or in other ways validated.

Radiopharmaceuticals can be divided into two distinctly different groups: therapeutic and diagnostic. The former rely on deposition of as much as possible of the energy of emitted particles from decaying atoms in the tissue and the latter on the reverse, i.e., as high penetration and low interaction with tissue as possible. The photons from PET and SPECT radionuclides penetrate the tissue and are detected by external detectors. In this chapter, the diagnostic applications will be discussed.

It is likely that diagnostic imaging will play a key role in locating and diagnosing diseases earlier, as well as provide us with more information about both normal and pathophysiological states. The PET technology, using radionuclides with high specific radioactivity and the opportunity to specifically label a compound in different positions by substituting a stable atom with its radioactive counterpart, combined with quantitative measurements of radioactivity, is thus the preferred modality for molecular imaging. These are key features where PET has an advantage over SPECT, where the latter is mainly dependent on analogues of endogenous compounds or pharmaceuticals whereas the PET chemist to a great extent can provide the structurally identical compound as a tracer.

Another aspect of PET is the short half-lives of the radionuclides, e.g., ^{15}O ($t_{1/2} =$ 2 min), ^{11}C ($t_{1/2} = 20$ min), ^{18}F ($t_{1/2} = 109$ min) and ^{68}Ga (68 min). This allows repeated investigations in the same subject with short time intervals. The patient or healthy volunteer can thus be used as its own reference following a pharmacological or other perturbation that affects a measurable in-vivo process.

This chapter will only address PET and molecular imaging will be the main key point discussed. The aim is not to cover all aspects of PET but to illustrate the strength of molecular imaging. The references are accordingly limited to the most relevant for the topics and examples discussed.

2 Molecular Imaging with PET

2.1 Background

Molecular imaging using PET may probe specific biochemical pathways and molecular targets through measurement of externally detected radiation in the form of photons. The detectors only measure the number of photons in a certain tissue volume without any information about the molecular structure the radiation emanated from. In this context is it worth mentioning the importance of labeling chemistry as a tool for elucidation of in-vivo biochemistry. By labeling a molecule in different positions and studying the dynamics of the different uptake patterns as a consequence of the labeled atom appearing in different metabolites of the administered tracer, it is possible to get insight into molecular events. Another important aspect is the possibility of obtaining quantitative data and thus relating the number of measured photons to the concentration of a specific molecule in the tissue of interest. The measured radioactivity can be related to biology by using sophisticated tracer molecules, and by combining the time-course of the tracer uptake with models for the interpretation of the data further functional information can be obtained. The understanding of PET data relies on several factors and we have to develop models simplifying the complex processes occurring in a living subject. Sensitivity and specificity are key words when developing molecular probes aimed at following a certain biochemical event in-vivo. Understanding the complex in-vivo chemistry in terms of biological functions is thus a difficult and challenging task. A multitude of processes affected by many factors and interpreted by measuring a radioactive signal makes the task difficult, but by approaching this challenge using multi-tracer protocols and repeated experiments, following perturbations, we may be able to collect the information.

PET and the concept of molecular imaging have also been shown to be useful in drug development. To achieve a better method for relating plasma pharmacokinetics to drug effect on target, PET can contribute by adding information on target pharmacokinetics (Bergström and Långström 2005) as well as pharmacodynamic measures such as drug receptor occupancy and enzyme inhibition. PET is also useful for assessment of the relation of the drug interaction with primary target and the therapeutic effect. Suitable labeled biomarkers for energy metabolism or other measures of downstream effects, such as FDG, can be used to monitor drug effects. Pharmacokinetic PET studies are not limited to intravenous administration of the labeled compound and deposition, and disposition studies following inhalation or via intranasal administration routes have also been performed.

2.2 Specific Radioactivity and Sensitivity Perspectives

The β^+-emitting PET radionuclides incorporated in molecules are our tools and the selection of the proper radionuclide with regard to the physical properties and production routes are important. An important aspect is the option of using radionuclides with half-lives ranging from a few minutes to several hours, which give us the opportunity to choose a radionuclide with a half-life that matches the time-frame of the biological process to be studied.

The choice of radionuclide is also important considering the achievable specific radioactivity. Specific radioactivity is a function of the physical half-life, and the neutron deficient PET radionuclides have short half-lives and thus theoretically very highly specific radioactivities can be obtained. However, isotopic dilution with stable isotopes occurs, in most cases to a significant extent, and the obtained specific radioactivity is far from theoretical level but still very high in comparison with, e.g., ^{14}C and ^3H. Table 1 shows a selection of suitable radionuclides, including the nuclear reaction and some physical characteristics.

The practical specific radioactivities of the tracers labeled with any of the above listed radionuclides differ from the theoretical due to isotopic dilution, either in the radionuclide production step or in the subsequent synthesis of a suitable reactive secondary precursor. For example, ^{11}C is susceptible to isotopic dilution due to presence of carbon in most materials and the use of reagents sensitive to atmospheric carbon dioxide. Typical specific radioactivity of ^{11}C at the end of radionuclide production is 2–3 TBq/μmol and generally results in tracers with specific radioactivities ranging 50–500 GBq/μmol at the end of synthesis. Although the isotopic dilution is

Table 1 Some examples of PET radionuclides

Radio-nuclide	$T_{1/2}$ [min]	Nuclear reaction	Decay	Specific radioactivity [GBq/μmol]
^{15}O	2.05	$^{14}N(d,n)^{15}O$	$\beta^+ > 99\%$	3.4×10^6
^{11}C	20.4	$^{14}N(p,\alpha)^{11}C$	$\beta^+ > 99\%$	3.4×10^5
^{68}Ga	68	$^{68}Ge/^{68}Ga$	$\beta^+ 90\%$	1.0×10^5
^{18}F	109	$^{18}O(p,n)^{18}F$	$\beta^+ 97\%$	6.3×10^4

extensive, on average for ^{11}C the ratio of $^{11}C/^{12}C$ in the radiopharmaceutical to be administered is about 1/7,000, it is still sufficiently high to make the tracers very sensitive probes for biochemical and physiological processes. For example, 400 MBq of a compound with a specific radioactivity of 100 GBq/μmol corresponds to 4 nmol, which is equivalent to 2 μg for a molecular weight of 500.

The sensitivity of PET is also related to the high efficiency of measuring the photons produced from the annihilation reaction between the positron emitted by the decaying nuclide and an electron in the surrounding tissue. The relation of radioactivity to concentration of a specific compound can easily be quantified by combining the decay correction of the radioactivity and initial specific radioactivity of the administered labeled compound. Another feature of a useful tracer is the specificity, which is dependent on the molecular structure and labeling position, and the importance of labeling synthesis needs to be acknowledged.

2.3 Interactions with Molecular Targets

The molecular interactions studied with the PET technique are between the tracer molecule and a biological target, e.g., a protein. The protein can be, for example, a cell surface receptor, a transporter moving compounds through membranes or an enzyme catalyzing a biochemical reaction.

In general, biochemical reactions are facilitated and catalyzed by enzymes and this opens up a wide variety of important processes to be studied in vivo. Enzymes can be found either distributed systemically or specifically in some cell types or organelles. It is, thus, possible to characterize cells and tissue depending on expression of specific enzymes and up or down regulation may be related to a certain pathophysiological disturbance. Tumor cells may over-express specific enzymes and examples of tracer sensing increased turnover by being a substrate have been developed. In neurological disorders, similar specific changes in enzymatic processes can also be traced and used for diagnosis and prognosis. Also in drug development targeting enzymes, PET may be an important modality due to the capability of measuring the inhibition of an enzyme in a dose-dependent way, following administration of a drug.

Today there are about a hundred neurotransmitters identified as acting on different receptor proteins. Many neurological disorders are associated with changes in the receptor expression or the neurotransmitter concentration. The development of specific tracers that can be used to measure regional receptor density and quantify occupancy by a drug or endogenous ligands has been a major interest in PET research in the last two decades.

The advantages of PET over SPECT are the diversity of available tracer molecules, with labeling synthesis one of the key influencers of utility. Developments in labeling chemistry, especially in the field of ^{11}C, are thus major drivers for PET. Although the majority of PET tracers are of exogenous origin, the use of endogenous compounds (e.g., amino acids, carbohydrates and fatty acids) is of interest.

The tracer concept is based on the labeled compounds used not to any measurable extent disturbing the system under study. Another criterion is the specificity of the signal in relation to the studied biochemical event. In order to fulfill these prerequisites for a successful tracer, a molecule with well-defined biological characteristics, such as specificity for the target molecule in the body and sufficient sensitivity, is required. The latter is a function of the radionuclide used and the achievable specific radioactivity, which together with the in-vivo concentration of the biological target determine the inherent sensitivity of the chosen molecular probe. As a rule of thumb, for example B_{max}/K_D, [the ratio of available receptor proteins (B_{max}) and dissociation equilibrium constant (K_D)] should preferably be higher than 2 to ensure that a sufficiently large signal is obtained, in order to detect changes in receptor occupancy following dosing with the study drug.

It is, however, of importance to realize that the affinity of a tracer for a target is only one of several important parameters. A very high affinity in combination with a high B_{max} may present a problem if the rate-limiting step in the process is shifted from interaction between target and tracer to transport to tissue by blood. This has been encountered, for example, in studies of enzyme-substrate interactions and can be exemplified by measurement of the inhibition of brain monoamino oxidase type B enzyme (MAO-B) following dosing with an enzyme antagonist, using the inhibitor L-[^{11}C]deprenyl as tracer. L-Deprenyl binds irreversibly to MAO-B by forming a covalent bond to the enzyme. It was found that the PET images represented mainly blood flow, and the reason was a combination of high MAO-B expression and high reaction rate between substrate and enzyme. This could be circumvented by fine-tuning the tracer characteristics, by substituting two hydrogens in L-deprenyl with deuterium in a position involved in the rate-limiting step in the formation of the covalent bond to the enzyme. The rate of reaction was lowered due to the induced kinetic isotope effect (Fowler et al. 1995) and the rate limiting step was shifted to MAO-B interacting with the ^{11}C-labeled L-(^{2}H)deprenyl.

In the following sections, some examples are discussed where the interaction between tracers and their molecular target can be turned into valuable biochemical information related to both normal and pathological states. The concept of molecular imaging is exemplified and the importance of labeling a compound in different positions emphasized.

2.3.1 Aromatic Amino Acid Decarboxylase

It is well established that dopamine is the neurotransmitter involved in Parkinson's disease and schizophrenia, for example, as discovered by Arvid Carlsson (Carlsson et al. 1957). The search for new selective drugs demanded tools for the measurement of drug and target interaction, resulting in a paradigm shift in drug development and leading to a more science-driven process, the learning-confirming concept. This approach can be exemplified with the investigation of the functional aspects of the dopaminergic neuron, schema tically outlined in Fig. 1, where PET tracers have

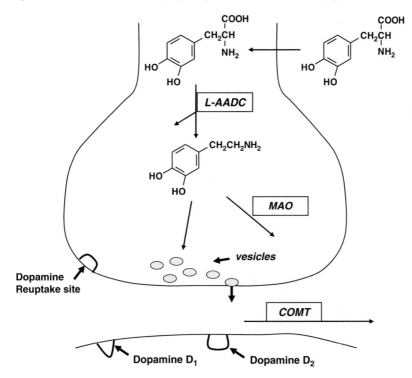

Fig. 1 Dopaminergic neuron and synapse

been developed that interact on several different receptors or enzymatic steps, as reviewed recently (Elsinga et al. 2006).

The processes in the dopaminergic neurotransmission can be investigated either on the presynaptic or postsynaptic level. The effect of dopamine is, for example, mediated by action on the postsynaptic dopamine D_1 and D_2 receptors and ^{11}C-labeled SCH23390 (Halldin et al. 1986) and N-methylspiperone (Wagner 1983) raclopride have been used successfully to measure receptor occupancy of drugs acting on these postsynaptic receptors. It is also possible to measure the endogenous level of dopamine by the dopamine D_2 antagonist raclopride (Farde et al. 1985) or agonist $(+)$[11]C]PHNO and study the effect of drugs changing dopamine levels in the brain (Hartvig et al. 1997; Ginovart et al. 2006). Challenge with amphetamine resulting in dopamine release reduces raclopride and PHNO binding to dopamine D_2 receptors due to competition with the endogenous receptor agonist.

The presynaptic dopaminergic system has also been studied by measuring the dopamine transporter, the re-uptake mechanism in striatum. Several tracers have been developed for that purpose, such as ^{11}C]nomifensine (Aquilonius et al. 1987; Tedroff et al. 1991), and the cocaine derivatives such as ^{11}C]β-CIT-FE (Halldin et al. 1996), ^{18}F]CFT (Rinne et al. 2001) and ^{18}F]β-CIT-FP (Lundkvist et al. 1997) have been applied in the study of drug binding to the dopamine transporter and the quantification of that may be used to determine the number of viable dopamine neurons. The quantitative use of PET can be exemplified by the use of $[^{11}C]\beta$-CIT-FE as a tool for the study of interaction of a drug with the dopamine transporter protein, as shown in Fig. 2 (Learned-Coughlin et al. 2003).

The dynamic information from the PET scanning can be translated by a suitable tracer kinetic modeling (Carson et al. 2003) to give information about the degree of drug-transporter protein binding in a quantitative fashion, as shown in Fig. 3. In this case, the cerebellum is used as a reference region assumed to be devoid of dopamine transporter proteins and thus not showing any specific binding of the tracer. In Fig. 3, the degree of blocking of the transporter, expressed as a percentage, is shown.

The enzyme aromatic amino acid decarboxylase (AADC) is predominantly found in catecholaminergic and serotonergic neurons, where it is responsible for converting 3,4-dihydroxy-L-phenylalanine(DOPA) and 5-hydroxytryptophan(HTP) to dopamine and serotonin, respectively. There are different opinions regarding the usefulness of diagnostic imaging using L-$[^{11}C]$DOPA and the fluoroanalogue

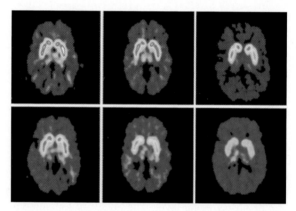

Fig. 2 PET images representing the uptake of $[^{11}C]\beta$-CIT-FE in striatum at baseline and after dosing with a drug. *Upper row*: baseline scans; *Lower row*: after dosing with different amounts of the drug

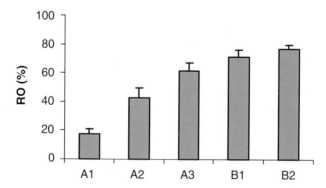

Fig. 3 Five different doses of drug showing increasing occupancy of the transporter as measured with the tracer L$[^{11}C]\beta$-CIT-FE

6-fluoro-[^{18}F]-L-DOPA to quantify AADC activity and storage capacity of dopamine (Garnett et al. 1983; Hartvig et al. 1991; Korf et al. 1978; Lindner 1995; Tedroff et al. 1992a) as a tool in clinical practice or as a surrogate endpoint in clinical trials (Ravina et al. 2005). However, some examples of functional imaging applied to the study of the dopaminergic system, including the use of position-specific labeling, will be presented.

Labeling a molecule in different positions can be used to provide evidence that a selective biochemical transformation such as decarboxylation occurs. L-[^{11}C]DOPA labeled either in the carboxylic or β-positions (Bjurling et al. 1990a, 1990b) undergoing in-vivo decarboxylation would produce different labeled products, [^{11}C]carbon dioxide and [^{11}C]dopamine, respectively, as shown in Scheme 1.

The use of PET to elucidate in-vivo biochemistry can be illustrated by use of L-[β-^{11}C]DOPA to compare striatal in-vivo dopamine synthesis in mild and advanced Parkinson's disease. The study was triggered by the well-known treatment-induced on-off side effect encountered in advanced Parkinson cases. Patients with either mild or advanced Parkinson's disease were examined before and after treatment with the mixed dopamine D_1/D_2 receptor agonist apomorphine. All patients showed clinical response to the treatment. The PET data was analyzed by reference Patlak plot (Patlak et al. 1985), where the slope of uptake in striatum K_i, denoted influx rate constant representing the rate for transport and conversion of L-[β-^{11}C]DOPA to [^{11}C]dopamine (Tedroff et al. 1992b). Patients with mild Parkinson's disease had decreased L-[β-^{11}C]DOPA influx in striatum in contrast to patients in advanced stages where the influx was independent of apomorphine treatment. The conclusion drawn was that the autoreceptor function providing feedback regulation of dopamine synthesis is subsensitive in the advanced stages of Parkinson's disease (Torstenson et al. 1997, 1998).

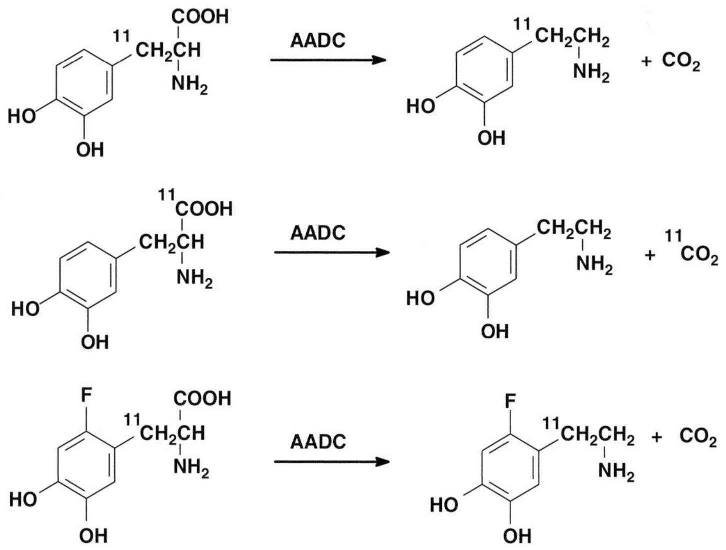

Scheme 1

Fig. 4 Compartmental model
for DOPA decarboxylation in
the dopaminergic neuron

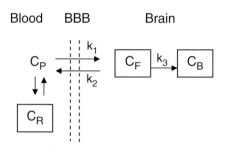

The influence of molecular structure on the biological characteristics of a compound can be well illustrated by comparing L-DOPA and 6-fluoro-L-DOPA. The endogenous L-[β-^{11}C]DOPA and the analogue 6-[^{18}F]fluoro-L-DOPA are both decarboxylated by AADC in vivo in the dopaminergic neuron, forming dopamine and 6-fluorodopamine, respectively (Scheme 1). The process studied in the neuron can be schematically outlined by the compartmental model shown in Fig. 4, where C_P, C_R, C_F and C_B denote L-DOPA or 6-fluoro-L-DOPA concentration in plasma, reference tissue, free fraction in target tissue and bound fraction (dopamine or 6-fluorodopamine) in target tissue, respectively.

The study was performed in rhesus monkeys with β-^{11}C-labeled L-DOPA and 6-fluoroDOPA as tracers. From PET data using a reference Patlak model, the striatal influx rate constant K_i could be determined, which at low tracer doses reflects the catalytic action of AADC and is thus a measure of the dopamine synthesis rate (k_3). A significant difference in K_i between L-DOPA and 6-fluoro-L-DOPA was found, with 6-fluoro-L-DOPA K_i values being 11% lower than for L-DOPA (Torstenson et al. 1999). One plausible explanation for the difference in K_i values could be the more prominent formation of the 3-O-methyl metabolite of 6-fluoro-L-DOPA, confirmed by metabolite analysis, which readily enters the brain and increases the background radioactivity level. The contribution of the radioactivity from the metabolite in the target tissue gives in the model a lower calculated K_i value. Affinity differences of the two compounds for the AADC enzyme may also contribute to the difference in K_i values (Cummings et al. 1988). These findings suggest that it may be difficult to detect changes in decarboxylation rate using 6-[^{18}F]fluoro-L-DOPA, whereas ^{11}C-labeling the endogenous compound L-DOPA may give a more accurate determination of enzyme activity. In a drug challenge study using 6-*R*-L-erythro-5,6,7,8-tetrahydrobiopterin, a cofactor for the enzyme tyrosin hydroxylase, an increase in the dopamine synthesis rate as measured by a higher K_i value was obtained for L-[β-^{11}C]DOPA but not for 6-[^{18}F]fluoro-L-DOPA (Tortenson et al. 1999).

2.4 Clinical Examples

In order to exemplify the molecular imaging concept and also point to the use of multi-tracer protocols in clinical routine applications as well as research, a few illustrative cases have been selected.

2.4.1 Neuroendocrine Tumors

L-[^{11}C]DOPA labeled in the carboxylic and β-positions was used to classify and visualize tumors over-expressing AADC. A patient with a pancreatic tumor, a gastrinoma, was examined with the two L-DOPA tracers differently labeled as shown in Fig. 5.

Significant decarboxylation (see Scheme 1) occurred in the tumor; and with L-[β-^{11}C]DOPA, high uptake of radioactivity — probably in the form of [^{11}C] dopamine — was found in the tumor, in contrast to L-[carboxy-^{11}C]DOPA where the radioactivity was rapidly eliminated, which would be the case for [^{11}C]carbon dioxide (Bergström et al. 1996). The kinetics of the uptake of L-[β-^{11}C]DOPA in the tumor also indicated trapping of the radioactivity during the time-frame of the investigation, which is consistent with dopamine being synthesized and stored in vesicles within the neuron (Eriksson et al. 1993). The same principle as discussed for DOPA applies to the use of 5-hydroxy-L-[^{11}C]tryptophan (HTP) as a tracer for endocrine tumors. PET using HTP, the endogenous precursor for serotonin, has shown to be of clinical relevance and 5-HTP has proved to be an excellent tracer for the detection and treatment follow-up of endocrine tumors such as carcinoid metastases. These serotonin-producing metastases are often found in the liver. Figure 6 shows PET images representing HTP uptake in a liver metastasis before and after medical treatment (Eriksson et al. 1993; Örlefors et al. 1998).

Carcinoid metastases can be visualized by CT, but with PET and HTP smaller tumors can be detected due to the very high contrast between tumor and surrounding tissue. It was concluded that PET resulted in better visualization compared with CT, and in one patient PET could also detect skeletal and pleural metastases not seen by CT.

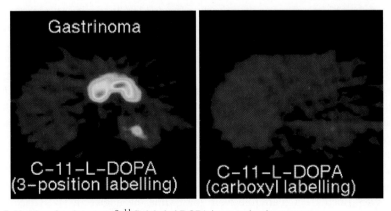

Fig. 5 Uptake of carboxy- or β-^{11}C- labeled DOPA in an endocrine tumor

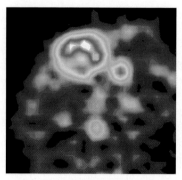 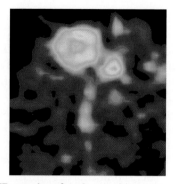

Uptake of HTP before treatment   HTP uptake after 3 month's treatment

Fig. 6 Uptake of 5-hydroxy-L-[β-^{11}C]tryptophan in a carcinoid metastasis in the liver. Ventral part of the right liver lobe is shown

2.4.2 Acetylcarnitine and Chronic Fatigue Syndrome

Position-specific labeling and labeling the same compound in different positions has already been discussed in relation to dopamine synthesis. Another example of where this approach bas been applied is in the field of fatigue science, with the aim of investigating the biochemical mechanism involved in chronic fatigue syndrome (CFS). The characteristic symptoms in CFS are diverse and have been defined as prolonged generalized fatigue, muscle weakness; myalgia and lymph node pain (Cho et al. 2006). The etiology for this disease is not known but a majority of CFS patients have a low serum level of acylcarnitines (Kuratsune et al. 1994) and symptomatic improvement correlates with recovered acylcarnitine levels. These observations led to an investigation of the coupling between CFS and acylcarnitines. There may be a connection between energy metabolism and carnitine. Carnitine is a transporter for long-chain fatty acids into the mitochondria and low levels of carnitine may result in decreased efficiency of energy metabolism. The main acylcarnitine found in plasma is acetylcarnitine, which serves not only as a precursor for acetyl-CoA that enters into the TCA cycle but also as an acetyl donor for in-vivo synthesis of acetylcholine and glutamate. A PET study was designed to investigate the biochemistry of acetylcarnitine in-vivo in a primate model (Kuratsune et al. 1997). Acetylcarnite was labeled by a multi-enzymatic synthesis in either of three different positions (Jacobsson et al. (1997)) and the uptake in rhesus monkey brain of the three labeled compounds studied using PET, as shown in Scheme 2 and Fig. 7, respectively.

The resulting PET images are shown in Fig. 7.

In summary, the results showed the uptake values of labeled acetylcarnitine into the brain were different depending on the labeling positions of ^{11}C. Brain levels of acetyl-L-[methyl-^{11}C]carnitine were low, while the uptake of [1-^{11}C]acetyl-L-carnitine was slightly higher and [2-^{11}C]acetyl-L-carnitine showed the highest uptake. The different uptake kinetics of three differently labeled acetyl-L-carnitine may to some extent be explained by exploring the biochemistry. With the label in the methyl carnitine there is no accumulation in the brain, where as when the ^{11}C-label

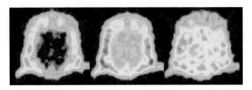

* denotes ^{11}C

Scheme 2

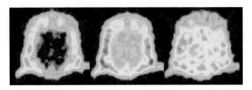

Fig. 7 Uptake of acetylcarnitine, labeled in different positions, in a rhesus monkey brain *From the left*: acetylcarnitine labeled in the [N-^{11}C-methyl], [1-^{11}C]acetyl and [2-^{11}C]acetyl group, respectively

is placed in either of the 2 positions in the acetyl group there is an uptake of radio-activity in the brain. The uptake suggest a process involving the TCA-cycle. The brain uptake [2-^{11}C]acetyl-L-carnitine could be suppressed by an intravenous admin-istration of glucose. These results suggest that endogenous serum acetyl-L-carnitine may be involved in the regulation of energy metabolism during an energy crisis by conveying an acetyl moiety into the brain. Further studies (Yamaguti 1996; Jacob-son 1997) have revealed the presence of ^{11}C-labeled aspartate and glutamate in the rat brain following administration of [2-^{11}C]acetyl-L-carnitine. It is thus likely that the acetyl moiety of acetylcarnitine taken up into the brain is used for the biosynthe-sis of neurotransmitters such as glutamate, aspartate and GABA. The preliminary results of a human PET study showed a distinct difference in global brain uptake of [2-^{11}C]acetyl-L-carnitine between CFS patients and age-matched healthy volun-teers. Altogether this might indicate abnormalities in neurotransmitter synthesis as one potential explanation for the chronic fatigue sensation.

2.4.3 Incidentalomas

Incidentalomas are lesions, seen as a mass at the site of the adrenal gland, typically discovered during a CT scan over the abdominal area. The frequency of enlargement of the adrenal gland is high. Around 2–5% of routine abdominal CT scans performed for other diagnostic reasons end up with the diagnosis of incidentaloma. This radio-logical finding requires an investigation to differentiate between a harmless, benign, hormonally inactive, adrenocortical adenoma and a cancer. In the latter case it can either be a primary tumor, such as pheochromocytoma originating from the chro-maffin cells, or a metastasis of nonadrenal origin. About 70–80% of the lesions are hormonally inactive adenomas, 15% metastases from tumors of nonadrenal origin and the rest adrenocortical cancer, e.g., pheochromocytoma. A multi-tracer PET

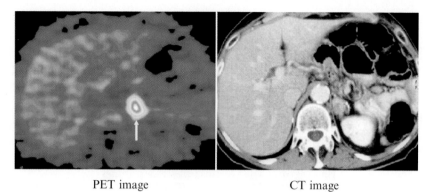

PET image   CT image

Fig. 8 Adrenocortical adenoma PET and CT images

protocol has been developed that provides a decision tree (Fig. 8) for how to use diagnostic imaging with the gathered information and more accurately select patients for surgical treatment.

The first tracer to be applied to this protocol is [11C]metomidate (MTO) (Bergström et al. 2000; Eriksson et al. 2005), a potent inhibitor of β-11-hydroxylase, the key enzyme in the adrenocortical synthesis of cortisol. MTO is the methyl ester analogue of etomidate, an anesthetic. From an imaging point of view etomidate may be preferred, but MTO synthesis is simpler and results in higher radiochemical yield and specific radioactivity. Figure 8 shows an example of MTO uptake in the adrenal gland.

Alternatively, [11C]etomidate or the fluoroanalogue [18F]fluoroethyletomidate can be used as tracers to study the functional aspects of the lesion (Bergström et al. 1998; Mitterhauser et al. 2006); followed by [11C]hydroxyephedrine (HED) and FDG (Shulkin et al. 1992, 1999; Trampal et al. 2004). Uptake of HED is related to presynaptic sympathetic innervations. The diagnostic decision tree is presented in Fig. 9.

The tracer [11C]MTO was found to be excellent for the visualization of adrenocortical tumors and to differentiate them from noncortical lesions. A positive MTO-PET manifested as elevated uptake in the adrenal cortex was used to determine the treatment (surgery or not) of that subgroup of patients; a negative MTO-PET was followed-up by a HED-PET to discriminate between a potential pheochromocytoma and other cancers of noncortical origin. A positive HED-PET was diagnosed with nearly 100% certainty as a pheochromocytoma and the patients accordingly subjected to surgical treatment. A negative HED-PET was followed-up with an FDG-PET, which if positive was diagnosed as a metastasis and if negative was categorized as other cancers. The clinical value of this functional imaging approach to incidentalomas has thus been verified (Hennings 2006) and resulted in improved patient handling.

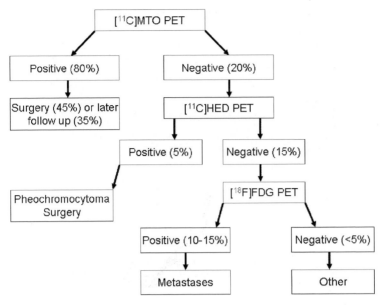

Fig. 9 Decision tree for investigation of incidentalomas

2.4.4 Pituitary Tumors

Tumors emanating from the pituitary gland can be diagnosed by CT and MRI investigations, and the progress or effect of treatment monitored. The tumors are surgically removed or, if possible, a dopamine agonist chemotherapy used. A simple method for selecting patients for chemotherapy is needed, since it is important to distinguish between responding and non-responding tumors and avoid unnecessary surgery. A wrong decision may lead to tumor growth negatively affecting the ophthalmic nerve, with the potential risk of damage to the visual pathway, leading to visual-field defects and blindness. A PET differential diagnosis (Bergström 1991; Muhr et al. 1991) has been developed, based on two characteristic features of the tumor. Increased metabolism, manifested as protein synthesis/amino acid transport, can be visualized by [^{11}C]methionine (MET) and be used both as a primary diagnostic tool and to study the effect of bromocriptine treatment. The differential diagnosis determining which tumors will respond to chemotherapy is performed by measuring the pituitary expression of dopamine D_2 receptors with the receptor antagonist [^{11}C]raclopride (RAC). As a negative control, to test the specificity of the raclopride binding, the inactive R-enantiomer of raclopride (RAR) was used. In Fig. 10, the resulting PET images are shown.

The inactive enantiomer R-raclopride does not accumulate in the tumor in contrast to the specific dopamine D_2 antagonist S-[^{11}C]raclopride (RAC). High uptake of RAC and the metabolism marker MET in the pituitary can thus be used as criteria for successful bromocriptine treatment. Response to treatment is very profound and within 3 h from start a significant reduction of protein synthesis is seen, as measured

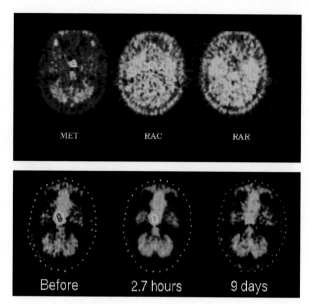

Fig. 10 Diagnosis and treatment follow up in pituitary tumors. The *upper row* shows [^{11}C]methionine, *S*-[^{11}C]raclopride and *R*-[^{11}C]raclopride uptake in the tumor and the lower row bromocriptine treatment follow-up using [^{11}C]methionine

with PET and MET. The functional imaging gives apparently an immediate measure of the in-vivo biochemistry, whereas the macroscopic changes as visualized by CT need several months to manifest the changes. It was concluded that PET with MET, as shown in over 400 patients with pituitary adenoma, can give valuable complementary information in the diagnosis of this tumor by adequately depicting viable tumor tissue in contrast to fibrosis, cysts and necrosis, and is a very useful and sensitive probe in the evaluation of the treatment. The use of RAC to characterize the degree of receptor binding can be used for selection of patients for dopamine agonist treatment.

3 PET in Drug Development

3.1 Pharmacodynamic Study Example

Plasma Pharmacokinetics is the traditional way of determining frequency of drug administration to achieve a steady state and relate that to clinical efficacy. Plasma pharmacokinetics are easily achieved experimentally, but there is a gap in knowledge as to how to relate that to mechanisms of action, such as interaction with target proteins. For a proper assignment of treatment regimen, dosage and dose interval, it is necessary to evaluate not only the plasma pharmacokinetics of the drug but also the duration of action on the target system. This can be achieved if a validated tracer is available which is binding to the same site as the drug on a receptor or enzyme protein. This concept is exemplified by the PET study of the antidepressant drug eusoprone acting by inhibiting the enzyme monoamino oxidase subtype A (MAO-A), as measured with [^{11}C]harmine. Since no validated tracer for measuring the inhibition of MAO-A in the brain was available, a tracer development project was initiated. Thus, [^{11}C]harmine and four other potential tracer candidates were evaluated in preclinical assays, followed by PET studies in rhesus monkeys. The kinetics of the uptake of [^{11}C]harmine in rhesus monkey brain with and without MAO-A inhibition was found to be compatible with a significant fraction of the tracer bound to MAO-A. Thus, [^{11}C]harmine was found to be a useful probe for the quantitative determination of brain MAO-A inhibition in a dose-dependent way (Bergström et al. 1997a). In the drug development PET study in healthy volunteers, interaction of the new antidepressant drug euseprone with MAO-A, as measured with [^{11}C]harmine, was investigated. The plasma kinetics indicated a drug half-life of about 3.5 h, whereas the brain kinetics measured an inhibiting effect of 14.5 h (Bergström et al. 1997b), as shown in Fig. 11.

The dosing frequency determined as MAO-A inhibition by the use of PET and [^{11}C]harmine gave more accurate information for establishing a dosing regimen than if the dose interval relied on plasma drug concentration. This may potentially lead to a dosing regimen with improved clinical efficacy and less side effects. This shows the potential of PET to determine dosing intervals and monitor drug effects directly on target proteins in the brain.

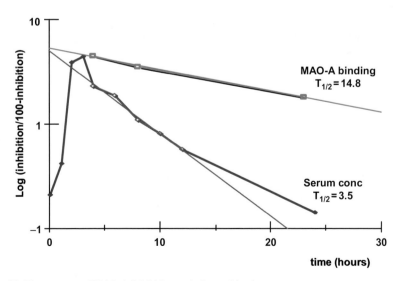

Fig. 11 Time-course of MAO-A inhibition and plasma kinetics

3.2 Pharmacokinetic Studies

Understanding the pharmacokinetics of a drug is a necessary component in the drug development process. Information on bio-distribution, particularly for a CNS drug for which knowledge of blood brain barrier (BBB) penetration is of immense importance, should preferably be available early in the drug development process. Whether or not a potential drug candidate reaches the target organ in sufficient amounts to achieve therapeutic effect is valuable information in the selection between different candidates. This type of information is usually obtained in animal experiments and the results extrapolated to human applications with the risk of interspecies differences, which might lead to wrong decisions. There is a complicated mechanism in drug-target interaction involving drug exchange between plasma and tissue and the next level where drug target protein kinetics mediates the first step in the therapeutic effect of the drug.

The discrepancy between the time-course of plasma and target protein kinetics discussed above is a general trend and typical curves for plasma and target kinetics are shown in Fig. 12.

A special case is drug deposition and disposition following oral, intranasal or inhalation administration routes. In these cases, PET is the only realistic molecular imaging alternative due to the opportunity of labeling the drug candidate with a suitable radionuclide and the quantitative determination of amount of radioactivity. One major limitation with local administration of radioactivity compared with intravenous is the low amount of radioactivity that can be given due to high local radiation dose. In studies where the labeled drug is administered by intranasal or inhalation routes, typically 10–50 MBq is given, and this usually precludes detailed information about brain or other organ kinetics.

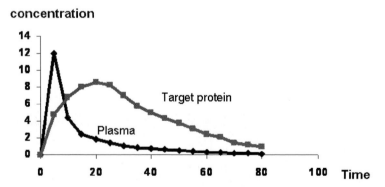

Fig. 12 Difference between plasma and target pharmacokinetics

3.2.1 [^{11}C]Nicotine Inhalation Study

An illustrative example of the use of PET to study deposition and disposition of drugs is the investigation of the smoking cessation device Nicorette®. This device consists of an inhalator with a porous plug impregnated with nicotine, and by sucking on it a suitable dose of nicotine, in the form of an aerosol, should be administered and relieve the withdrawal symptoms. In this study, the deposition and disposition was compared between the Nicorette® device and an ordinary cigarette, both labeled with [^{11}C]nicotine. The levels of radioactivity in arterial blood, assumed to represent [^{11}C]nicotine was also measured. In Fig. 13, distribution of the radioactive nicotine is visualized.

As shown in Fig. 13, the nicotine from the inhaler was not distributed to the lungs and at early time-points was mainly found in the large bronchi, and later in the esophagus and stomach. This was in contrast to nicotine from the cigarette, which was found to be in the lungs. A plausible explanation for the differences could be that the nicotine from the cigarette is particle-bound, whereas from the inhaler an aerosol is formed, which deposits nicotine on surfaces in the upper respiratory tract (Bergström et al. 1995; Lunell et al. 1996) and apparently does not reach the lungs. The time-course of labeled-nicotine appearing in arterial blood also differed significantly, as shown in Fig. 14.

From the cigarette, a very fast appearance of nicotine in blood — with a distinct peak at around 2–3 min from the start of smoking — was obtained, whereas the inhaler showed much slower kinetics, with a constant increase over time. The differences in nicotine blood kinetics are explained by a fast transfer from lung to blood when smoking a cigarette and a slow passage from esophagus and stomach using the inhaler. The peak seen in the blood kinetics from the cigarette may represent what the smoker is seeking, rapid increase of the nicotine level in the brain leading to the "kick" after uptake of nicotine.

3.2.2 Intranasal Administration of [^{11}C]zolmitriptan

Another educational example of a deposition-disposition study is the intranasal administration of the antimigraine drug zolmitriptan. Zolmitriptan is a 5-HT$_{1B/1D}$

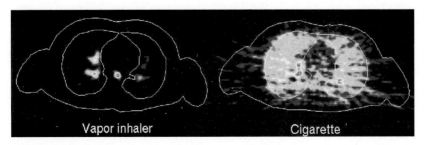

Fig. 13 Deposition of [^{11}C]nicotine

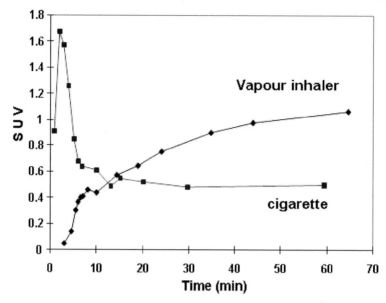

Fig. 14 Deposition of zolmitriptan in the nasal cavity following intranasal administration of [methyl-^{11}C]zolmitriptan

agonist taken orally. The antimigraine action of zolmitriptan is due to activation of vascular 5-HT receptors as well as the trigeminal nucleus, and higher pain centers in the brain may also be involved. Thus, the therapeutic activity may be mediated by both central and peripheral mechanisms. The intranasal formulation administered via a spray device was designed with the expectation of faster relief of symptoms by quick transport from the nasal mucosa to blood. Also, the nausea and vomiting found in connection with a migraine attack, which makes it difficult to swallow a tablet, could be circumvented by an intranasal administration route. Zolmitriptan was labeled in different positions, as shown in Scheme 3 (Antoni et al. 2006). The methyl labeling was used in the first study and [carbonyl-^{11}C]zolmitriptan in the follow-up study.

In the first part of the study, [methyl-^{11}C]zolmitriptan was mixed with the therapeutic amount of zolmitriptan and administered by an intranasal route using a spray device (Yates et al. 2005). In Fig. 15, the deposition of zolmitriptan in the nasal cavity is shown.

In this study, deposition and disposition data for intranasally administered zolmitriptan was obtained. Due to the low amount of radioactivity given (around 25 MBq), the counting statistics from brain tissue was too low to give significant data.

The following study was designed partly based on the results from the blood pharmacokinetics data obtained from intranasal administration. In the follow-up study, a therapeutic dose of zolmitriptan was given by the intranasal route, followed by intravenous administration of 300–400 MBq of [carbonyl-^{11}C]zolmitriptan. By the latter protocol it was possible to achieve sufficient brain radioactivity levels to

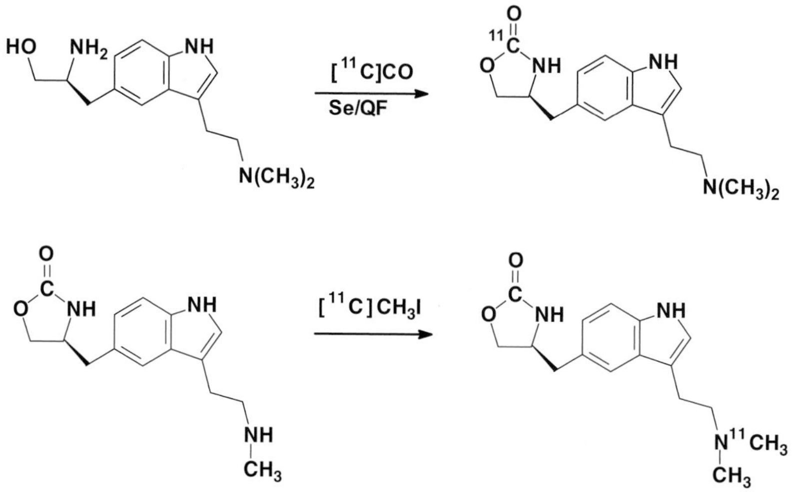

Scheme 3

Fig. 15 Time-course of [^{11}C]nicotine in arterial blood. Overlay of PET and MRI images at 0.5 and 20 min following intranasal administration of [^{11}C]zolmitriptan

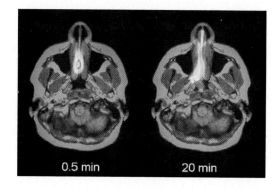

0.5 min   20 min

quantitatively determine the concentration of zolmitriptan in brain (Bergström et al. 2006; Wall et al. 2006). The relationship between arterial and venous tracer concentrations, respectively between the brain and arterial tracer concentrations were calculated. This was followed by recalculating plasma PK data using the impulse response functions derived from the PET studies to estimate the brain zolmitriptan concentration after a nasal administration of a therapeutic dose. By the use of a dynamic PET investigation and PK modeling, it was possible to quantify the brain concentration of the drug after nasal administration of a therapeutic dose and to extend the time window beyond the typical 4–5 half-lives of the radionuclide (approximately 90 min for ^{11}C). It was concluded that zolmitriptan entered the brain in sufficient amount to suggest a central action and the data support rapid brain availability after intranasal administration.

4 Conclusions

The examples presented show that we can interpret a radioactive signal, measured with a PET camera, in terms of specific biochemical reactions. The understanding of the complex interactions between a tracer molecule and a molecular target in a living organism is a challenging task. The toolbox and methodology consists of choice of radionuclide, labeling position and development of tracer kinetic models. The use of position-specific labeling is a powerful tool to elucidate in-vivo biochemistry. A multi-tracer protocol is an alternative way to evaluate complex biological processes and has proved useful in both biomedical research and in clinical applications. PET and molecular imaging is increasingly applied to acquire knowledge of how the human body is regulated at the molecular level, giving insight into both pathophysiological and normal conditions. The use of molecular imaging in drug development is a field of research where PET will contribute, potentially leading to the development and use of improved drugs in a cost-effective way. The development of methods and techniques for the labeling of molecules either as tracers for drugs or as potential tracer tools in the last years is significant and especially the use of ^{11}C-carbon monoxide as a building block in labeling synthesis is worth mentioning (Långström et al. 2007). In the light of this, we advocate that PET has a role in the implementation of the personalized medicine concept into the healthcare system, for the benefit of the individual as well as society.

We have barely scratched the surface of knowledge in the field of in-vivo molecular interactions and the future holds almost unlimited, challenging research opportunities in the field of molecular imaging.

Acknowledgements The examples discussed in this chapter are the results of many scientists' joint efforts, mainly past and present members of Uppsala University PET Centre/Uppsala Imanet GEHC, which we acknowledge.

References

Antoni G, Gustavsson SÅ, Kihlberg T, Warren K, Långström B (2006) Synthesis of [carbonyl-^{11}C]zolmitriptan by selenium mediated carbonylation. Internal communication, Uppsala Imanet AB

Aquilonius SM, Bergström K, Eckernäs SA, Hartvig P, Leenders KL, Lundquist H, Antoni G, Gee A, Rimland A, Ulin J, Långström B (1987) In vivo evaluation of striatal dopamine reuptake sites using ^{11}C-nomifensine and positron emission tomography. Acta Neurol Scand 76: 283–287

Bergström M, Muhr C, Lundberg PO, Långström B (1991) PET as a tool in the clinical evaluation of pituitary adenomas. J Nucl Med 32:610–615

Bergström M, Nordberg A, Lunell E, Antoni G, Långström B (1995) Regional deposition of inhaled ^{11}C-nicotine vapor in the human airway as visualized by positron emission tomography. Clin Pharmacol Ther 57:309–317

Bergström M, Eriksson B, Öberg K, Sundin A, Ahlström H, Lindner KJ, Bjurling P, Långström B (1996) In vivo demonstration of of enzymatic activity in endocrine pancreatic tumours – decarboxylation of ^{11}C-DOPA to dopamine. J Nucl Med 37:32–37

Bergström M, Westerberg G, Kihlberg T, Långström B (1997a) Synthesis of some ^{11}C-labelled MAO-A inhibitors and their in vivo uptake kinetics in rhesus monkey. Nucl Med Biol 24: 381–388

Bergström M, Westerberg G, Nemeth G, Traut M, Gross G, Greger G, Muller-Peltzer H, Safer A, Eckernas SA, Grahner A, Langstrom B (1997b) MAO-A inhibition in brain after dosing with esuprone, moclobemide and placebo in healthy volunteers: in vivo studies with positron emission tomography. Eur J Clin Pharmacol. 52:121–128

Bergström M, Bonasera T, Li L, Bergström E, Backlin C, Juhlin C, Långström B (1998) In vitro and in vivo primate validation of ^{11}C-etomidate and metomidate as potential tracers for the adrenal cortex and its tumours. J Nucl Med 39:982–989

Bergström M, Juhlin C, Bonasera TA, Sundin A, Rastad J, Åkerström G, Långström B (2000) PET imaging of adrenal cortical tumors with the 11-β–hydroxylase tracer ^{11}C-metomidate. J Nucl Med 41:275–282

Bergström M, Långström B (2005) Pharmacokinetic studies with PET. In: Rudin M (ed) Progress in drug research, vol 62. Birkhauser, Basel

Bergström M, Yates R, Wall A, Kagedal M, Syvänen S, Långström B (2006) Blood-brain barrier penetration of zolmitriptan – modelling of positron emission tomography data. J Pharmacokinet Pharmacodyn 33:75–91

Bjurling P, Antoni G, Watanabe Y, Långström B (1990a) Enzymatic synthesis of carboxy-^{11}C-labelled L-tyrosine, L-DOPA, L-tryptophan, and 5-hydroxy-tryptophan. Acta Chem Scand 44:178–182

Bjurling P, Watanabe Y, Oka S, Nagasawa T, Yamada H, Långströn B (1990b) Multi-enzymatic synthesis of β-^{11}C labeled L-tyrosine, and L-DOPA. Acta Chem Scand 44:183–188

Carlsson A, Lindqvist M, Magnusson T (1957) 3,4-dihydroxyphenylalanine and 5-hydroxy-tryptophanas reserpine antagonist. Nature 180:1200–1201

Carson RE (2003) Tracer kinetic modeling in PET. In: Valk PE, Bailey DL, Townsend DE, Maisey MN (eds) Positron Emission Tomography – basic science and clinical practice. Springer, London

Cho HJ, Skowera A, Cleare A, Wessely S (2006) Chronic fatigue syndrome: an update on phenomenology and patophysiology. Curr Opin Psychiatry 19:67–73

Cummings P, Hausser M, Martin WR, Grierson J, Adam MJ, Ruth TJ, McGeer EG (1988) Kinetics of in vitro decarboxylation and the in vivo metabolism of 2-[18]F- and 6-^{18}F-fluorodopa in the hooded rat. Biochem Pharmacol 37:247–250

Elsinga PH, Hatano K, Ishiwata K (2006) PET tracers for imaging of the dopaminergic system. Curr Med 13:2139–2153

Eriksson B, Lilja A, Ahlström H, Långström B (1993) Positron emission tomography in neuroendocrine gastrointestinal tumours. Acta Oncologia Suppl 32:189–196

Eriksson B, Örlefors H, Öberg K, Sundin A, Bergström M, Långström B (2005) Developments in PET for the detection of endocrine tumours. Best Prac Res Clin Endocrinol Metab 19:311–324

Farde L, Ehrin E, Eriksson L, Greitz T, Hall H, Hedstrom CG, Litton JE, Sedvall G (1985) Substituted benzamides as ligands for visualization of dopamine receptor binding in the human brain by positron emission tomography. Proc Natl Acad Sci USA 82:3863–3867

Fowler JS, Wang GJ, Logan J, Xie S, Volkov ND, MacGregor RR, Schlyer DJ, Pappas N, Alexoff DL, Patlak C, Wolf AP (1995) Selective reduction of radiotracer trapping by deuterium substitution: comparison of carbon-11 L-deprenyl and carbon-11 deprenyl-D2 for MAO-B mapping. J Nucl Med 36:1255–1262

Garnett ES, Firnau G, Nahmias C (1983) Dopamine visualized in the basal ganglia of living man. Nature 305:137–138

Ginovart N, Galineau L, Willeit M, Mizrahi R, Bloomfield PM, Seeman P, Houle S, Kapur S, Wilson AA (2006) Binding characteristics and sensitivity to endogenous dopamine of [11C]-(+)-PHNO, a new agonist radiotracer for imaging the high-affinity state of D2 receptors in vivo using positron emission tomography. J Neurochem 97:1089–1103

Halldin C, Stone-Elander S, Farde L, Fasth KJ, Långström B, Sedvall L (1986) Preparation of ^{11}C-labelled SCH23390 for the in vivo study of dopamine D_1 receptors using positron emission tomography. Appl Radiat Isot 40:557–561

Halldin C, Farde L, Lundkvist C, Ginovart N, Nakashima Y, Karslsson P, Swahn CG (1996) [11C]-β-CIT-FE, a radioligand for quantitation of the dopamine transporter in the living brain isung positron emission tomography. Synapse 22:386–390

Hartvig P, Ågren H, Reibring L, Tedroff J, Bjurling P, Kihlberg T, Långström B (1991) Brain kinetics of L-[β-11C]dopa in humans studied by positron emission tomography. J Neural Transm 86:25–41

Hartvig P, Torstenson R, Tedroff J, Watanabe Y, Fasth KJ, Bjurling P, Långström B (1997) Amphetamine effects on dopamine release and synthesis rate studied in the rhesus monkey barin by positron emission tomography. J Neural Transm 104:329–339

Hennings J, Lindhe Ö, Bergström M, Långström B, Sundin A, Hellman P (2006) [11C]metomidate positron emission tomography of adrenocortical tumors in correlation with histopathological findings J Clin Endocrinol Metab 91:1410–1414

Hoffman EJ, Phelps ME (1986) Positron emission tomography: principles and quantitation In: Phelps ME, Mazziotta J, Schelbert (eds) Positron emission tomography and autoradiography: principles and applications for the brain and heart. Raven Press, New York

Jacobson GB, Moulder R, Lu L, Bergström M, Markides KE, Långström B (1997) Supercritical Fluid Extraction of 11C-Labelled Metabolites in Tissue using Supercritical Ammonia. Analytical Chem 69(3):275–280

Jazczak RJ, Tsui BM (1995) Single photon emission computed tomography (SPECT) In: Wagner HN, Szabo Z (eds) Principle of nuclear medicine. Saunders, Philadelphia

Korf J, Reiffers S, Beerling van der molen HD, Lakke JP, Paans AM, Valburg W, Woldring MG (1978) Rapid decarboxylation of carbon-11 labelled DL-dopa in the brain: a potential approach for external detection of nervous structures. Brain Res 145:59–67

Kuratsune H, Yamagushi K, Takahashi M, Misaki H, Tagawa S, Kitani T (1994) Acylcarnitine deficiency in chronic fatigue syndrome. Clin Infect Dis 18(Suppl 1):62–67

Kuratsune H, Watanabe Y, Yamaguti K, Jacobsson G, Takahashi M, Machii T, Onoe H, Onoe K, Matsumara K, Valind S, Katani K, Långström B (1997) High uptake of [2-11C]acetyl-L-carnitine into the brain: a PET study. Biochem Biophys Res Commun. 231:488–493

Långström B, Itsenko O, Rahman O (2007) 11C-Carbonmonoxide, a versatile and useful precursor in labeling chemistry for PET-ligand development. J Lab Comp Radiopharmaceutic 50: 794–810

Learned-Coughlin SM, Bergström M, Savitcheva I, Ascher J, Schmith VD, Långström B (2003) In vivo activity of buproprion at the human dopamine transporter as measured by positron emission tomography. Biol Psychiatry 54:800–805

Lindner KJ, Hartvig P, Tedroff J, Ljunsgtröm A, Bjurling P, Långström B (1995) Liquid chromatographic analysis of brain homogenates and microdialysates for the quantification of L-[β-11C]DOPA and its metabolites for the validation of positron emission tomography studies. J Pharm Biomed Anal 13:361–367

Lundkvist C, Halldin C, Ginovart N, Swahn CG, Farde L (1997) [18F]-CIT-FP is superior to [11C]-CIT-FP for quantitation of the dopamine transporter. Nucl Med Biol 24:621–627

Lunell E, Bergström M, Antoni G, Långström B, Nordberg A (1996) Nicotine deposition and body distribution froma nicotine inhaler and a cigarette with positron emission tomography. Clin Pharmacol Ther 593–594

Muhr C, Bergström M (1991) Positron emission tomography applied in the study of pituitary adenomas. J Endocrinol Invest 14:509–528

Örlefors H, Sundin A, Ahlström H, Bjurling P, Bergström M, Lilja A, Långström B, Öberg K, Eriksson B (1998) PET with 5-hydroxytryptophan in endocrine tumours. J Clin Oncol 7: 2534–2542

Patlak CS, Blasberg RG (1985) graphical evaluation of blood-to-brain transfer constants from multiple-time uptake data. Generalizations. J Cereb Blood Flow Metab 5:584–590

Ravina B, Eidelberg D, Ahlskog JE, Albin RL, Brooks DJ, Carbon M, Dhawan V, Feigin A, Fahn S, Guttman M, Gwinn-Hardy K, McFarland H, Innis R, Katz RG, Kieburtz K, Kish SJ, Lange N, Langston JW, Marek K, Morin L, Moy C, Murphy D, Oertel WH, Oliver G, Palesch Y,

Powers W, Seibyl J, Sethi KD, Shults CW, Sheehy P, Stoessl AJ, Holloway R (2005) The role of radiotracer imaging in Parkinson disease. Neurology 25:208–215

Rinne OJ, Nurmi E, Ruottinen HM, Bergman J, Eskola O, Solin O (2001) [18F]FDOPA and [18F]CFT are both sensitive markers to detect presynaptic hypofunction in early Parkinson's disease. Synapse 40:193–200

Shulkin BL, Wieland DM, Schwaiger M, Thompsson NW, Francis IR, Haka MS, Rosenspire B, Sisson JC, Kuhl DE (1992) An approach to the localization of pheochromocytoma. J Nuc Med 33:1125–1131

Shulkin BL, Thompson NW, Shapiro B, Francis IR, Sisson JC (1999) Pheochromocytoma: imaging with 2-[fluorine-18]fluoro-2-deoxy-D-glucose PET. Radiology 212:35–41

Sonnewald U, Gribbestad IS, Westergaard N, Nielsen G, Unsgard G, Schousboe A, Petersen SB (1994) Nuclear magnetic resonance spectroscopy: biochemical evaluation of brain function in vivo and in vitro. Neurotoxicology 15:579–590

Tedroff J, Aquilonius SM, Laihinen A, Rinne U, HArtvig P, Andersson J, Lundquist H, Haaparanta M, Solin O, Antoni G, Ulin J, Långström B (1990) Striatal kinetics of [11C]-(+)nomifensine and 6-[18F]fluoro-L-dopa in Parkinson's disease measured with positron emission tomography. Acta Neurol Scand 8:24–30

Tedroff J, Aquilonius SM, Hartvig P, Bredberg E, Bjurling P, Långström B (1992a) Cerebral uptake and utilization of therapeutic [beta-11C]-L-DOPA in Parkinson's disease measured by positron emission tomography. Relation to motor response. Acta Neurol Scand 85:95–102

Tedroff J, Aquilonius SM, Hartvig P, Lundqvist H, Bjurling P, Långström B (1992b) estimation of regional cerebral utilization of [11C]-L-3,4-dihydroxyphenylalanine (DOPA) in the primate by positron emission tomography. Acta Neurol Scand 85:166–173

Torstenson R, Hartvig P, Långström B, Westerberg G, Tedroff J (1997) Differential effects of levodopa on dopaminergic function in early and advanced Parkinson's disease. Ann Neurol 41:334–340

Torstenson R, Hartvig P, Långström B, Bastami S, Antoni G, Tedroff J (1998) Effect of apomorphine infusion on dopamine synthesis rate relates to dopaminergic tone. Neuropharmacology 37:989–995

Torstenson R, Tedroff J, Hartvig P, Fasth KJ, Lånsgtröm B (1999) A comparison of 11C-labelled L-DOPA and L-fluoroDOPA as PET tracers for the presynaptic dopaminergic system. J Cereb Blood Flow 19:1142–1149

Trampal C, Engler H, Juhlin C, Bergström M, Långström B (2004) Pheochromocytoma: detection with 11C-hydroxyephedrine PET. Radiology 230:423–428

Valk PE, Bailey DL, Townsend DE, Maisey MN (eds) (2003) Positron Emission Tomography – basic science and clinical practice. Springer, London

Wadsal W, Mitterhauser M, Rendl G, Schuetz M, Mien LK, Ettlinger DE, Dudczak R, Kletter K, Karanikas G (2006) [18F]FETO for adrenocortical PET imaging; a pilot study in healthy volunteers. Eur J Nucl Med Mol Imaging 33:928–931

Wagner jr, HN, Burns D, Dannals RF, Wong D, Långström B, Duelfer T, Frost JJ, Ravert HT, Links JM, Rosenbloom SB, Lukas SF, Kramer AW, Kuhar MJ (1983) Assessment of dopamine receptor activity in the human brain with 11C-labelled N-methylspiperone. Science 221:1264–1266

Wall A, Bergström M, Jacobsson E, Nilsson D, Antoni G, Frandberg P, Gustavsson SA, Långström B, Yates R (2005) Distribution of zolmitriptan into the CNS in healthy volunteers: a positron emission tomography study. Drugs R D 6:139–147

Yamaguti K, Kuratsune H, Watanabe Y, Takahashi M, Nakamoto I, Machii T, Jacobson G, Onoe H, Matsumura K, Valind S, Långström B (1996) Acylcarnitine metabolism during fasting and after refeeding. Biochem Biophys Res Commun 225:740–746

Yates R, Sorensen J, Bergström M, Antoni G, Nairn K, Kemp J, Långström B, Dane A (2005) Distribution of intranasal 11C-zolmitriptan assessed by positron emission tomography. Cephalalgia 25:1103–1109

Optical Agents

Kai Licha(✉), Michael Schirner, and Gavin Henry

Abstract Optical imaging is an emerging modality in the growing field of bio-medical diagnostics. The past decade has witnessed the development of a variety of promising strategies for optical imaging techniques. Fundamental to these techniques is the design and application of novel fluorescent markers to allow molecular level in-vivo studies of disease in animal models in the laboratory and eventually in human clinical studies.

This review surveys the range of fluorophores employed in these probes and the alternative probe systems in which they are used: non-specific, targeted and activatable; recent developments in the area of fluorescent nanoprobes and multimodality constructs are also reviewed.

1 Introduction

The field of optical imaging is experiencing a period of rapid expansion and increased attention. The reasons for this growing interest include the growth of the clinical diagnosis market and the rise of molecular imaging, which offers insights

Kai Licha

migenion GmbH, Robert-Koch-Platz 4-8, 10115 Berlin, Germany

licha@migenion.com

W. Semmler and M. Schwaiger (eds.), *Molecular Imaging I.*

Handbook of Experimental Pharmacology 185/I.

© Springer-Verlag Berlin Heidelberg 2008

into the workings of biological processes at a molecular level and is of particular interest for drug development. The goal of observing molecular processes drives the development of specific probes to report on particular molecular interactions.

Optical imaging distinguishes itself from other diagnostic modalities by several key characteristics. It provides high instrumental sensitivity for detection, it is a non-radiative method and only low dosages are required, allowing repeated dosing. Imaging instrumentation is relatively inexpensive and generally easy to apply. Also useful is the direct correlation between results obtained in bioanalytical research, e.g. by fluorescence microscopy, with those from macroscopic and in-vivo imaging. The key properties sought for imaging probes are that they are biocompatible, injectable and detectable at a sensitivity level which is determined by the molecular mechanism to be studied.

The most evident challenge is the limitation given by the penetration and scattering of light in the tissue, deteriorating the ability to localise the spatial origin of fluorescence with increasing distance from tissue surfaces. On surfaces, however, fluorescence can be visualised with high accuracy, as apparent in microscopy. Accordingly, the location and type of tissue abnormality in the body requires dedicated instrumental approaches adapted to the specific imaging problem. This is reflected in the broad range of fluorphore types applied to design molecular probes, either based on organic fluorophores or on anorganic nanoparticles, covering a broad range of photophysical and chemical characteristics.

This chapter reviews the range of optical agents published and summarises the different targeting principles incorporated into the design of these probes.

2 Optical Probes Based on Organic Dyes

2.1 Properties of Different Fluorophore Classes

The photophysical properties of fluorescent imaging probes lie at the heart of optical imaging and provide a fitting starting point for this review. These key properties include: typical absorption wavelengths and fluorescence emission, fluorescence quantum yields and lifetimes, and potential photodynamic characteristics. For diagnostic applications, the most common fluorophores of an organic nature have been polymethine dyes (carbocyanine dyes), tetrapyrroles (porphyrins, chlorins, bacteriochlorins), rare earth metal chelates (terbium and europium complexes) and xanthene dyes, including fluorescein- and rhodamine-type fluorophores. In order to select a probe suitable for a specific research or clinical application, the basic features of these fluorophores have to taken into account. In Fig. 1, typical spectra of these fluorophores are illustrated. Cyanine dyes are perhaps the most widespread and versatile fluorophores in the area of biological imaging. They are available at practically each desired absorption wavelength from the visible (VIS) to

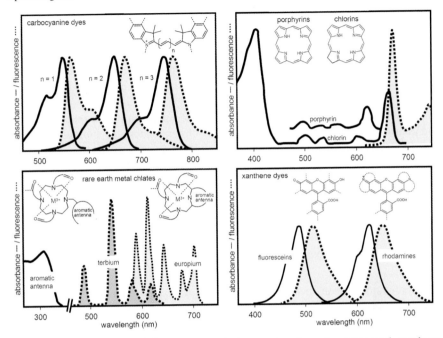

Fig. 1 Typical absorption and fluorescence emission spectra of cyanine, tetrapyrrol, xanthene and lanthanide chelate fluorophores. The graphs include structure sketches of the basic chromophore types

near-infrared spectral range making them useful for both superficial and deep tissue imaging (Licha 2002); they have short fluorescence lifetimes ($\sim$1 ns), high molar extinction coefficients and moderate fluorescence quantum yields. Drawbacks such as chemical instability and photobleaching have been addressed with novel stabilised derivatives (Ballou et al. 2005). Tetrapyrrol chromophores, such as porphyrins, chlorins, benzochlorins, bacteriochlorins and phthalocyanines, are well established for photodynamic therapy, as these structures have the ability to generate singlet oxygen and radicals from their long-lived triplet excited states, leading to cell-toxic events (Nyman and Hynninen 2004). To review the therapeutic aspects is beyond the scope of this chapter, but many tetrapyrroles have red-shifted absorption and reasonable fluorescence emission (lifetime $\sim$10 ns), making them applicable for diagnostic purposes (see also Sect. 2.4.2).

Lanthanide chelates, particularly with terbium and europium, are interesting because of their long fluorescence lifetimes up to the millisecond range. The fluorescence derives from the metal ion, which intramolecularly receives excitation energy from an aromatic system in close proximity. As a result, these complexes exhibit large Stokes' shifts but also very short excitation wavelengths determined by the aromatic moiety (UV to VIS), thus making them primarily useful for superficial examinations.

Xanthene dyes encompass derivatives of fluorescein and rhodamine, which are essential tools in bioanalytics. They are particularly advantageous for microscopy and other equipment for cell analysis, since they exhibit very high fluorescence quantum yields (near 100%). It is difficult to tune these structures to absorb in the near-infrared region, so that for in-vivo imaging preference has been given to cyanine dyes.

Many of these dyes have undergone synthetic modifications to meet chemical and pharmacological requirements or are part of conjugates with biological targeting units, e.g. antibodies, proteins, peptides, small molecules, or enzyme-activatable constructs. The following chapters group the dyes according to their mode of action: non-specific dyes (passive targeting), target-specific probes (reporters of protein structure and expression) and activatable systems (reporters of protein function).

2.2 Non-specific Dyes (Passive Targeting)

The application of non-specific contrast agents that achieve contrast enhancement based on morphological and physiological properties of tumor tissue is daily medical routine in X-ray, CT and MR imaging. In principle, the knowledge that exists here can be exploited for optical contrast agents and has led to the development of several probes mainly studied as fluorescent contrast agents for tumours.

The carbocyanine dye indocyanine green (ICG, absorption ~780–800 nm) is the only clinically applicable near-infrared dye; it was approved in the 1960s as a diagnostic drug for the assessment of hepatic function and cardiac output (rapid liver uptake with blood half life of ~10 min), and re-discovered later in the 1990s as an imaging agent. ICG has been studied as a potential near-infrared contrast agent for the detection of tumours both in animals and patients (Licha et al. 2000; Gurfinkel et al. 2000; Ntziachristos et al. 2000), and is meanwhile a frequently applied dye for fluorescence angiography of vascular disorders in ophthalmology (Richards et al. 1998). Novel indotricarbocyanines have been synthesised with substantially increased hydrophilicity and reduced plasma protein binding, thus increasing the circulation and tissue retention times, which is particularly important for optical imaging procedures of longer duration (e.g. optical breast scans or intraoperative procedures). Examples are the dye SIDAG (Licha et al. 2000; Ebert et al. 2001), a bis-glucamine derivatized carbocyanine, and TSC, a tetrasulfonated alternative (Perlitz et al. 2005), both of which having demonstrated potential for the detection of tumours (absorption at ~750 nm/emission >780 nm). Similar approaches were followed by decorating near-infrared carbocyanines with sugars such as galactose (Zhang and Achilefu 2004) or even multivalent dendritic glucosamine arrays (glucosamine cypates; Ye et al. 2005). The near-infrared cyanine dye IRDye78-CA, employing sulfonate and carboxylic acid moieties, has been applied for the intraoperative visualisation of myocardial blood flow and perfusion (Nakayama et al. 2002). A pyclen-based macrocyclic complex with terbium has been studied as a diagnostic imaging probe for the detection of animal tumours on tissue surfaces

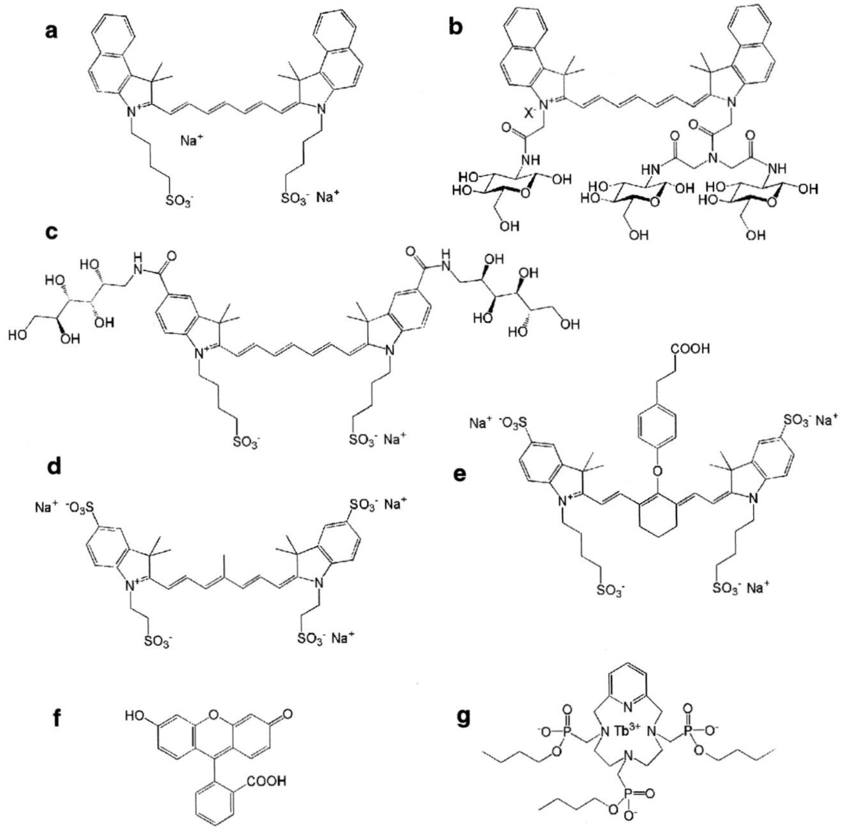

Fig. 2 a–g Chemical structures of non-targeted fluorescence imaging agents. **a** Indocyanine green, **b** tris-glucosamine cypate, **c** SIDAG, **d** TSC, **e** IRDye78-CA, **f** fluorescein, and **g** Tb-PCTMB

with simple UV illumination (Tb-PCTMB; Bornhop et al. 2003). The xanthene-type dye fluorescein is one of the few that is clinically approved and today it is the most widespread fluorophore in medical imaging, routinely applied as a probe drug for fluorescence angiography in ophthalmology (Hogan and Zimmerman 1997). The chemical structures of probes discussed in this chapter are depicted in Fig. 2.

By attaching fluorescent dyes like cyanines and fluoresceins to methoxy(poly-ethylene)glycols (MPEGs) of different molecular weights (Riefke et al. 1998) or to biological macromolecules such as transferrin or human serum albumin (Becker et al. 2000; Kremer et al. 2000), increased blood circulation times and pronounced tumour uptake were observed. These probes enable the creation of in-vivo contrast by the enhanced permeability of tumour vasculature or inflammatory processes compared with normal tissues.

2.3 Target-specific Conjugates

2.3.1 Conjugates with Peptide Ligands

Following the approaches of radiodiagnostic imaging, target-specific optical agents have been designed by utilising low molecular weight peptide ligands as vehicles for the delivery of fluorophores. Many tumours are known to overexpress receptors [mostly studied are G-protein coupled receptors (GPCRs)] for specific peptide ligands with diverse regulatory function, e.g. somatostatin (SST), vasoactive intestinal peptide (VIP) or bombesin. For example, the pharmacologically optimised SST analogue octreotate internalizes receptor-mediated into cells with virtually every payload, ranging from radiochelates to fluorophores. Imaging agents such as ITCC-octreotate (Becker et al. 2001), cypate-octreotate (Bugaj et al. 2001), and sulforhodamin B-octreotate analogue (Mier et al. 2002) demonstrate the utility of this approach and provide a broad spectrum of in-vitro and in-vivo biochemical data. Similarly, the conjugate Cybesin, targeting the bombesin receptor (Pu et al. 2005), and a cyanine-labelled, stabilised derivative of vasoactive intestinal peptide (Bhargava et al. 2002) have been studied. Some cell adhesion molecules, in particular the integrins αvß3 and αvß5, have been proposed as markers for angiogenesis in tumours. The well-known peptide ligand containing the RGD-motif was used as targeting vehicle for fluorescence imaging (Aina et al. 2005; Wang et al. 2004). Cy5.5-RGD peptide uptake could be inhibited in vivo by free peptide, suggesting specific interaction with integrins (Achilefu et al. 2005; Chen et al. 2004).

In Fig. 3, selected structures of fluorescent peptide probes are depicted, and they are summarised by Table 1. General advantages of peptide conjugates are that they can be readily synthesised as defined and robust structures, are not immunogenic as antibodies might be (see Sect. 2.3.2) and have favourable pharmacokinetics in terms of reasonably rapid blood clearance and decreasing background fluorescence.

2.3.2 Conjugates with Antibodies and Protein Ligands

Advances in biotechnology created powerful targeting systems based on antibodies and their bioengineered analogues, such as antibody fragments, diabodies or minibodies. The strategy of coupling cyanine dye labels to antibodies for in-vivo imaging was first followed by Folli et al. (1994) and Ballou et al. (1995), and was later reinforced by Neri and co-workers, who described affinity-maturated single-chain antibody fragments directed against an angiogenesis-specific oncofetal isoform of fibronectin (ED-B fibronectin). After injection of Cy7 or Cy5.5-labeled antibody fragments, the expression of ED-B-fibronectin was visualised in tumour-bearing mice (Birchler et al. 1999a), in a mouse atherosclerosis model (Matter et al. 2004), and in angiogenesis induced in the cornea of rabbits (Birchler et al. 1999b), impressively demonstrating the relevance of ED-B-fibronectin as a marker of angiogenetic processes.

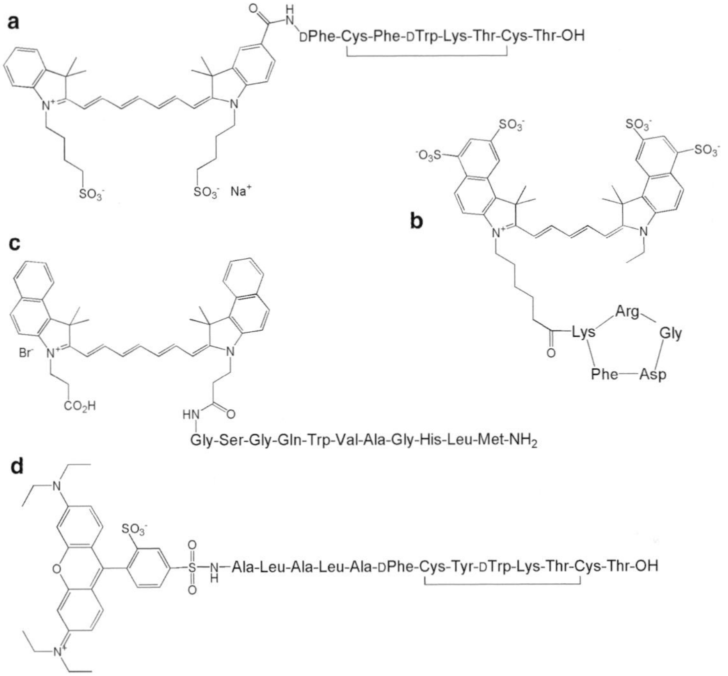

Fig. 3 a–d Chemical structures of receptor-targeted peptide conjugates. **a** ITCC-octreotate, **b** Cy5.5-RGD peptide, **c** cypate bombesin analogue Cybesin, and **d** sulphorhodamine B-ALALA-octreotate

The utilisation of the apoptosis marker annexin V conjugated to a near-infrared fluorophore to assess cell death in vivo was first demonstrated by Petrovsky et al. (2003) and furthermore studied to assess pharmacological responses of cancer chemotherapy in animals (Schellenberger et al. 2003). Labelling of annexin V highlighted a typical pitfall of antibody and protein conjugation chemistry: above labelling ratios of 2, protein functionality was drastically hampered due to covalent attachment of fluorophores in the active binding region of the protein (Schellenberger et al. 2004).

Other examples for antibody- and protein-based ligands are cyanine conjugates with epidermal growth factor EGF (Ke et al. 2003), endostatin (Citrin et al. 2004), and an IgM antibody targeting the endothelial expression of glycoproteins for the optical imaging of inflammation and lymph nodes (Licha et al. 2005). A summary of the content of this chapter is included in Table 1.

2.3.3 Conjugates with Small Molecule Ligands

Small molecule ligands can mediate specific target interaction and uptake into tumour cells, even when the diagnostic molecule is considerably larger than the

Table 1 Targeted fluorescent probes

Targeting vehicle	Target	Dye	Disease	Reference
Somatostatin peptides	GPCR	Cyanines, rhodamins, fluoresceins	Tumours	Achilefu et al. 2002, Becker et al. 2001, Bugaj et al. 2001, Mier et al. 2002
Bombesin peptides	GPCR	Cyanines, fluoresceins	Tumours	Pu et al. 2005, Bugaj et al. 2001
Vasoactive intestinal peptides	GPCR	Cyanines	Tumours	Bhargava et al. 2002
RGD peptides	Integrins ($\alpha_V\beta_3$)	Cyanines	Tumours	Achilefu et al. 2005, Aina et al. 2005, Chen et al. 2004, Wang et al. 2004
Annexin A5	Apoptotic cell	Cyanines	Tumours, metastases atherosclerosis	Schellenberger et al. 2003, Schellenberger et al. 2004, Petrovsky et al. 2003
Endostatin	Endothelial cell	Cyanines	Tumours	Citrin et al. 2004
EGF	Glycoprotein on tumor cell	Cyanines	Tumours	Ke et al. 2003
Anti-ED-B-fibronectin single chain antibody	Matrix protein ED-B-fibronectin	Cyanines	Tumours, atherosclerosis, ocular diseases	Birchler et al. 1999a, b, Matter et al. 2004
Various monoclonal antibodies (IgM, IgG)	Several cellular targets	Cyanines	Tumours, inflammation	Folli et al. 1994, Ballou et al. 1995, Tadatsu et al. 2003, Licha et al. 2005
Bis-phosphonates pamidronate/ alendronate	Hydroxyapatite	Cyanines, fluoresceins	Tumours (breast), microcalcification, skeletal disease	Zaheer et al. 2001, Wang et al. 2003, Lenkinski et al. 2003
Folic acid	Folate receptor	Cyanines	Tumours, rheumatoid Arthritis	Tung et al. 2002, Moon et al. 2003
Cobalamin (Vit B$_{12}$)	Cellular transporter	Cyanines	Tumours, sentinel lymph nodes	McGreevy et al. 2003
Cholesteryl lipids	LDL receptor	Cyanines, chlorins	Tumours	Zheng et al. 2002a, b
PSMA ligands	PSMA	Cyanines	Tumours (prostate)	Humblet et al. 2005
Progesterone receptor antagonst (mifepristone)	Progesterone receptor	Fluoresceins	Tumours	Hödl et al. 2004
Glucose derivatives	Glucose transporter	Cyanines, chlorins	Tumours	Chen et al. 2003, Li et al. 2004, Ye et al. 2005, Zhang et al. 2003, Zhang et al. 2004, Zhang and Achilefu 2004
1-(2-chlorophenyl) isochino-line-3-carboxyl PBR ligand	PBR receptor	Europium chelate	Tumours, metastases	Manning et al. 2004
Oxazine dye	ß-Amyloid plaques	Oxazine dye	Alzheimer's disease	Hintersteiner et al. 2005

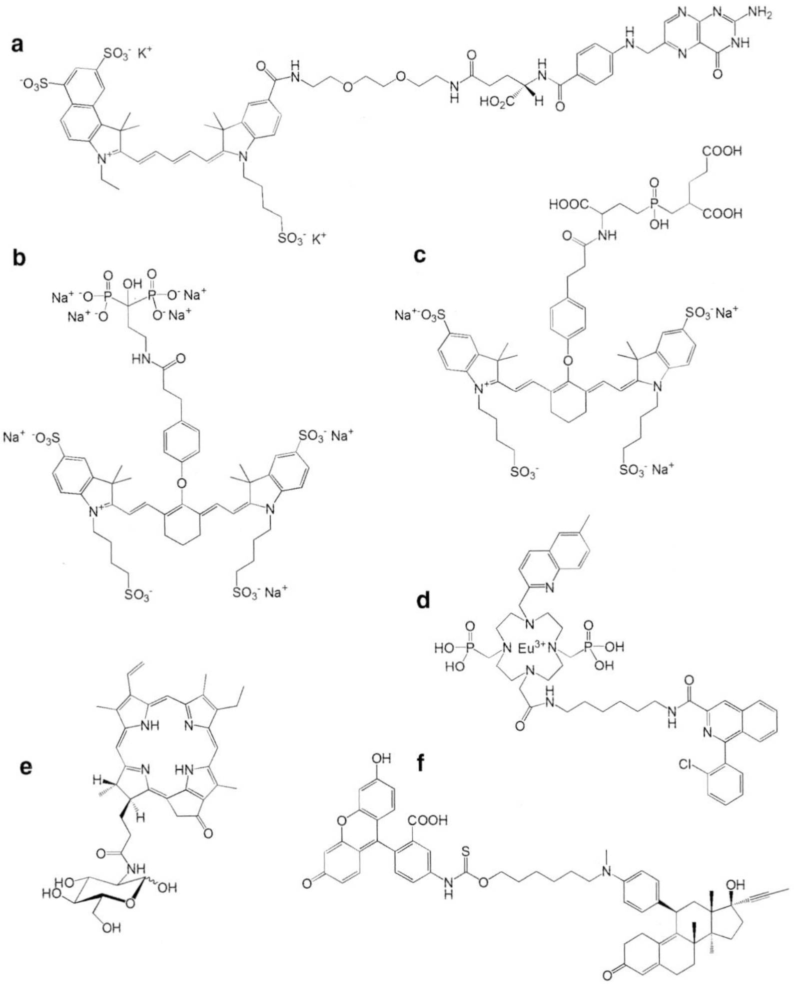

Fig. 4 a–f Chemical structures of fluorophore conjugates with small molecule ligands. **a** Cy5.5-folate conjugate, **b** bone-targeted IRDye78 pamidronate Pam78, **c** IRDye78 conjugate with PSMA-ligand GPI, **d** europium chelate conjugate with PBR-ligand (Eu-PK11195), **e** pyropheophorbide a glucosamine conjugate Pyro-2DG, and **f** progesterone receptor antagonist mifepristone labeled with fluorescein isothiocyanate

carrier. As illustrated by Table 1, a large variety of such agents have been synthesised and successfully validated as targeted probes. A selected panel of agents is depicted in Fig. 4 and discussed in the following paragraph.

The vitamin folic acid has been utilised as carrier molecule to target the abundant folate receptor on proliferating cells and activated macrophages. After derivatization of folic acid with the cyanine dye Cy5.5 or NIR2, uptake studies demonstrated convincing imaging properties in cancer models (Tung et al. 2002; Moon et al. 2003) similar to peptide-based ligands and showed utility for the early detection of inflammatory disease in a rheumatoid arthritis model (Chen et al. 2005). Vitamin B12 linked to Cy5 (CobalaFluor) was elucidated as a surgical tool for lymphatic mapping (McGreevy et al. 2003).

Glucose transporters (GLUTs) facilitate the internalization of the carbohydrate into proliferating cells more pronounced than into normal cells. Thus, ^{18}F-radiolabelled 2-fluorodeoxyglucose (FDG) is used to detect cancers in humans. Chen et al. (2003) and Ye et al. (2005) conjugated glucosamine to a near-infrared carbocyanine dye similar to already published derivatives (Licha et al. 2000). Furthermore, a glucosamine derivative of pyropheophorbid a, an often employed PDT chromophore, was synthesised (Pyro-2DG; Zhang et al. 2003). The uptake of these conjugates could be inhibited by the addition of glucose. These results suggest near-infrared versions of ^{18}F-FDG, which function via GLUTs (Zhang et al. 2004).

The feasibility to specifically target microcalcification has been shown in a suitable breast cancer model with a cyanine dye-pamidronate derivative, Pam78 (Lenkinski et al. 2003). Bisphosphonates such as pamidronate or alendronate are ligands to hydroxyapatite, an indicative component of microcalc formation. The functionality after covalent linkage to cyanine dyes or fluoresceins was proven in animal models of osteoblastic activity (Zaheer et al. 2001; Wang et al. 2003).

Targeting of the receptor for low-density lipoprotein (LDLr) was achieved by coupling a cyanine dye to a cholesteryl laurate which is known to incorporate into the lipid region of the receptor ligand LDL. Similarly, the PDT agent pyropheophorbide linked to a respective oleate was internalized into tumour cells by way of LDL formulation (Zheng et al. 2002a, 2002b).

The successful localisation of the fluorescein-labelled progesterone receptor antagonist mifepristone into cell nuclei demonstrated for the first time the capability to image progesterone receptor-positive cells in vitro, suggesting near-infrared analogues for in-vivo applications (Hödl et al. 2004).

A ligand to the peripheral benzodiazepine receptor (PBR) was employed for fluorescence imaging by means of fluorescent lanthanide chelates. The PBR-ligand conjugate with a europium macrocycle (Eu-PK11195) was evaluated for early cancer lesion detection (Manning et al. 2004).

Finally, it was shown that an oxazine-type fluorophore is capable of acting by itself as a specific ligand for a binding site in ß-amyloid plaques (Hintersteiner et al. 2005), demonstrating the potential for fluorescence detection of Alzheimer plaques, with the proviso that longer wavelengths will certainly be crucial for studies in organisms larger than laboratory animals.

2.4 Activatable and Biosynthetic Probes

2.4.1 Enzyme-activatable Conjugates

Fluorescence activation involves the conversion of a fluorophore from a quenched, non-emitting state into a free state where it is capable of emitting fluorescence light upon excitation. The ability to control the fluorescence output of dyes by changing their local chemical environment is unique for optical techniques. The idea of a sophisticated poly(L-lysine)/poly(ethylene gylcol) graft polymer labelled with a high number of cyanine dyes (in most cases Cy5.5 with an excitation/emission maximum at ~680nm/710nm) allowed Weissleder and co-workers to establish a versatile molecular imaging platform. Attachment of the fluorophores either directly or via cleavable peptide sequences in close proximity to each other causes strong fluorescence quenching. As illustrated in Fig. 5, enzymatic cleavage converts the probe from a quenched, non-detectable to a fluorescent state by liberating single dye-loaded fragments either through backbone cleavage of the lysine-lysine amide bonds (Weissleder et al. 1999) or cleavage at the peptide sequences by proteolytic enzymes (various peptides as substrates possible, see Fig. 5). Broad utility has been demonstrated for many disease models, including cancers, atherosclerosis, rheumatoid arthritis, and thrombosis (see Fig. 5 for references) and by elucidating enzyme activity as indicator for therapeutic efficacy. A more simple design employed dimeric constructs consisting of an enzyme-cleavable peptide flanked by either two different self-quenching cyanine dyes (MMP-7 cleavable; Pham et al. 2004) or a quencher/dye pair (Caspase-3 cleavable; Pham et al. 2002). In both cases, an approximately fourfold increase in fluorescence was reached, whereas the polymeric carrier system described above leads to factors greater than 100.

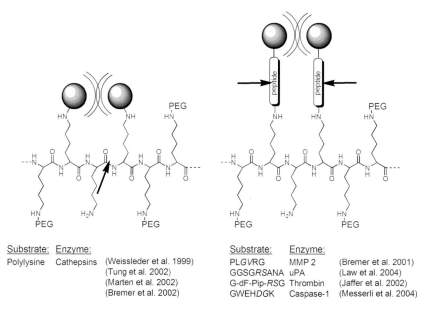

Substrate:	Enzyme:	
Polylysine	Cathepsins	(Weissleder et al. 1999)
		(Tung et al. 2002)
		(Marten et al. 2002)
		(Bremer et al. 2002)

Substrate:	Enzyme:	
PLGVRG	MMP 2	(Bremer et al. 2001)
GGSGRSANA	uPA	(Law et al. 2004)
G-dF-Pip-RSG	Thrombin	(Jaffer et al. 2002)
GWEHDGK	Caspase-1	(Messerli et al. 2004)

Fig. 5 Illustration of the active structural elements of activatable probes. Backbone-cleavable polylysine-poly(ethylene glycol) graft polymer (*left*) and peptide substrate-derivatized graft polymer (*right*). The bulbs represent fluorophores (e.g. Cy5.5) which become fluoroescent upon cleavage from the polymer. *Arrows* indicate cleavage sites. Cleavage occurs between amino acids typed *italic*

2.4.2 Biosynthetic Precursor 5-ALA

5-Aminolevulinic acid (ALA) has been thoroughly studied as an imaging agent. ALA is not fluorescent per se, but as a biosynthetic precursor in the heme synthetic pathway stimulates the intracellular synthesis of the fluorescent heme intermediate protoporphyrin IX (PpIX) with a certain selectivity for tumours. Accordingly, PpIX fluorescence allows the visualisation of tumours and other tissue abnormalities in a large variety of clinical applications after administration of ALA — intraveneously, topically or orally. A recent insight into ALA applications was, for example, published by Fukuda et al. (2005). Beyond ALA, several derivatives have been designed with the primary objective of improving bioavailability, uptake kinetics and phototherapeutic efficacy. Some alkyl esters of different alkyl chain length (Lange et al. 1997; Uehlinger et al. 2000), ethylene glycol esters and amino acid conjugates (Berger et al. 2000) which are converted into free ALA through ester cleavage by esterases, have shown superior properties. Approximately 30- to 150-fold lower drug concentrations were required to create comparable amounts of PpIX. Depending on the alkyl chain length used, the highest benefit was obtained with the n-hexyl ester, which recently underwent clinical approval (HexVix from PhotoCure, Norway) for the photodiagnosis of bladder cancer (Witjes et al. 2005).

3 Optical Probes Based on Inorganic Nanoparticles

3.1 Semiconductor Nanocrystals or Quantum Dots

Quantum dots (QDs) are semiconductor nanocrystals consisting of atoms such as Cd, Se, Te, S and Zn. These materials have been extensively studied as fluorescent probes and are primarily gaining interest as fluorescent tags for biological molecules due to their large quantum yield and photostability (Chan et al. 2002; Michalet et al. 2005). They can be prepared with high monodispersity at 2–10 nm in diameter carrying different organic shells, e.g. phospholipids (Dubertret et al. 2002), and are already commercially available (e.g. Quantum Dot Corporation). The size of the QDs can be synthetically controlled such that fluorescence emission bands of narrow bandwith ($\sim$30 nm) covering the VIS to near-infrared spectral range can be obtained (Lim et al. 2003). Figure 6 illustrates the typical broad-band absorption and narrow fluorescence profile of four different QD sizes. Increase in size and modifications to the metal content by incorporating In, As and P into the alloy has lead to a remarkable red-shift of fluorescence beyond 750 nm (Kim et al. 2004, 2005; Zimmer 2006).

QDs have an outstanding potential for cellular high-resolution imaging, single-molecule detection studies on ligand-protein interactions, cell trafficking and molecular diagnostics. In recent publications, different ways to alter the solubility and biocompatibility of QDs and improve their in-vivo properties were addressed, on

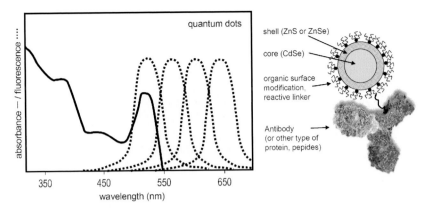

Fig. 6 Illustration of a typical absorption and fluorescence emission pattern of quantum dots. Sketch of the composition of a quantum dot, including the option to attach a reactive linker and conjugate the particle with an antibody

the one hand by surface modifications, such as hydrophilic groups, PEGs, and block polymers (Ballou et al. 2004; Kim and Bawendi 2003; Gao et al. 2004) and on the other hand by adding reactive moieties for bioconjugation with targeting vectors, such as antibodies (Michalet et al. 2005; Wu et al. 2003) and peptides (Akerman et al. 2002). An extensively explored research field has been the use of QDs for the highly sensitive fluorescence guidance to sentinel lymph nodes, pioneered by Frangioni and co-workers, who showed not only a proof of principle but also furthered the instrumental understanding (e.g. aspects of colour coding and image fusion) (Kim et al. 2004; Parungo et al. 2005; Soltesz et al. 2005).

While in-vivo imaging of QDs has shown to be highly efficacious at the animal level, their future as drugs approved for human use is questionable as major issues have still to be addressed, particularly due to the potential long-term toxic effects generated by traces of heavy metals. Therefore, metal-free systems would be beneficial, provided that they exhibit comparable photo-optical properties.

3.2 Other Nanomaterials

Fluorescent nanoparticles based on materials which are either metal-free or have matrices that allow doping with metal atoms are interesting materials (Santra et al. 2004), e.g. ruthenium-doped silica nanoparticles (Santra et al. 2001). Fluorescent dye-loaded nanospheres based on polystyrene have been explored for sentinel node detection (Nakajima et al. 2005) similarly to the application of QDs described above in Sect. 3.1. Targeted gold nanoparticles that are heated up by laser pulses, leading to cell damage, provide a potential extension into therapeutic applications (Pitsillides et al. 2003). Other novel nanoarchitectures are gold nanorods that produced a strong two-photon luminescence, which has shown utility for the imaging of superficial vessels in an animal model (Wang et al. 2005), or surface-modified nanodiamonds, which are extremely photostable and have been used in cellular imaging (Yu et al. 2005).

4 Multi-modality Probes

This section of the review deals with chemical probes which, in addition to being used for optical imaging, have another function, either as an imaging agent in a second diagnostic technique or as a photosensitizer for photodynamic therapy.

A small body of literature exists at the present time to represent this new growing field. It seems natural, with the present optimistic outlook and the expected rapid growth in the field of diagnostic contrast agents, that cross-fertilization between techniques will increase, giving rise to new multimodality probes, which, in contrast to monofunctional probes, potentially offer higher diagnostic value and added product differentiation in the marketplace as competition increases.

These first multimodality probes with relevance to optical imaging have combined fluorescent dyes with imaging ability for MRI based on iron oxide nanoparticle techniques (Koch et al. 2003; Huh et al. 2005; Veiseh et al. 2005). Based on this technology, target-specific delivery via molecular vehicles attached to the coating of the multimodal particle has been extensively elucidated, taking advantage

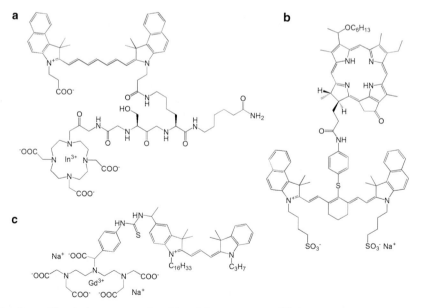

Fig. 7 a–c Chemical structures of multimodality probes. **a** In^{111}-DOTA radiolabeled cyanine dye probe, **b** photosensitizer cyanine dye conjugate and **c** Gd-DTPA cyanine dye for dual MRI/fluorescence

of the dual character, e.g. by correlating cellular fluorescence microscopy with in-vivo MRI and optical imaging (Funovics et al. 2005; Weissleder et al. 2005; Quinti et al. 2006). Other systems comprise radioisotope/PET entities (Pandey et al. 2005; Achilefu et al. 2005; Zhang et al. 2005), and structures for photodynamic therapy (Pandey et al. 2005). Other work by Pandey and co-workers instead combines photodynamic therapy with MRI imaging (Li et al. 2005).

Selected examples of these probes are illustrated in Fig. 7, including work on the imaging of low-density lipoprotein receptors using a probe with a GdDTPA moiety for MRI and a cyanine dye for fluorescent confocal microscopy (Li et al. 2004), a monomolecular agent consisting of a heptamethine carbocyanine and a ^{111}In-DOTA chelate which acts as an antenna for optical and radioisotope imaging (Achilefu et al. 2005; Zhang et al. 2005), and a derivitized pheophorbide photosensitizer that was conjugated with a cyanine dye which showed both efficient tumour imaging and photosensitization (Chen Y et al. 2005).

5 Summary and Conclusion

This review summarises the current state of research in the area of fluorescent probes for optical imaging. It is targeted at readers with a wide range of backgrounds in this subject and, as such, a closer consideration of the probes described should be possible based on any of the following properties of the imaging agent: the photophysical nature (absorption and fluorescence properties), the chemical origin (e.g. biomolecules, small molecules, nanoparticles and combinations thereof), the mode of action (non-targeted, targeted, activatable) of the imaging agent or the disease mechanism (angiogenesis, inflammation, apoptosis, etc.).

As apparent in this and many other articles, there is a large and growing range of optical agents available for biomedical imaging at the research level; this growth being driven in part by the ongoing discovery of new molecular disease targets.

In the field of optical imaging, rapid development is predicted for the future, bringing with it an even greater variety of probes and the foreseeable entry of some of these moieties into the clinical scenario, in the face of increasing challenges to pharmaceutical development. This review documents the proof of utility of the concepts of optical imaging, which provides a solid foundation for its application and future impact on the medical landscape.

References

Achilefu S, Jimenez HN, Dorshow RB, Bugaj JE, Webb EG, Wilhelm RR, Rajagopalan R, Johler J, Erion JL (2002) Synthesis, in vitro receptor binding, and in vivo evaluation of fluorescein and carbocyanine peptide-based optical contrast agents. J Med Chem 45:2003–2015

Achilefu S, Bloch S, Markiewicz MA, Zhong T, Ye Y, Dorshow R, Chance B, Liang K (2005) Synergistic effects of light-emitting probesand peptides for targeting and monitoring integrin expression. Proc Natl Acad Sci USA 102:7976–7981

Aina OH, Marik J, Gandour-Edwards R, Lam KT (2005) Near-infrared optical imaging of ovarian cancer xenografts with novel A3-integrin binding peptide 'OA02'. Mol Imaging 4:439–447

Akerman ME, Chan WC, Laakkonen P, Bhatia SN, Ruoslahti E (2002) Nanocrystal targeting in vivo. Proc Natl Acad Sci USA 99:12617–12621

Ballou B, Fisher GW, Waggoner AS, Farkas DL, Reiland JM, Jaffe R, Mujumdar RB, Mujumdar SR, Hakala TR (1995) Tumor labeling in vivo using cyanine-conjugated monoclonal antibodies. Cancer Immunol Immunother 41:257–263

Ballou B, Lagerholm BC, Ernst LA, Bruchez MP, Waggoner AS (2004) Noninvasive imaging of quantum dots in mice. Bioconjugate Chem 15:79–86

Ballou B, Ernst LA, Waggoner AS (2005) Fluorescence imaging of tumors in vivo. Curr Med Chem 12:795–805

Becker A, Ebert B, Sukowski U, Rinneberg H, Semmler W, Licha K (2000) Macromolecular contrast agents for optical imaging of tumors: indotricarbocyanine-labeled humans serum albumin and transferrin. Photochem Photobiol 72:234–241

Becker A, Hessenius C, Licha K, Ebert B, Sukowski U, Semmler W, Wiedenmann B, Grötzinger C (2001) Receptor-targeted optical imaging of tumors with near-infrared fluorescent ligands. Nat Biotechnol 19:327–331

Berger Y, Greppi A, Siri O, Neier R, Juillerat-Jeanneret L. (2000) Ethylene glycol and amino acid derivatives of 5-aminolevulinic acid as new photosensitizing precursors of protoporphyrin IX in cells. J Med Chem 43:4738–4746

Bhargava S, Licha K, Knaute T, Ebert B, Becker A, Grötzinger C, Hessenius C, Wiedenmann B, Schneider-Mergener J, Volkmer-Engert R (2002) A complete substitutional analysis of VIP for better tumor imaging properties. J Mol Recognit 15:145–153

Birchler M, Neri G, Tarli L, Halin C, Viti F, Neri D (1999a) Infrared photodetection for the in vivo localisation of phage-derived antibodies directed against angiogenic markers. J Immunol Methods 231:239–248

Birchler M, Viti F, Zardi L, Spiess B, Neri D (1999b) Selective targeting and photocoagulation of ocular angiogenesis mediated by a phage-derived human antibody fragment. Nat Biotechnol 17:984–988

Bornhop DJ, Griffin JM, Goebel TS, Sudduth MR, Bell B, Motamedi M (2003) Luminescent lanthanide chelate contrast agents and detection of lesions in the hamster oral cancer model. Appl Spectr 57:1216–1222

Bremer C, Tung CH, Weissleder R (2001) In vivo molecular target assessment of matrix metalloproteinase inhibition. Nat Med 7:743–748

Bremer C, Tung CH, Bogdanov Jr A, Weissleder R (2002) Imaging of differential protease expression in breast cancers for detection of aggressive tumor phenotypes. Radiology 222:814–818

Bugaj JE, Achilefu S, Dorshow RB, Rajagopalan R. (2001) Novel fluorescent contrast agents for optical imaging of in vivo tumors based on a receptor-targeted dye-peptide conjugate platform. J Biomed Opt 6:122–133

Chan WC, Maxwell DJ, Gao X, Bailey RE, Han M, Nie S (2002) Luminescent quantum dots for multiplexed biological detection and imaging. Curr Opin Biotechnol 13:40–46

Chen WT, Mahmood U, Weissleder R, Tung CH (2005) Arthritis imaging using a near-infrared fluorescence folate-targeted probe. Arthritis Res Ther 7:R310–R317

Chen X, Conti PS, Moats RA (2004) In vivo near-infrared fluorescence imaging of integrin $\alpha v\beta 3$ in brain tumor xenografts. Cancer Res 64:8009–8014

Chen Y, Zheng G, Zhang ZH, Blessington D, Zhang M, Li H, Liu Q, Zhou L, Intes X (2003) Metabolism-enhanced tumor localization by fluorescence imaging: in vivo animal studies. Opt Lett 28:2070–2072

Chen Y, Gryshuk A, Achilefu S, Ohulchansky T, Potter W, Zhong T, Morgan J, Chance B, Prasad PN, Henderson BW, Oseroff A, Pandey RK (2005) A novel approach to a bifunctional photosensitizer for tumor imaging and phototherapy. Bioconjugate Chem 16:1264–1274

Citrin D, Scott T, Sproull M, Menard C, Tofilo PJ, Camphausen K (2004) In vivo tumor imaging using a near-infrared-labeled endostatin molecule. Int J Radiation Oncology Biol Phys 58:536–541

Dubertret B, Skourides P, Norris DJ, Noireaux V, Brivanlou AH, Libchaber A (2002) In vivo imaging of quantum dots encapsulated in phospholipid micelles. Science 298:1759–1762

Ebert B, Sukowski U, Grosenick D, Wabnitz H, Moesta KT, Licha K, Becker A, Semmler W, Schlag PM, Rinneberg H (2001) Near-infrared fluorescent dyes for enhanced contrast in optical mammography: phantom experiments. J Biomed Opt 6:134–140

Folli S, Westermann P, Braichotte D, Pelegrin A, Wagnieres G, van den Bergh H, Mach JP, (1994) Antibody-indocyanin conjugates for immunophotodetection of human squamous cell carcinoma in nude mice. Cancer Res 54:2643–2649

Fukuda H, Casas A, Batlle A (2005) Aminolevulinic acid: from its unique biological function to its star role in photodynamic therapy. Int J Biochem Cell Biol 37:272–276

Funovics M, Montet X, Reynolds F, Weissleder R, Josephson L (2005) Nanoparticles for the optical imaging of tumor E-selectin. Neoplasia 7:904–911

Gao X, Cui Y, Levenson RM, Chung LW, Nie S (2004) In vivo cancer targeting and imaging with semiconductor quantum dots. Nat Biotechnol 22:969–976

Gurfinkel M, Thompson AB, Ralston W, Troy TL, Moore AL, Moore TA, Gust JD, Tatman D, Reynolds JS, Muggenburg B, Nikula K, Pandey R, Mayer RH, Hawrysz DJ, Sevick-Muraca EM (2000) Pharmacokinetics of ICG and HPPH-car for the detection of normal and tumor tissue using fluorescence, near-infrared reflectance imaging: a case study. Photochem Photobiol 72:94–102

Hintersteiner M, Enz A, Frey P, Jaton AL, Kinzy W, Kneuer R, Neumann U, Rudin M, Staufenbriel M, Stoeckli M, Wiederholt KH, Gremlich HU (2005) In vivo detection of amyloid-beta deposits by near-infrared imaging using an oxazine-derivative probe. Nat Biotechnol 23:577–583

Hödl C, Strauss WSL, Sailer R, Heger C, Steiner R, Haslinger E, Schramm HW (2004) A novel, high-affinity, fluorescent progesterone receptor antagonist: synthesis and in vitro studies. Bioconjug Chem 15:359–365

Hogan RN, Zimmerman CF (1997) Sodium fluorescein and other tissue dyes. In: Zimmerman TJ (ed) Textbook of ocular pharmacology. Lippincott-Raven, Philadelphia, p 849

Huh YM, Jun YW, Song HT, Kim S, Choi JS, Lee JH, Yoon S, Kim KS, Shin JS, Suh JS, Cheon J (2005) In vivo magnetic resonance detection of cancer by using multifunctional magnetic nanocrystals. J Am Chem Soc 127:12387–12391

Humblet V, Lapidus R, Williams LR, Tsukamoto T, Rojas C, Majer P, Hin B, Ohnishi S, De Grand AM, Zaheer A, Renze JT, Nakayama A, Slusher BS, Frangioni JV (2005) High-affinity near-infrared fluorescent small-molecule contrast agents for in vivo imaging of prostate-specific membrane antigen. Mol Imaging 4:448–462

Hyman ES, Hynninen PH (2004) Research advances in the use of tetrapyrrolic photosensitizers for photodynamic therapy. J Photochem Photobiol B: Biol 73:1–28

Jaffer FH, Tung CH, Gerszten RE, Weissleder R (2002) In vivo imaging of thrombin activity in experimental thrombi with thrombin-sensitive near-infrared molecular probe. Arterioscler Thromb Vasc Biol 22:1929–1935

Josephson L, Kircher MF, Mahmood U, Tang Y, Weissleder R (2002) Near-infrared fluorescent nanoparticles as combined MR/optical imaging probes. Bioconjugate Chem. 13:554–560

Ke S, Wen X, Gurfinkel M, Charnsangarvej C, Wallace S, Sevick-Muraca EM, Li C (2003) Near-infrared optical imaging of epidermal growth factor receptor in breast cancer xenographs. Cancer Res 63:7870–7875

Kim SW, Bawendi MG (2003) Oligomeric ligands for luminescent and stable nanocrystal quantum dots. J Am Chem Soc 125:14652–14653

Kim SW, Lim YT, Soltesz EG, DeGrand AM, Lee J, Nakayama A, Parker JA, Mihaljevic T, Laurence RG, Dor DM, Cohn LH, Bawendi RG, Frangioni JV (2004) Near-infrared fluorescent type II qunatum dots for sentinel lymph node mapping. Nat Biotechnol 22:93–97

Kim SW, Zimmer JP, Ohnishi S, Tracy JB, Frangioni JV, Bawendi MG (2005) Engineering InAs(x)P(1-x)/InP/ZnSe III-V alloyed core/shell quantum dots for the near-infrared. J Am Chem Soc 127:10526–10532

Koch AM, Reynolds F, Kircher MF, Merkle HP, Weissleder R, Josephson L (2003) Uptake and metabolism of a dual fluorochrome Tat-nanoparticle in HeLa cells. Bioconjugate Chem 14:1115–1121

Kremer P, Wunder A, Sinn H, Haase T, Rheinwald M, Zillmann U, Albert FK, Kunze S (2000) Laser-induced fluorescence detection of malignant gliomas using fluorescein-labeled serum albumin: experimental and preliminary clinical results. Neurol Res 22:481–489

Lange N, Jichlinski P, Zellweger M, Forrer M, Marti A, Guillou L, Kucera P, Wagnières G, van den Bergh H (1997) Photodetection of early human bladder cancer based on the fluorescence of 5-aminolaevulinic acid hexylester-induced protoporphyrin IX: a pilot study. Br J Cancer 80:185–193

Law B, Curino A, Bugge TH, Weissleder R, Tung CH (2004) Design, synthesis, and Characterization of urokinase plasminogen-activator-sensitive near-infrared reporter. Chem Biol 11:99–106

Lenkinski RE, Ahmed M, Zaheer A, Frangioni JV, Goldberg SN (2003) Near-infrared fluorescence imaging of microcalcification in an animal model of breast cancer. Acad Radiol 10:1159–1164

Li G, Slansky A, Dobhal MP, Goswami LN, Graham A, Chen Y, Kanter P, Alberico RA, Spernyak J, Morgan J, Mazurchuk R, Oseroff A, Grossman Z, Pandey RK (2005) Chlorophyll-a analogues conjugated with aminobenzyl-DTPA as potential bifunctional agents for magnetic resonance imaging and photodynamic therapy. Bioconjugate Chem 16:32–42

Li H, Chen J, Zhang M, Zhang Z, Benaron D, Chance B, Glickson J, Zheng G (2004) NIR optical probes targeting glucose transporters. Proc SPIE 5329:254–261

Li H, Gray BD, Corbin I, Lebherz C, Choi H, Lund-Katz S, Wilson JM, Glickson JD, Zhou R (2004) MR and fluorescent imaging of low-density lipoprotein receptors. Acad Radiol 11:1251–1259

Licha K (2002) Contrast agents for optical imaging. In: Krause W (ed) Topics in current chemistry, vol 222. Springer, Heidelberg, pp 1–29

Licha K, Riefke B, Ntziachristos V, Becker A, Chance B. Semmler W (2000) Hydrophilic cyanine dyes as contrast agents for near-infrared tumor imaging: synthesis, photophysical properties and spectroscopic in vivo characterization. Photochem Photobiol 72:392–398

Licha K, Debus N, Ebert B, Vollmer-Emig S, Hasbach M, Sydow S, Stibenz D, Semmler W, Bührer C, Schirner M, Tauber R (2005) Optical molecular imaging of lymph nodes using a targeted vascular contrast agent. J Biomed Optics 10(4), 041205

Lim YT, Kim S, Nakayama A, Stott NE, Bawendi MG, Frangioni JV (2003) Selection of quantum dot wavelengths for biomedical assays and imaging. Mol Imaging 2:50–64

Manning HC, Goebel T, Thompson RC, Price RR, Lee H, Bornhop DJ (2004) Targeted molecular imaging agents for cellular-scale bimodal imaging. Bioconjug Chem 15:1488–1495

Marten K, Bremer C, Khazaie K, Sameni M, Sloane B, Tung CH, Weissleder R (2002) Detection of dysplastic intestinal adenomas using enzyme-sensing molecular beacons in mice. Gastroenterol 122:406–414

Matter CM, Schuler PK, Alessi P, Meier P, Ricci R, Zhang D, Halin C, Castellani P, Zardi L, Hofer CK, Montani M, Neri D, Luscher TF (2004) Molecular imaging of atherosclerotic plaques using a human antibody against the extra-domain B of fibronectin. Circ Res 95:1225–1233

McGreevy JM, Cannon MJ, Grissom CB (2003) Minimally invasive lymphatic mapping using fluorescently labeled vitamin B12. J Surg Res 111:38–44

Messerli SH, Prabhakar S, Tang Y, Shah K, Cortes M, Murthy V, Weissleder R, Breakefield SO, Tung CH (2004) A novel method for imaging of apopthosis using a caspase-1 near-infrared fluorescent probe. Neoplasia 6:95–105

Michalet X, Pinaud FF, Bentolila LA, Tsay JM, Doose S, Li JJ, Sundaresan G, Wu AM, Gambhir SS, Weiss S (2005) Quantum dots for live cells, in vivo imaging, and diagnostics. Science 307:538–544

Mier W, Beijer B, Graham K, Hull WE (2002) Fluorescent somatostatin receptor probes for the intraoperative detection of tumor tissue with long-wavelength visible light. Bioorg Med Chem 10:2543–2552

Moon WK, Lin Y, O'Loughlin T, Tang Y, Kim DE, Weissleder R, Tung CH (2003) Enhanced tumor detection using a folate receptor-targeted near-infrared fluorochrome conjugate, Bioconjug Chem 14:539–545

Nakayama A, del Monte F, Hajjar RJ, Frangioni JV (2002) Functional near-infrared fluorescence imaging for cardiac surgery and targeted gene therapy. Mol Imaging 1:365–377

Nakajima M, Takeda M, Kobayashi M, Suzuki S, Ohuchi N (2005) Nano-sized fluorescent particles as new tracers for sentinel node detection: experimental model for decision of appropriate size and wavelength. Cancer Sci 96:353–356

Ntziachristos V, Yodh AG, Schnall M, Chance B (2000) Concurrent MRI and diffuse optical tomography of breast after indocyanine green enhancement. Proc Natl Acad Sci USA 97: 2767–2772

Nyman ES, Hynninen PH (2004) Research advances in the use of tetrapyrrolic photosensitizers for photodynamic therapy. J Photochem Photobiol B 73:1–28

Pandey SK, Gryshuk AL, Sajjad M, Zheng X, Chen Y, Abouzeid MM, Morgan J, Charamisinau I, Nabi HA, Oseroff A, Pandey RK (2005) Multimodality agents for tumor imaging (PET, fluorescence) and photodynamic therapy. A possible "see and treat" approach. J Med Chem 48:6286–6295

Parungo CP, Ohnishi S, Kim SW, Kim S, Laurence RG, Soltesz EG, Chen FY, Colson YL, Cohn LH, Bawendi MG, Frangioni JV (2005) Intraoperative identification of esophageal sentinel lymph nodes with near-infrared fluorescence imaging. J Thorac Cardiovasc Surg 129:844–850

Perlitz C, Licha K, Scholle FD, Ebert B, Bahner M, Hauff P, Moesta KT, Schirner M (2005) Comparison of two carbocyanine-based dyes for fluorescence optical imaging. J Fluoresc 15: 443–454

Petrovsky A, Schellenberger E, Josephson L, Weissleder R, Bogdanov A Jr (2003) Near-infrared fluorescent imaging of tumor apoptosis. Cancer Res 63:1936–1942

Pham W, Weissleder R, Tung CH (2002) An azulene dimer as a near-infrared quencher. Angew Chem Int Ed 41:3659–3662

Pham W, Choi Y, Weissleder R, Tung CH (2004) Developing a peptide-based near-infrared molecular probe for protease sensing. Bioconjug Chem 15:1403–1407

Pitsillides CM, Joe EK, Wei X, Anderson RR, Lin CP (2003) Selective cell targeting with light-absorbing microparticles and nanoparticles. Biophys J 84:4023–4032

Pu Y, Wang WB, Tang GC, Zeng F, Achilefu S, Vitenson JH, Sawczuk I, Peters S, Lombardo JM, Alfano RR (2005) Spectral polarization imaging of human prostate cancer tissue using a near-infrared receptor-targeted contrast agent. Technol Cancer Res Treat 4:429–436

Quinti L, Weissleder R, Tung CH (2006) A fluorescent nanosensor for apoptotic cells. Nano Lett 6:488–490

Richard G, Soubrane G, Yanuzzi L (eds) (1998) Fluorescein and ICG angiography. Thieme, Stuttgart

Riefke B, Licha K, Nolte D, Ebert B, Rinneberg H, Semmler W (1998) Tumor detection with cyanine dye-poly(ethylene glycol) conjugates as contrast agents for near-infrared imaging. Proceedings of SPIE 3196:103–110

Santra S, Zhang P, Wang K, Tapec R, Tan W (2001) Conjugation of biomolecules with luminophore-doped silica nanoparticles for photostable biomarkers. Anal Chem 73:4988–4993

Santra S, Xu J, Wang K, Tan W (2004) Luminescent nanoparticle probes for bioimaging. J Nanosci Nanotechnol 4:590–599

Schellenberger EA, Bogdanov Jr A, Petrovsky A, Ntziachristos V, Weissleder R, Josephson L (2003) Optical imaging of apoptosis as a biomarker of tumor response to chemotherapy. Neoplasia 5:187–192

Schellenberger EA, Weissleder R, Josephson L (2004) Optimal modification of annexin V with fluorescent dyes. Chembiochem 4:271–274

Soltesz EG, Kim S, Laurence RG, DeGrand AM, Parungo CP, Dor DM, Cohn LH, Bawendi MG, Frangioni JV, Mihaljevic T (2005) Intraoperative sentinel lymph node mapping of the lung using near-infrared fluorescent quantum dots. Ann Thorac Surg 79:269–277

Tadatsu M, Ito S, Muguruma N, Kusaka Y, Inayama K, Bandu T, Tadatsu Y, Okamoto K, Ii K, Nagao Y, Sano S, Taue H (2003) A new infrared fluorescent-labeling agent and labeled antibody for diagnosing microcancers. Bioorg Med Chem 11:3289–3294

Tung CH, Lin Y, Moon WK, Weissleder R (2002) A receptor-targeted near-infrared fluorescence probe for in vivo tumor imaging. Chembiochem 3:784–786

Uehlinger P, Zellweger M, Wagnières G, Juillerat-Jeanneret L, van den Bergh H, Lange N (2000) 5-Aminolevulinic acid and its derivatives: physical chemical properties and protoporphyrin IX formation in cultured cells. J Photochem Photobiol 54:72–80

Veiseh O, Sun C, Gunn J, Kohler N, Gabikian P, Lee D, Bhattarai N, Ellenbogen R, Sze R, Hallahan A, Olson J, Zhang M (2005) Optical and MRI multifunctional nanoprobe for targeting gliomas. Nano Lett. 5:1003–1008

Wang D, Miller S, Sima M, Kopecková P, Kopecek J (2003) Synthesis and evaluation of water-soluble polymeric bone-targeted drug delivery systems. Bioconjug Chem 14:853–859

Wang H, Huff TB, Zweifel DA, He W, Low PS, Wei A, Cheng JX (2005) In vitro and in vivo two-photon luminescence imaging of single gold nanorods. Proc Natl Acad Sci USA 102: 15752–15756

Wang W, Ke K, Wu Q, Charnsangavej C, Gurfinkel M, Gelovani JG, JameAbbruzzese JL, Sevick-Muraca EM, Li C (2004) Near-infrared optical imaging of integrin αvß3 in human tumor xenografts. Mol Imaging 3:343–351

Weissleder R, Tung CH, Mahmood U, Bognanov A (1999) In vivo imaging of tumors with protease-activated near-infrared fluorescent probes. Nat Biotech 17:375–378

Weissleder R, Kelly K, Sun EY, Shtatland T, Josephson L (2005) Cell-specific targeting of nanoparticles by multivalent attachment of small molecules. Nat Biotechnol 23:1418–1423

Witjes JA, Moonen PM, van der Heijden AG (2005) Comparison of hexaminolevulinate based flexible and rigid fluorescence cystoscopy with rigid white light cystoscopy in bladder cancer: results of a prospective Phase II study. Eur Urol 47:319–322

Wu X, Liu H, Liu J, Haley KN, Treadway JA, Larson JP, Ge N, Peale F, Bruchez MP (2003) Immunofluorescent labeling of cancer marker Her2 and other cellular targets with semiconductor quantum dots. Nat Biotechnol 21:41–46

Ye Y, Bloch S, Kao J, Achilefu S (2005) Multivalent carbocyanine molecular probes: synthesis and applications. Bioconjug Chem 16:51–61

Yu SJ, Kang MW, Chang HC, Chen KM, Yu YC (2005) Bright fluorescent nanodiamonds: no photobleaching and low cytotoxicity. J Am Chem Soc 127:17604–17605

Zaheer A, Lenkinski RE, Mahmood A, Jones AG, Cantley LC, Frangioni JV (2001) In vivo near-infrared fluorescence imaging of osteoblastic activity. Nat Biotechnol 19:1148–1154

Zhang M, Zhang Z, Blessington B, Li H, Busch TM, Madrak V, Miles J, Chance B, Glickson JD, Zheng G (2003) Pyropheophorbide 2-deoxyglucosamide: A new photosensitizer targeting glucose transporters. Bioconjug Chem 14:709–714

Zhang Z, Achilefu S (2004) Synthesis and evaluation of polyhydroxylated near-infrared carbocyanine molecular probes. Org Lett 6:2067–2070

Zhang Z, Li H, Lui Q, Zhou L, Zhang M, Luo Q, Glickson J, Chance B, Zheng G (2004) Metabolic imaging of tumors using intrinsic and extrinsic fluorescent markers. Biosens Bioelectron 20:643–650

Zhang Z, Liang K, Bloch S, Berezin M, Achilefu S (2005) Monomolecular multimodal fluorescence-radioisotope imaging agents. Bioconjugate Chem. 16:1232–1239

Zheng G, Li H, Yang K, Blessington D, Licha K, Lund-Katz S, Chance B, Glickson JD (2002a) Tricarbocyanine cholesteryl laurates labeled LDL: new near infrared fluorescent probes (NIRFs) for monitoring tumors and gene therapy of familial hypercholesterolemia. Bioorg Med Chem Lett 12:1485–1488

Zheng G, Li H, Zhang M, Lund-Katz S, Chance B, Glickson JD (2002b) Low-density lipoprotein reconstituted by pyropheophorbide cholesteryl oleate as target-specific photosensitizer. Bioconjug Chem 13:392–396

Zimmer JP, Kim SW, Ohnishi S, Tanaka E, Frangioni JV, Bawendi MG (2006) Size series of small indium arsenide-zinc selenide core-shell nanocrystals and their application to in vivo imaging. J Am Chem Soc 128:2526–2527

Ultrasound Contrast Agents
for Molecular Imaging

Peter Hauff(✉), Michael Reinhardt, and Stuart Foster

Abstract The successful use of targeted ultrasound contrast agents (USCAs) for qualitative US-based imaging has been shown by several academic and industrial research groups in different animal models. Furthermore, techniques have been developed that enable the in-vivo quantification of targeted microbubbles (MBs). USCAs for quantitative functional and molecular imaging in small animals can be used for a more detailed characterization of new and established disease models and provide quantitative biological insights into the interaction between drug and target or target and disease in living animals.

The advantages of such contrast agents in research and development are seen to be as follows:

- new functional or molecular findings in the complex biology of disease development
- these findings can lead to new therapeutic strategies or drug candidates
- a better understanding of the treatment effects of new and existing drug candidates

Peter Hauff

Global Drug Discovery, Bayer Schering Pharma AG, 13342 Berlin, Germany

peter.hauff@bayerhealthcare.com

W. Semmler and M. Schwaiger (eds.), *Molecular Imaging I.*
Handbook of Experimental Pharmacology 185/I.
© Springer-Verlag Berlin Heidelberg 2008

- a more sensitive and specific characterization of early treatment effects in living animals
- identification of in-vivo biomarkers for translational medicine

Further outcomes are seen in speeding up the evaluation of new drug compounds and in a reduction of the number of animals used for biomedical research.

1 Introduction

The term "molecular imaging" describes a relatively new and fascinating technology that opens the possibility for the noninvasive examination of molecular mechanisms. The in-vivo imaging of processes at the cellular and molecular level is an important part in better understanding physiological and pathophysiological procedures at the molecular level and offers new opportunities for diagnosing and treating oncological, cardiovascular and other illnesses (Weissleder and Mahmood 2001). Molecular imaging shifts the focus of diagnostics from macrophysiological processes and structural changes at the organ level toward initial changes at the molecular and cellular level. This form of imaging does, however, have two rudimentary requirements: on the one hand, specific probes ("molecular probes") are needed, which interact with molecular target structures ("molecular targets") and thereby labeling them. On the other hand, these probes have to possess the ability of being visualized by appropriate imaging procedures. Apart from these requirements, there are further specifications to be met by the molecular imaging, such as high sensitivity, high specificity of the probes for the molecular target, the highest possible spatial resolution and the possibility of quantifying the signals of target-bound probes. PET and SPECT are already well established molecular imaging technologies in clinical diagnostics by the detection of radioactively labeled probes. However, these procedures still have a low spatial resolution. Nonetheless, using image fusion techniques in combination with high-resolution imaging procedures, such as CT or MRT with PET or SPECT images, presently improves the anatomical assignment of molecular information. The suitability of molecular imaging has already been established at the preclinical level for other procedures, such as optical, magnetic and ultrasound imaging technologies.

2 Ultrasound Contrast Agents (USCAs)

Even the word combination "ultrasound contrast agent" indicates that it is a medium which results in contrast when used with ultrasonic waves. Contrast actually defines the intensity ratio of two neighboring pixels, shown in the image replication. This also means, in the broader sense of ultrasonic imaging, the echogenicity ratio of two neighboring anatomical structures. If neighboring structures in the B-mode possess the same echogenicity, then we talk about isodense contrast and discrimination between these structures being impossible in such situations. On the other hand, neighboring structures can be differentiated sonographically very well in the B-mode if they exhibit different echogenicities. The structure with the higher echogenicity is also called hyperdense and that with the lesser echogenicity is referred to as hypodense. Unfortunately, many pathologies cannot be discriminated from the surrounding tissue due to their isodensity. However, such a lesion would become visible if either the signal of the tumor itself or the signal intensity (SI) of the surrounding tissue could be changed in any direction. This becomes possible with USCA in many cases, because the kinetics of USCA is sometimes different for a pathology compared with the surrounding tissue. Thus, the concentration of the USCA is then quite different for the adjacent tissues.

2.1 Overview

Gas bubbles have proven to be particularly advantageous as a USCA, since gases possess low acoustic impedance (low density and thus a low acoustic wave propagation speed) when compared with the surrounding tissue. The large differences in acoustic impedance between gases and tissue lead to an intensified reflection of acoustic waves, the impedance jump, at their interface. This phenomenon was first described by Gramiak and Shah in 1968, when they observed intensified reflections in the ultrasonic image following the intraaortal administration of physiological saline solution to a patient. They discovered that minuscule, highly reflexive air bubbles in the injected liquid were responsible for this observation. As a result of this observation, various solutions (saline solutions, plasma expanders, X-ray contrast agents or albumin solutions), which had to be shaken or treated mechanically in order to form gas bubbles, were tested and/or clinically used in order to improve sonography, mainly in cardiology (Chiang et al. 1986; Berwing and Schleppe 1988; Keller 1988) but also in other indications such as the liver (Mattrey 1983) and brain (Simon et al. 1990). The gas bubbles that resulted from these aforementioned manual methods, however, had poorly defined sizes and were hardly characterized in their acoustic behavior with respect to various ultrasonic parameters. Since these procedures were not standardized, there were also problems with reproducibility of the ultrasound contrast effects (Lange 1986). The above-mentioned preparations also lacked toxicological safety testing; adverse reactions were also reported in individual cases (Lee and Ginzton 1983). Due to the high potential benefit of such gas bubbles for an improved clinical sonography, the pharmaceutical industry decided on the focused development of a USCA as a diagnostic product. Accordingly, it was in 1991 when Echovist (Schering), the first standardized USCA, was made commercially available for use in right-heart diagnosis (Schlief 1997), after which further indications were to follow. The rapid research and development in this area led to new USCA formulations and the identification of many possible uses in the areas of anatomical, functional and molecular diagnostics. Apart from the diagnostic use of USCAs, their use in therapeutic approaches was and is being additionally examined (Hauff et al. 2005). According to the current point of view, the various USCA formulations can be divided into six categories based on their morphology, how they function and their indication (cf. Table 1).

In principle, USCAs are minuscule gas microbubbles with a size in the vicinity of 1–5 µm, which are stabilized with a thin shell (cf. Fig. 1). Various shell-forming materials and gases provide these USCAs with varying acoustic characteristics and ranges of application.

Due to their size, the USCA bubbles cannot leave the intravascular space and, therefore, remain in the blood pool for several minutes following intravenous injection. There, they are destroyed either by ultrasonic effect or metabolic processes, whereby the gas set free dissolves and/or the gases are exhaled through the lungs when slightly soluble gases have been used. The shell material is metabolized. Since

Table 1 Organization of the USCA formulation into categories on the basis of their research and development as related to time

Category	Formulation	Characteristics
1	Free gas bubble	Dissolves rapidly in blood and does not pass the capillary bed of the lung (right-heart CA)
2	Encapsulated gas bubble with a soft elastic lipid or protein shell (soft shell)	Stabilized gas bubble, which can pass the capillary bed of the lung (CA for the entire cardiovascular system)
3	Encapsulated soft-shell gas bubble, for which slightly soluble gases are used (e.g., perfluoro gases)	Gases with longer acoustic life span in the cardiovascular-system
4	Encapsulated gas bubble with a stable shell consisting of biodegradable polymers such as polylactide or cyanoacrylate (hard shell)	Gas bubbles with longer half-live and specific acoustic characteristics, such as stimulated acoustic emission (SAE)
5	Encapsulated gas bubble with target-specific ligands on the shell surface	USCA for molecular imaging
6	Gas bubbles as carriers of therapeutic substances	Gas bubbles as drug delivery system (DDS)

Ultrasound Contrast Agent (USCA)

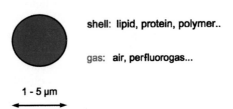

shell: lipid, protein, polymer..

gas: air, perfluorogas...

1 - 5 µm

Fig. 1 Schematic diagram demonstrating the possible compositions of USCA bubbles

the gas microbubbles (MBs) have a smaller diameter than do erythrocytes, there is no danger of capillary embolization.

2.2 USCA for Molecular Imaging – Mode of Action

The molecular imaging with ultrasound requires the use of specially modified MBs, which can label molecular targets as probes. There are two described methods for MB targeting of appropriate targets: (1) passive targeting and (2) active targeting. *Passive targeting* is a rather nonspecific target enhancement by MBs without the use of antibodies. In contrast to this, *active targeting* attaches special ligands, such as antibodies, peptides, polysaccharides or aptamers to the surface of the MBs, which make it possible to selectively bind these MBs to the desired cellular epitopes or receptors (Lanza and Wickline 2001; Dayton and Ferrara 2002).

2.2.1 Passive Targeting

Passive targeting is a nonspecific accumulation of MBs at the target site after their administration which does not require a shell-labeling with specific ligands. The desired mechanism of passive targeting can be specified by a targeted modulation of the MBs' morphology, such as size, chemical properties and electrical charge of the shell, as well as the type of encapsulated gas, but also via the route of injection and by physiological processes of the immune system (cf. Fig. 2).

Thus far, there have been three principal mechanisms described for passive targeting:

- Phagocytosis
- Interaction with cell membranes and
- Lymph flow transport

passive targeting with microbubbles (MBs)

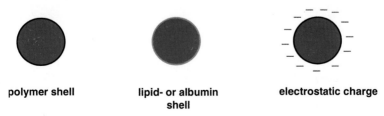

polymer shell   lipid- or albumin   electrostatic charge
                              shell

Fig. 2 Principle of passively targeted MBs

2.2.2 Active Targeting

With active targeting, as opposed to passive targeting, special molecular structures are targeted by specific binding partners. On the one hand, this requires knowledge of the molecular targets within the living organism in certain physiological and pathophysiological situations, and on the other hand, the possibility of producing specific signal emitters that are capable of recognizing appropriate molecular structures and bind strongly with them. The revolutionary progress made in biotechnology, such as in the finalization of the Human Genome Project and the associated intensive research in the area of proteomics, as well as in bioinformatics, has led to an improved understanding of the molecular processes at the core of disease. Building thereupon, modern medicinal products already selectively intervene in certain key molecular processes. Aside from their use in treatment, these new findings are also suited for the further development of diagnostic imaging. With molecular imaging, new paths are opening for the diagnosis of disease years before the occurrence of anatomical and physiological changes. In relation to this, treatment can be better targeted and therapeutic effect better monitored. Also, the use of molecular imaging in biomedical research for discovering pathophysiological mechanisms in the emergence and development of disease processes in appropriate animal models, and the possibility of thereby developing new therapeutic approaches, is not to be underestimated.

The manufacture of specific USCAs for active targeting has only become successful in the past decade and their diagnostic potential is presently being intensively examined, exclusively in the area of preclinical application. Specific USCAs generally consist of a signal-emitting element, a stabilized gas bubble (signaling moiety) and ligands, which target molecular structures (targeting moiety) that are fastened to the surface of the MBs' encasement (MB shell). Depending on the molecular target, these ligands can be antibodies, peptides, polysaccharides or aptamers (cf. Fig. 3).

Apart from the possible differences in the morphology of the signal emitters, such as the use of various gases or shell materials, there are also different strategies for

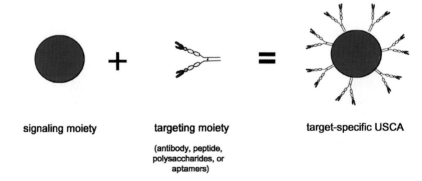

signaling moiety   targeting moiety   target-specific USCA

(antibody, peptide,
polysaccharides, or
aptamers)

Fig. 3 Principle of actively targeted MBs. The conjunction of a targeting moiety with the signaling moiety results in target-specific MBs

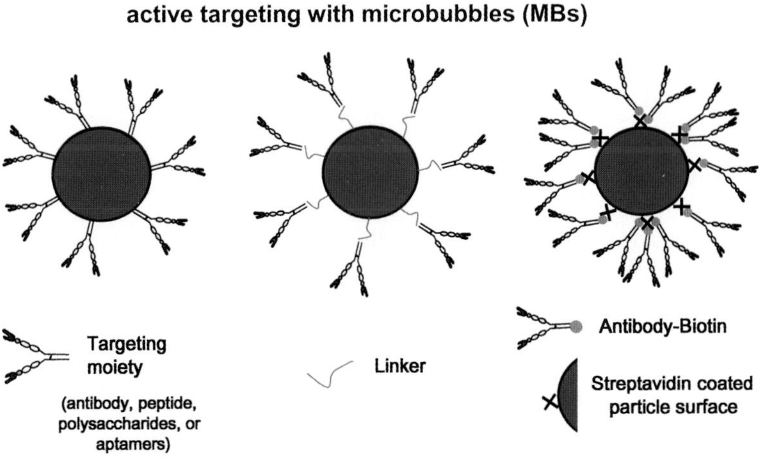

active targeting with microbubbles (MBs)

Targeting moiety
(antibody, peptide, polysaccharides, or aptamers)

Linker

Antibody-Biotin

Streptavidin coated particle surface

Fig. 4 Strategies for active targeted MBs. Actively targeted MBs can be produced by different coupling strategies depending on the targeting moiety (e.g., antibodies, peptides, polysaccharides, or aptamers)

producing a connection of ligands to the MBs' shell. Usually, this strategy depends on the physicochemical characteristics of the shell material (cf. Fig. 4). In principle, there are two coupling strategies: (1) the direct and (2) the indirect connection of the ligands to the covering material. In the case of the indirect connection, a so-called linker is connected between the MB shell and the ligands. This is necessary in such cases, where there is no direct coupling between MB shell and ligands possible or when the ligand does not extend far enough from the encasement into the outside environment after direct coupling and thus is not in a position to connect to the molecular targets structures. In this case, the linker works as a spacer to the MB's surface. In both the coupling strategies, the linker or ligand can either be integrated during the production process of a stabilized MB into the shell or after manufacture of the MBs, it can be attached through covalent or noncovalent procedures (Klibanov 1999, 2005).

The biotin-streptavidin system is also used in the majority of preclinical trials with specific USCAs. The particular advantages are in the high flexibility in using various biotinylated ligands, which bind firmly to streptavidin-carrying MBs due to the high affinity between biotin and streptavidin. Even if this type of formulation is not suitable for clinical use, due to the allergic risk that streptavidin presents to humans, above all in the case of repeated use, this modular system does, however, offer a broad field of application for various indications in biomedical research.

3 Applications for Molecular Ultrasound Imaging

3.1 Passively Targeted

3.1.1 Phagocytosis

Macrophages and microphages of the cellular immune system have, among other things, the task of freeing the human and animal organism by means of phagocytosis of corpuscle components, such as foreign matter, microorganisms or the body's own cells, which have died. By using this physiological process, a selective enhancement of MBs in organs of the reticuloendothelial system (RES) can be attained following intravascular administration. In order to be able to maintain the acoustic activity of phagocyted MBs for as long a time as possible, they should have a relatively stable encapsulation, preferably made of a biodegradable polymer, to avoid rapid lysis in the phagolysosomes. One such USCA is particularly well suited for use in the sonographic detection of isodense, neoplastic change in the liver, since it contains hardly any phagocyting cells (Hauff et al. 1997; Bauer et al. 1999). Additionally, Lindner et al. (2000) were able to show that activated neutrophil granulocytes engulf and absorb MBs, which are surrounded with an albumin or a lipid shell, particularly well during inflammatory processes. As an explanation for this, they were able to detect adhesion caused by ß$_2$-integrin Mac-1 (in MBs with an albumin encasement) or a C3 complement (in MBs with a lipid encasement). In more extensive in-vivo experiments with inflammation models in mice (using TNF-α), in rats (ischemia-reperfusion of the kidneys) or in dogs (ischemia-reperfusion of the myocardium) it could also be shown that the MBs containing leukocytes deposit on activated endothelial cells and are sonographically detectable (Lindner et al. 2000; Christiansen et al. 2002). Moreover, the process of the leukocyte adhesion of lipid-encased MBs was able to be clearly strengthened by the addition of the phospholipid phosphatidylserine, a constituent of cell membranes during the production of MBs. In the end, this caused an increased phagocytosis of MBs, therefore resulting in a stronger signal yield and/or imaging of inflammatory processes.

The examples mentioned here impressively demonstrate the potential of USCA for the diagnostics of neoplasias in organs of the reticuloendothelial system and of inflammatory processes.

3.1.2 Interaction with Cell Membranes

Aside from the adhesion of lipid or albumin-encapsulated MBs to activated leukocytes caused by ß$_2$-integrin, Mac 1 and C3 complement as described above, tests were also conducted with reference to the MBs' surface charge and the interaction with cell membranes. For this purpose, Fischer et al. (2002) manufactured lipid encapsulated MBs with negative and neutral surface charges and, in a preliminary study using intravital microscopy, examined the intravascular behavior of MBs in the cremaster muscle of wild-type and C3-deficient mice. Here, negatively charged MBs showed significant retention in the blood vessels of the cremaster muscle, which was not observed with the neutral MBs. This retention was clearly less in C3-deficient mice, so that the C3-mediated complement reaction was postulated as an essential mechanism of the retention and could be confirmed in vitro. In a subsequent ultrasonic investigation in the myocardium of dogs, a myocardial contrast could only be achieved with the negatively charged MBs 10 min after intravenous injection. The neutral MBs did not show any contrast enhancement in this case. These data support the results of the intravital microscopy and underline the meaning of the MBs' surface charge on the pharmacokinetic behavior.

3.1.3 Lymph Flow Transport

A further possibility for passive targeting is to alter the route of administration for USCAs. Injecting MBs subcutaneously or intracutaneously allows them access to initial lymphatic vessels (= lymphatic capillaries and precollectors) and via interendothelial openings (open junctions or flutter valves) or by transcellular endocytosis or exocytosis and are transported with the lymph flow into the nearest lymph nodes. The size of the MB seems to be of crucial importance. Oussoren et al. (1997) examined the influence of the size of liposomes with respect to their transport from the injection site into the lymphatic vessels and their enhancement in regional lymph nodes (popliteal lymph nodes and iliac lymph nodes) in rats during the period of 52 h after subcutaneous injection above the foot of the right hind leg. Accordingly, they found, for example, that after 52 h only 26% of the liposomes with a size of 40 nm were present; however, there were still 95% of the liposomes with a size of 400 nm in the area of the injection site. In contrast to this, the difference in enhancement was not as clear in the regional lymph nodes, which indicates that larger liposomes become more enhanced in the lymph node than do smaller ones. Hauff et al. (1994) conducted early pilot studies on the possible use of a USCA as an indirect lymphographic agent. These were air bubbles of about 1 μm in the size, which had been stabilized with a biodegradable polymer encasement (polybutyl-cyanoacrylic acid) (Sonavist). Undertaking to clarify this question, dogs were injected with this USCA intracutaneously in several small depots in the distal area of the rear extremities. The sonographic examination took place after 2 h of the animals moving about freely, in order to promote lymph flow and consequently the transport of the MBs. The sonographic examination took place in the color Doppler mode at high mechanical index (MI) while utilizing highly sensitive SAE effect (*see* Sect. 2.3, in the Chapter "Ultrasound Basics" by us in this volume). As proof of MB enhancement, a homogeneous color-coded imaging of all popliteal lymph nodes could be shown. This procedure also made it possible to find popliteal lymph nodes, which could not previously be found using sonography, due to their isodense signals. Additionally, a displacement process was simulated in the lymph nodes of a dog by the intranodal administration of a small volume of an echo-poor substance (ultrasound gel). After USCA administration, this region did not exhibit any MB-induced SAE effects and was, therefore, able to be clearly defined in a size of 2 mm within the lymph node that was contrasted. The signals caused by MBs in the lymph nodes could be shown repeatedly several times by refreshing the MBs from the lymphatic vessel system. In other examinations, Mattrey et al. (2002) as well as Choi et al. (2004) tested an USCA for the indirect lymphography in a VX-2 tumor-bearing (thigh) rabbit. In this case, they were perfluorohexane bubbles in size of between 1 and 3 μm, which had been stabilized with a phospholipid encasement (Imagent). After subcutaneous injection in different regions of the leg with the VX-2 tumor, they were able to depict sonographically in the harmonic B-mode both the MBs during their transport in lymphatic vessels and after their accumulation in the regional lymph node (popliteal node and iliac node). Additionally, they were able to define metastases of the VX-2 tumor in lymph nodes by their lack of contrast.

Although the MBs of both USCAs clearly exceeded the size of the liposomes described by Oussoren et al. (1997), their subcutaneous and/or intracutaneous injection did lead to their enhancement in the regional lymph nodes. Even if a quantity of the MBs transported there remained unidentified, this was sufficient, however, to obtain complete imaging of the lymph nodes, as well as the discrimination of space-filling processes in these lymph nodes.

As a result, USCAs represent an additional alternative for the indirect lymphography as regards the detection and characterization of regional lymph nodes or for finding sentinel lymph nodes in the area of neoplastic change.

3.2 Actively Targeted

The areas of use of actively targeted USCAs are limited to the intravascular region by the size of the MBs (1–5 μm), since they possibly cannot exit the vascular system without assistance following phagocytosis by macrophages. Whether phagocytized MBs actually can gain access to the surrounding tissue by macrophage migration through the vascular endothelia has not yet been sufficiently examined. On the other hand, the endothelial cells of the blood vessels do offer a broad range of indications for molecular ultrasound diagnostics (Hauff et al. 2003), which, among other things, exchange various biological information (e.g., inflammation → immune response) between local tissues and organs and the entire organism . Although the endothelial cells only line the luminal side of vessels as a single cell layer, their estimated total quantity amounts in an adult human to a considerable 6×10^{13} with an estimated total mass of 1 kg and, as such, approximately corresponds to the size of a liver (Simionescu 2000).

Depending on the MBs' morphology and the dose administered, stabilized MBs are completely eliminated from the circulatory system via the reticuloendothelial system within 10–20 min following intravascular injection. In the case of specific MBs, this has the large advantage that the unbound portion is filtered relatively quickly out of the cardiovascular system and that the MB signals then received at the target do come exclusively from specifically bound MBs. This physiological detail results in a high signal-to-noise ratio of target-bound MBs, from just a few minutes after their injection (Hauff et al. 2004).

Active targeting of various molecules was able to be represented in preclinical trials for indications such as tumor angiogenesis, inflammation, thrombosis and lymphography.

3.2.1 Neoangiogenesis

The process of tumor neoangiogenesis has meanwhile been sufficiently described and there is detailed information on molecular interactions of stimulating and inhibiting tissue factors (Schirner et al. 2004). There is also a set of well-known indicative label molecules that are postembryonically expressed specifically on the endothelium of the tumor vessel or the surrounding stromal tissue and that can be regarded as a potential target for the molecular tumor diagnostics with USCA. Accordingly, Korpanty et al. (2005) were able to show in cell cultures that antibody-carrying MBs which are targeting the tumor endothelial cell marker, endoglin (CD105), specifically deposit on the polyoma virus middle-t transfomed endothelial cells of the mouse brain. Thereby, a mouse fibroblast cell line (3T3) served as an endoglin-negative control. In another study, Leong-Poi et al. (2003) could confirm, using a Matrigel model, which contained an active substance (FGF-2 = fibroblast growth factor and heparin) to stimulate vessel growth and which was implanted subcutaneously in mice, that it resulted in a specific enhancement of antibody (= echistatin)-carrying MBs, which are targeted at the $\alpha_v\beta_3$-integrin of the new vessels, formed in Matrigel. Moreover, they were able to prove a close correlation between the MBs' signal strength and the extent of the formation of the new vessel. The results from the Matrigel trial were able to be verified in the same laboratory in a subsequent in-vivo trial in tumor-carrying mice (intracerebrally implanted human glioblastoma). Here, the examinations took place 14 and 28 days after implanting the tumors. During this period, there was a significant increase in the size of the tumors, as well as to a distinct rise in the tumor blood volume. Equally, a significant rise in the measured sonographic signal strength pointed to the administration of echistatin-carrying MBs (Ellegala et al. 2003). Weller et al. (2005) examined the possibility of using small peptides directed against the endothelial cells of tumor vessels for the molecular imaging of tumor neoangiogenesis. In order to do this, they used the tripeptide arginine-arginine-leucine, which was coupled on the surface of phospholipid-encased MBs containing perfluoro gas. Cells of a human pancreatic carcinoma (PC3) and stable transfected FGF-secreting mouse fibroblasts (NIH3T3) were implanted subcutaneously in athymic nude mice. In both tumor models, there was a significant signal enhancement seen after administration of the specific MBs when compared with various controls (control MBs and the myocardium as control organ), indicating that small peptides directed against tumor-vessel endothelia are suitable as ligands for molecular imaging with ultrasound.

3.2.2 Inflammation

In inflammatory processes, various selectins and adhesion molecules are up-regulated onto the surface of endothelial cells to induce and accomplish immunological defense (attracting and activating leukocytes). This process can be used very well for molecular imaging by coupling appropriate antibodies on the surface of the MBs. In an in-vitro experiment on human coronary endothelial cells activated with interleukin-1, there was an unambiguous accumulation of MBs loaded with anti-ICAM-1 antibodies on up-regulated ICAM-1 when compared with control MBs or nonactivated endothelial cells (Villanueva et al. 1998). In a later in-vivo study conducted with cardiac-transplanted rats, where donor and receiver animals were used from the same inbred species (isotransplant) or from different inbred species (allotransplant), the ultrasound-signal intensity was clearly higher in the allotransplanted hearts when compared with the isotransplanted hearts following the intravenous injection of MBs loaded with anti-ICAM-1 antibodies. The following histomorphological evaluation of the hearts after euthanizing the animals showed among the allotransplants a Group III to IV rejection reaction, evaluated according to the criteria of the International Society for Heart and Lung Transplantation, as well as a strong ICAM-1 immune coloring. In the case of the isotransplants, none or only a marginal sign of any rejection reaction was observed (without any information as to the grade). The ICAM-1 immunohistology was also negative (Weller et al. 2003). These results confirm the specificity of the anti-ICAM-1 MBs and show that ultrasound procedures, even when evaluating transplant rejection reactions, can possess a potential in future clinical application, which should not be underestimated. Tests on the sonographic representation of inflammatory changes in the brain were conducted in an animal model for multiple sclerosis (MS), the EAE (experimental autoimmune encephalomyelitis) rat model (Mäurer et al. 2003, 2005). In human MS, as is the case in experimental autoimmune encephalomyelitis of the rat, the immigration of inflammatory cells depends to a large extent on the expression of adhesion molecules on the endothelial cells of the blood-brain barrier (Fox and Ransohoff 2004). In various experiments, Reinhardt et al. (2005a) as well as Linker et al. (2005) were able to specifically represent sonographically the expression of the adhesion molecules ICAM-1 (intercellular adhesion molecule) and VCAM-1 (vascular cell adhesion molecule) in the rat brain, first ex vivo and later in vivo by using MBs that carry anti-ICAM-1 antibodies and anti-VCAM-1 antibodies. The controls that were used (healthy rats, control MBs and unloaded or IgG-isotype-loaded MBs) were negative in all cases or showed significantly smaller echo signal enhancement, which could be proven to have been caused by MBs still freely circulating in the bloodstream.

In another experiment in postischemic kidneys (ischemia reperfusion model) of wild-type and P-selectin-deficient mice, the administration of anti-P-selectin MBs led to an unambiguous ultrasonic signal in kidneys changed by postischemic inflammation in wild-type mice. Likewise, the immunohistology of the kidneys showed an unambiguous color reaction when testing for P-selectin in these animals.

As opposed to this, the signal in the P-selectin-deficient mice was relatively weak, as was the ultrasonic signal obtained when using the nonspecific control MBs (Lindner et al. 2001).

3.2.3 Thrombosis

Vascular endothelial injuries cause an immediate accumulation and activation of thrombocytes, which finally lead to the formation of a thrombus. Thrombocyte activation results in the exposition of a receptor complex from the thrombocyte membrane, glycoprotein (GP) IIb/IIIa, which is necessary for subsequent binding to fibrinogen and thrombospondin. Wright et al. (1998) as well as Wu et al. (1998) coupled the peptide sequence of fibrinogen, arginine-lysine-aspartat, which is responsible for binding to the GP IIb/IIIa of the thrombocytic membrane, on the surface of the MBs, in order to conduct sonographic thrombus detection using specific MBs. Compared with unloaded control MBs (no specific signal enhancement) they were able to measure in vitro a clear specific ultrasonic signal enhancement in a thrombus-containing flow model after administration of thrombus-specific MBs. This formulation, which is designated as MRX 408, was tested for specificity subsequently in vivo in dogs with an artificially induced thrombus in the iliac artery. When compared with a parallel nonspecific control MB formulation, the administration of MRX 408 led to a significant echo enhancement of the thrombus and made it additionally possible to achieve a substantially better discrimination and determination of the size of the thrombus within the artery. Takeuchi et al. (1999) attained the same test results in another study on artificially induced thrombi in dogs, which were set in the area of the inferior vena cava in the one group and in another group in the area of the left atrium (left atrial appendage thrombus), following the administration of MRX 408 and nonspecific control MBs. Schumann et al. (2002) used the same peptide sequence for the production of their own thrombus-specific MB formulation and tested it for specificity in vitro (1) microscopically on activated thrombocytes and (2) sonographically on thrombi in a flow model, as well as in vivo by means of intravital microscopy on artificially induced thrombi in venoles and arterioles in the cremaster muscle of mice. The microscopic examination of specific MB and nonspecific control MBs showed a clear binding of specific MB to activated thrombocytes, which increased linearly with the addition of greater amounts of MBs. No enhancement or only isolated MBs could be determined after the addition of nonspecific MBs. These results were able to be verified in the flow model, where there was a clear echo signal enhancement in the thrombi, which was also substantially better defined and the size of which better measured, following administration of the specific MBs. In the ensuing in-vivo study, a substantially stronger thrombus enrichment of specific MBs could be observed compared with that of nonspecific ones. It was proven that the cause of the low enhancement of the nonspecific MBs was their adhesion to activated leukocytes that accompanied the thrombus.

3.2.4 Lymphography

Hauff et al. (2004) described in a feasibility study the active targeting of specific MBs in normal, not pathologically changed peripheral lymph nodes. To do this, they chose the ligands for L-selectin. The postcapillary network of the lymph nodes is lined with special endothelial cells [so-called HEV (high endothelial venules)], which, on the surface, continuously carry ligands for L-selectin, a glycoprotein, which is found on virtually all white blood cells (leukocytes). Certain leukocytes (lymphocytes) immigrate via these ligands from the bloodstream to the interior of the lymph nodes. This continuously running physiologically process is also called homing (Streeter et al. 1988). L-Selectin ligands are presented on all other endothelial cells only during an inflammatory reaction. The antibody, MECA-79, was used as the anti-L-selectin ligand for the manufacture of the specific MBs. This antibody is cross-reactive for several animal species (including mouse and dog) and available on the open market. In the study on mice, three awake animals each received intravenously administered either MECA-79 MBs, unloaded control MBs or IgMκ-loaded MBs as isotype control. All animals were euthanized 30 min after the MB injection and the cervical, inguinal, axillaries, popliteal and mesenteric lymph nodes removed, as well as the spleen as positive control and the kidney as blood-pool negative control and examined ex vivo in a water bath for MB-specific signals. This examination had to be conducted ex vivo due to the small size of mice and the necessity of using a clinical ultrasound device. To confirm that each mouse was injected with MBs, the spleen was examined as positive control. Since the spleen contains phagocyting cells of the reticuloendothelial system, there has to be inevitably an enhancement of MBs in the spleens of all groups of mice (see also passive targeting), independently of whether they are specific or nonspecific. The kidneys do not belong to the organs of the reticuloendothelial system and serve as negative controls in order to verify that at the time of the organ removals there were no more MBs in the bloodstream and that MB signals from the lymph nodes could only have come from specifically bound MBs. The highly sensitive SAE effect was used for MB detection, in which the destruction of the MBs in the color Doppler leads to characteristic color pixels on the monitor of the ultrasound device. The results of the ex vivo ultrasonic investigation show unambiguous SAE effects in all the spleens of the three groups of mice as proof of the fact that all animals were injected with MBs. On the other hand, there were no MB-induced SAE effects found in the kidneys of any of the animals, which led to the conclusion that at the time of the organ removals there were no MBs circulating in the bloodstream. The results of the lymph node examination showed unambiguous SAE effects in all of the lymph nodes of all of the mice that were injected with specific (MECA-79) MBs, compared with all of the lymph nodes of the mice in both control groups (unloaded and IgMκ-loaded control MBs) that were SAE negative. In a subsequent in-vivo study in dogs, where the same MB formulations were used and also the positive and negative organ controls ran parallel, these results could be verified using popliteal lymph nodes. The distribution of the SAE signals corresponded thereby with the immunohistological pattern of the L-selectin-ligand expression. These results open interesting perspectives for the development and use of an indirect target-specific lymphographic contrast agent to the evaluation of macroscopically changed lymph nodes or four the detection of sentinel lymph nodes in tumor diagnostics.

The examples of active targeting show that the endovascular visualization of molecules with specific USCAs is possible and offer various practice-relevant applications in branches of medicine. However, only qualitative statements about their expression can be made with these USCA bubbles that can be used for various vascular molecules. Their quantitative representation is desirable, however, beside the purely qualitative detection of certain molecular structures. This would, for example, make possible the identification of completely new disease-associated molecular markers. Moreover, it would be possible to initiate a temporally guided mapping of known and newly identified disease-associated molecular markers in the entire organism during pathogenesis in vivo and, from this gained knowledge, new therapeutic medicinal products and/or treatment strategies could be derived. Additionally, a highly sensitive monitoring of treatment effects would be possible at the molecular level.

4 Quantitative Molecular Imaging with Ultrasound

4.1 High-resolution Imaging: Microultrasound

High-resolution molecular imaging with microultrasound is performed using the instrumentation described by us in Chapter "Ultrasound Basics" of this volume (*see* Sect. 3.1). Cine loops of approximately 800 frames are acquired for each experiment at a frame rate of 15 Hz post contrast injection. Mice are placed prone on the imaging stage (*see* Fig. 6 in Chapter "Ultrasound Basics" of , this volume) and the area to be imaged stabilized to minimize respiration motion. The scanhead is held fixed with the integrated small animal rail system (VisualSonics, Toronto). MBs (VisualSonics MicroMarker, Toronto) bearing a target ligand, such as anti-VEGFR-2 antibody or an isotype control antibody, are administered via a jugular cannula consisting of PE-20 tubing or by tail vein injection. MBs are typically administered as a bolus of 5×10^7 particles in $\sim$100 ul, followed by a 20- to 50-μl saline flush. MB wash-in within the target tissue is verified by imaging at low power (10%) immediately following administration. Imaging at low power is important to minimize destruction of the agent by the imaging beam. Subsequently, imaging is paused for 4 min to allow circulating MBs to attach to the molecular target. Following the 4-min accumulation period, imaging recommences at a power of 50%. After approximately 200 frames, a high-power destructive pulse sequence with a center frequency of 10 MHz is applied to destroy MBs within the beam elevation. Immediately after the destruction sequence, imaging at a power of 50% continues for 600 frames to observe any residual circulating MBs.

The "molecular" signal is visualized by a destruction-subtraction imaging scheme, as described below. It is assumed that the pixel amplitude within the target immediately before the destruction sequence is due to the acoustic response of tissue, adherent MBs, and circulating (nonstationary) MBs. The destruction sequence eliminates MBs in the beam elevation, and within several seconds post destruction the pixel amplitude is assumed to be due to tissue and any circulating MBs that have replenished the beam. The postdestruction frames therefore represent a reference that can subsequently be subtracted from the predestruction frames to yield the "molecular" signal. The effects of tissue motion are minimized by searching the data sets for optimally correlated reference frames before subtraction. The molecular signal is then encoded as a colored mask that can be overlaid (usually in green) on the B-mode imaging data. Scanner software allows the molecular signal to be tracked in a region of interest to quantify relative levels of molecular expression.

Examples of high frequency molecular studies are given in Figs. 5 and 6.

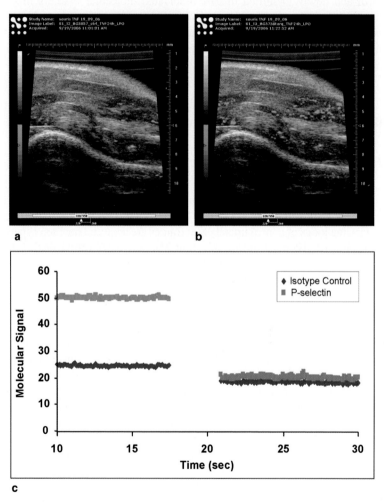

Fig. 5 a–c TNFα model of inflammation. **a** Predestruction molecular images of isotype control antibody labeled MicroMarker contrast MBs and **b** P-selectin antibody labeled MicroMarker contrast MBs. The molecular signal is plotted in **c** through the destruction sequence. Approximately 5×10^7 MBs in 100 µl of saline were injected

Figure 5 shows P-selectin expression in the hind limb 24 h after the induction of inflammation via TNFα injection. Binding of control antibody-labeled MBs (cf. Fig. 5a) is considerably lower than the targeted P-selectin labeled antibody MBs (cf. Fig. 5b) before MB destruction. Post destruction, similar levels of residual signal are achieved for both MB populations, indicating the disruption of stationary bound MBs. A more quantitative view of the P-selectin molecular signal is given in Fig. 5c. Similar findings are evident in a melanoma xenograft (Mewo) that is expressing VEGFR-2 in its periphery (cf. Fig. 6).

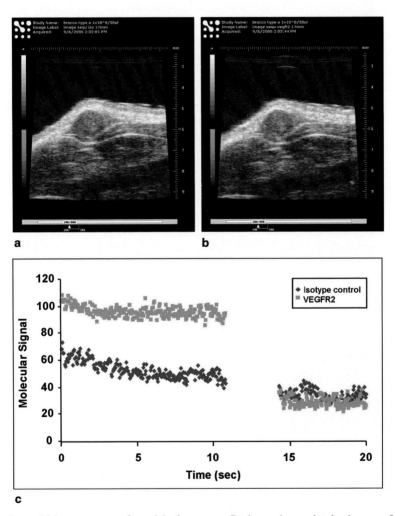

Fig. 6 a–c Melanoma xenograft model of cancer. **a** Predestruction molecular images of isotype control and **b** VEGFR-2 labeled MBs demonstrating peripheral binding and expression of VEGFR-2. The molecular signal is plotted in **c** through the destruction sequence. Approximately 5×10^7 MBs in 100 μl of saline were injected

Detailed results for VEGFR-2 imaging are reported in (Rychak 2007). The unique ability of microultrasound to provide resolution of <100 μm in molecular imaging studies of the mouse offers many exciting opportunities for preclinical imaging.

4.2 Sensitive Particle Acoustic Quantification (SPAQ)

Technical details of the 3D-SPAQ principle are described by these authors earlier in this volume (*see* Part I Instrumentation, Sect. 3.2). In this chapter, we describe the in-vitro, ex-vivo and in-vivo evaluation of this new technology.

First, the SPAQ method was tested in an agar phantom with 30,000 bubbles/ml with different SPAQ resolution (10–100 μm) (many times higher than the MB concentration that can be quantified with conventional ultrasonic methods). In the results, a linear correlation ($r = 0.9918$) could be demonstrated between the thickness of the ultrasonic (cross-)sectional views and the SAE signals measured therein, and the number of MBs could be determined with a virtually exact accuracy at $28,720 \pm 3,412$ MBs (cf. Fig. 7).

These results were verified in a rat-liver experiment. In this examination, two groups of rats received different doses (1×10^7 and 1×10^8 MB/kg bodyweight) of nonspecific MBs. Following uptake of the MBs in their livers (30 min after intravenous injection), the animals were euthanized, their livers removed and examined ex vivo with both the conventional technique and SPAQ. With the conventional technique, the livers of all animals showed up completely color-saturated, not permitting any difference between both dose groups. In comparison, by using the SPAQ method, the livers could be accurately assigned to the respective dose groups through the quantification of the MBs, as illustrated in Fig. 8 (Reinhardt et al. 2005b).

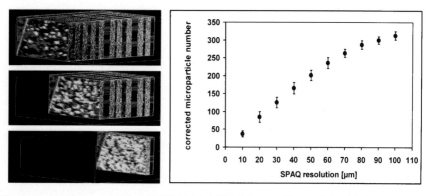

Fig. 7 Agar phantom containing 30,000 MBs/ml. SPAQ shows a linear relationship between SAE-slice-thickness (SPAQ-resolution) and the number of particles

Group 1, 1*10^7 MB/kg   **Group 2, 1*10^8 MB/kg**

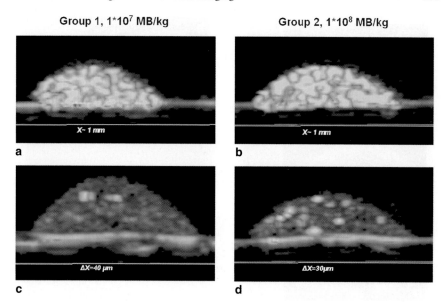

Fig. 8 a–d Rat-livers ex vivo. **a, b** Without SPAQ, there is no difference visible between both rats regardless of the tenfold different particle dose they received. **c, d** With the higher resolution of SPAQ, a clear difference in the number of particles is visible, reflecting the dose difference between the animals

Subsequently, there was a series of ex-vivo and in-vivo examinations conducted in the EAE rat model, in which the disease process is associated with an up-regulation of ICAM-1 to the endothelia of the blood-brain barrier. With the aid of SPAQ in these examinations, the sensitivity and specificity of the molecular imaging with ultrasound could be confirmed using anti-ICAM-1-specific USCA bubbles.

Specificity could be demonstrated by pretreating the diseased animals with anti-ICAM-1, where, after subsequent administration of anti-ICAM-1-MBs, there were significantly less specifically enhanced MBs measured ($p < 0.05$) in the brain and spinal cord of the pretreated animals, compared with the diseased animals that were not pretreated (cf. Fig. 9). The sensitivity of this method was confirmed by premedicating the animals with cortisone (2 days after the induction of EAE). None of the rats treated with cortisone presented any clinical symptoms of EAE and the SPAQ measurements resulted in a significantly smaller enhancement of anti-ICAM-1-MBs ($p < 0.008$) in the brain of the treated animals when compared with the untreated EAE control rats (Reinhardt et al. 2005a; Linker et al. 2005).

In summary, it can be stated that substantial preconditions for molecular imaging with ultrasound have been created based on the specific MBs and the SPAQ method, such as:

- high sensitivity and specificity
- quantifiability
- high spatial resolution.

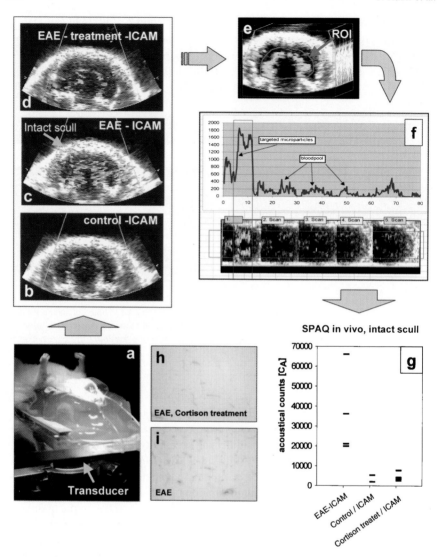

Fig. 9 a–g SPAQ for the measurement of ICAM-1 in the AT-EAE model in rats in vivo. **a** A rat is scanned on the SPAQ device. **b, c, d** The density of targeted MBs in the periventricular area of the rat-brains is clearly different between all investigated groups. **e** The 3D data were analysed by defining a region of interest (ROI) within all brains. **f** For the quantification of solely the targeted bubbles, all other bubbles that still remain within the blood pool were substracted from the first peak. **g** The graph shows, that ICAM-1 was clearly up-regulated in the untreated EAE-rats compared with the control group, whereas the cortisone treatment in the other group led to a strong down-regulation of ICAM-1. (It should be noted here, that the measurement was conducted through the intact scull, which leads to a marked absorption of the transmitted signal. However, the remaining signal was still sufficient to gain SAE signals)

Both as regards the attainable spatial resolution and the slice thickness of the individual ultrasonic images (layer thickness of up to 10 µm), as well as with reference to the fact that, with this procedure, various binding molecules can be specifically detected, one could also characterize this procedure as "sono-immuno-histology." When compared with immunohistochemistry, however, this procedure does have crucial advantages, such as:

- the specifically targeted MBs can be quantified very exactly in the living animal ("in-vivo sono-immuno-histology")
- the vascular expression molecules can be investigated and quantified in the same animal over a long period of time
- with one ultrasound scan, serial sonographic (cross-)sectional views of organs, tumors or other tissue regions are recorded and evaluated within a few seconds
- in contrast to immunohistochemistry, where only a few representative (more or less) slices are evaluated, SPAQ allows the assessment of the complete tissue of interest
- aside from that quantitative determination of expression molecules, even these anatomical regions can be categorized, since the sonographic image is automatically provided with its relatively high detail resolution.

Additionally, the specific MBs and SPAQ provide a contribution to animal protection which should not be underestimated. Since this procedure can be used in vivo several times on the same animal, one can significantly minimize the number of study groups in the case of particular vascular questions, which, up to the present time, can only be answered by using many study groups (euthanizing a certain number of animals at different points in time during the course of pathogenesis, histological processing and microscopic evaluation of the samples). A further advantage consists of the fact that there is not the large expenditure of time and manpower related to histology. The quantitative in-vivo data are available on the same day.

References

Bauer A, Blomley M, Leen E et al (1999) Liver-specific imaging with SHU 563 A: Diagnostic potential of a new class of ultrasound contrast media. Eur Radiol 9(Suppl 3):S349–S352

Berwing K, Schleppe M (1988) Echocardiographic imaging of the left ventricle by peripheral intravenous injection of echo contrast agent. Amer Heart 115:399–408

Chiang CW, Lin FC, Fu M et al (1986) Importance of adequate gas-mixing in contrast echocardiography. Chest 89:723–726

Choi SH, Kono Y, Corbeil J et al (2004) Model to quantify lymph node enhancement on indirect sonographic lymphography. AJR Am J Roentgenol 183:513–517

Christiansen JP, Leong-Poi H, Klibanov AL et al (2002) Noninvasive imaging of myocardial reperfusion injury using leukocyte-targeted contrast echocardiography. Circulation 105:1764–1767

Cosgrove D (1996) Warum brauchen wir Kontrastmittel für den Ultraschall? Clin Radiol 51(Suppl 1):1–4

Dayton PA, Ferrara KW (2002) Targeted imaging using ultrasound. J Magn Reson Imaging 16:362–377

De Jong N (1997) Physics of microbubble scattering. In: Nanda NC, Schlief R, Goldberg BB (eds) Advances in echo imaging using contrast enhancement, 2nd edn. Kluwer, Dordrecht, pp 39–64

Ellegala DB, Leong-Poi H, Carpenter JE et al (2003) Imaging tumor angiogenesis with contrast ultrasound and microbubbles targeted to $\alpha_v\beta_3$. Circulation 108:336–341

Fischer NG, Christiansen JP, Klibanov AL et al (2002) Influence of microbubble surface charge on capillary transit and myocardial contrast enhancement. J Am Coll Cardiol 40:811–819

Fox RJ, Ransohoff RM (2004) New directions in MS therapeutics: vehicles of hope. Trends Immunol 25:632–636

Gramiak R, Shah P (1968) Echocardiography of the aortic root. Invest Radiol 3:356–366

Hauff P, Reinhardt M, Jeschke J et al (1994) Indirekte Lymphographie mit einem neuen Ultra-schallkontrastmittel (USKM). Ultraschalldiagnostik '94, Drei-Länder-Treffen, Basel, Schweiz, 26–29.10.1994. Bildgebung/Imaging 61(Suppl 2):17

Hauff P, Fritzsch T, Reinhardt M et al (1997) Delineation of experimental liver tumors in rabbits by a new ultrasound contrast agent and stimulated acoustic emission. Invest Radiol 32:94–99

Hauff P, Stephens A, Bräutigam M (2003) New imaging probes. In: Debatin JF, Hricak H, Niendorf HP (eds) MRI: from current knowledge to new horizon. Excerpta Medica, pp 259–268

Hauff P, Reinhardt M, Briel A et al (2004) Molecular targeting of lymph nodes with L-selectin ligand-specific us contrast agent: a feasibility study in mice and dogs. Radiology 231:667–673

Hauff P, Seemann S, Reszka R et al (2005) Evaluation of gas-filled microparticles and sonoporation as gene delivery system: Feasibility study in rodent tumor model. Radiology 236:572–578

Keller MW, Glasheen W, Teja K et al (1988) Myocardial contrast echocardiography without signif-icant hemodynamic effects or reactive hyperemia: a major advantage in the imaging of regional myocardial perfusion. J Amer Coll Cardiol 12:1039–1047

Klibanov AL (1999) Targeted delivery of gas-filled microspheres, contrast agents for ultrasound imaging. Adv Drug Deliv Rev 37:139–157

Klibanov AL (2005) Ligand-carrying gas-filed microbubbles: ultrasound contrast agents for tar-geted molecular imaging. Bioconjugate Chem 16:9–17

Korpanty G, Grayburn PA, Shohet RV et al (2005) Targeting vascular endothelium with avidin microbubbles. Ultrasound Med Biol 31:1279–1283

Lange L, Fritzsch T, Hillmann J et al (1986) Right-heart echocontrast in the anesthetized dog after i.v. administration of a new standardized sonographic agent, 3rd communication: Comparison of various contrast agents employed in contrast echocardiography. Arzneim-Forsch 36: 1037–1040

Lanza GM and Wickline SA (2001) Targeted ultrasonic contrast agents for molecular imaging and therapy. Prog Cardiovasc Dis 44:13–31

Lee F and Ginzton L (1983) A central nervous system complication of contrast echocardiography. J Clin Ultrasound 11:292–294

Leong-Poi H, Christiansen J, Klibanov AL et al (2003) Noninvasive Assessment of Angiogenesis by Ultrasound and Microbubbles Targeted to α_v-Integrins. Circulation 107:455–460

Lindner JR, Coggins MP, Kaul S et al (2000) Microbubble persistence in the microcirculation during ischemia/reperfusion and inflammation is caused by integrin- and complement-mediated adherence to activated leukocytes. Circulation 101:668–675

Lindner JR, Dayton PA, Coggins MP et al (2000) Noninvasive imaging of inflammation by ultra-sound detection of phagocytosed microbubbles. Circulation 102:531–538

Lindner JR, Song J, Xu F et al (2000) Noninvasive ultrasound imaging of inflammation using microbubbles targeted to activated leukocytes. Circulation 102:2745–2750

Lindner JR, Song J, Christiansen J et al (2001) Ultrasound assessment of inflammation and renal tissue injury with microbubbles targeted to P-selectin. Circulation 104:2107–2112

Linker R, Reinhardt M, Bendszus M et al (2005) In vivo molecular imaging of adhesion molecules in experimental autoimmune encephalomyelitis (EAE). J Autoimmunity 25:199–205

Mäurer M, Linker R, Hauff P et al (2003) Imaging of ICAM-1 in experimental autoimmune ene-cephalomyelitis (EAE) with a specific ultrasound contrast agent. Neurology 60:A423

Mäurer M, Linker R, Reinhardt M et al (2005) Möglichkeiten target-spezifischer molekularer Bildgebung mit Ultraschallkontrastmitteln. Radiologe 45:560–568

Mattrey RF (1983) Perfluorochemicals as liver- and spleen-seeking ultrasound contrast agents. J Ultrasound Med 2:173–176

Mattrey RF, Kono Y, Baker K et al (2002) Sentinel lymph node imaging with microbubble ultrasound contrast Material. Acad Radiol 9(Suppl 1):S231–S235

Oussoren C, Zuidema J, Crommelin DJ et al (1997) Lymphatic uptake and biodistribution of liposomes after subcutaneous injection. II. Influence of liposomal size, lipid composition and lipid dose. Biochim Biophys Acta 1328:261–272

Reinhardt M, Fritzsch T, Heldmann D et al (1993) Use of microcapsules as contrasting agents in colour Doppler sonography. WO 93/25241

Reinhardt M, Hauff P, Linker RA et al (2005a) Ultrasound derived imaging and quantification of cell adhesion molecules in experimental autoimmune encephalomyelitis (EAE) by Sensitive Particle Acoustic Quantification (SPAQ). Neuroimage 27:267–278

Reinhardt M, Hauff P, Briel A et al (2005b) Sensitive Particle Acoustic Quantification (SPAQ): a new ultrasound-based approach for the quantification of ultrasound contrast media in high concentrations. Invest Radiol 40:2–7

Rychak JJ et al (2007) Microultrasound molecular imaging of vascular endothelial growth factor receptor 2 in a mouse model of tumor angiogenesis. Mol Imaging 6:289–296

Schirner M, Menrad A, Stephens A et al (2004) Molecular imaging of tumor angiogenesis. Ann N Y Acad Sci 1014:67–75

Schlief R (1997) Echo-enhancing agents: their physics and pharmacology. In: Nanda NC, Schlief R, Goldberg BB (eds) Advances in echo imaging using contrast enhancement, 2nd edn. Kluwer, Dordrecht, pp 85–113

Schrope V, Newhouse VL, Uhlendorf V (1992) Simulated capillary blood flow measurement using a non-linear ultrasonic contrast agent. Ultrasonic Imaging 14:134–158

Schumann PA, Christiansen JP, Quigley RM et al (2002) Targeted-microbubble binding selectively to GPIIb IIIa receptors of platelet thrombi. Invest Radiol 37:587–593

Simionescu M (2000) Structural, biochemical and functional differentiation of the vascular endothelium. In: Risau W, Rubanyi GM (eds) Morphogenesis of the endothelium. Harwood, Amsterdam, pp 1–22

Simon RH, Ho SY, D'Arrigo J et al (1990) Lipid-coated ultrastable microbubbles as a contrast agent in neuro-sonography. Invest Radiol 25:1300–1304

Streeter PR, Rouse BT, Butcher EC (1988) Immunohistologic and functional characterization of a vascular addressing involved in lymphocyte homing into peripheral lymph nodes. J Cell Biol 107:1853–1862

Takeuchi M, Ogunyanki K, Pandian NG et al (1999) Enhanced visualization of intravascular and left atrial appendage thrombus with the use of a thrombus-targeting ultrasonographic contrast agent (MRX-408A1): in vivo experimental echocardiographic studies. J Am Soc Echocardiogr 12:1015–1021

Tiemann K, Pohl C, Schlosser T et al (2000) Stimulated acoustic emission: pseudo-Doppler shifts seen during the destruction of non-moving microbubbles. Ultrasound Med Biol 26:1161–1167

Uhlendorf V, Hoffmann C (1994) Nonlinear acoustic response of coated microbubbles in diagnostic ultrasound. Ultrasonics Symposium, Cannes, France, pp 1559–1562

Villanueva FS, Jankowski RJ, Klibanov S et al (1998) Microbubbles targeted to intercellular adhesion molecule-1 bind to activated coronary artery endothelial cells. Circulation 98:1–5

Weissleder R, Mahmood U (2001) Molecular imaging. Radiology 219:316–333

Weller GER, Lu E, Csikari MM (2003) ultrasound imaging of acute cardiac transplant rejection with microbubbles targeted to intercellular adhesion molecule-1. Circulation 108:218–224

Weller GER, Wong MKK, Modzelewski RA et al (2005) Ultrasonic imaging of tumor angiogenesis using contrast microbubbles targeted via the tumor-binding peptide arginine-arginine-leucine. Cancer Res 65:533–539

Wright WH, McCreery TP, Krupinski EA et al (1998) Evaluation of new thrombus-specific ultrasound contrast agent. Acad Radiol 5(Suppl 1):S240–S242

Wu Y, Unger EC, McCreery TP et al (1998) Binding and lysing of blood clots using MRX-408. Invest Radiol 33:880–885

Agents for Polarization Enhancement in MRI

Silvio Aime(✉), Walter Dastrù, Roberto Gobetto, Daniela Santelia,
and Alessandra Viale

Abstract The intrinsic low sensitivity of the NMR phenomenon can be overcome thanks to hyperpolarization procedures that break the limits of the Boltzmann equilibrium and may increase the NMR signal by a factor of 10^5. Hyperpolarization procedures have been applied to enhance the signal from noble gases, such as ^{3}He and ^{129}Xe, and small ^{13}C-containing molecules. For the latter class, attention has been focused on the use of methods based on dynamic nuclear polarization (DNP) and para-hydrogen induced polarization (PHIP). After discussion of the basics of the methods, an overview of the main applications with ^{13}C-containing molecules is presented. This includes pre-clinical MR investigations of vascular imaging, perfusion and catheter tracking as well as molecular imaging protocols that allow the development of highly innovative studies in the field of metabolic imaging.

Silvio Aime

Dipartimento di Chimica I.F.M, Università degli Studi di Torino, V. P. Giuria 7, 10125 Torino, Italy

silvio.aime@unito.it

W. Semmler and M. Schwaiger (eds.), *Molecular Imaging I.*

Handbook of Experimental Pharmacology 185/I.

© Springer-Verlag Berlin Heidelberg 2008

1 Introduction

Magnetic resonance imaging (MRI) has gained a primary role in diagnostic clinical medicine and biomedical research, because it allows the obtainment of anatomic images of the body in its various parts and functional information (flow, perfusion, etc). It is based (as NMR) on the interaction of atomic nuclei possessing a non-zero spin quantum number with an external magnetic field, and may therefore in principle make use of any of these nuclei [for example, ^{1}H, ^{13}C, ^{31}P (endogenous) or ^{129}Xe, ^{3}He (exogenous)]. Nevertheless, up to present the clinical use of MRI has been restricted to ^{1}H due to sensitivity problems. In fact, the NMR signal intensity depends upon the concentration of the active nucleus and its polarization, which is defined according to (1):

$$P = \frac{|N_+ - N_-|}{N_+ + N_-} = \tanh\left(\frac{\gamma \hbar B_0}{2k_B T}\right) \tag{1}$$

where N_+ and N_- represent the number of spins having up and down orientations with respect to the magnetic field, respectively, γ is the gyromagnetic ratio of the observed nucleus, B_0 is the magnetic field strength, k_B is the Boltzmann constant and T is the temperature. Under thermal equilibrium conditions, the population difference, and P, as a consequence, is very low and therefore low intensity signals are detected.

The diagnostic quality of MR images strongly depends upon the signal-to-noise ratio (SNR), since it is a measure of what resolution is needed to separate the signal deriving from a region of interest from the background noise in the image.

^{1}H gives raise to quite intense signals with respect to other nuclei due to its higher gyromagnetic ratio and its high concentration in tissues, and is therefore the most used for MRI purposes. The various tissues are differentiated in proton imaging on the basis of relaxation times (T_1 and T_2) or proton density. ^{1}H contrast agents are based on the same principle: they are usually paramagnetic or superparamagnetic substances, which increase the relaxation rates of adjacent protons thus enhancing their signal in the image.

Among the magnetically active endogenous nuclei, ^{31}P has also been considered mainly for localized spectroscopic investigations, thanks to its relative high concentration (mM range) and its relevance to describe basic metabolic pathways (Ortidge et al. 2000; Brown 2000; Lamerichs and Luyten 2000).

For other nuclei, it is necessary to increase the polarization in order to use them for MRI. This can be done by creating a non-equilibrium state in which the population difference between the up and down states is increased: this state is the "hyperpolarized" state and various techniques aimed to achieving the goal have been developed in recent years. As the hyperpolarization process is carried out before the administration of the agent to the patient/animal, a general rule is to deal with species characterized by very long relaxation times. The heteronuclei-based images are generated simply by the heteronucleus signal corresponding to the distribution of the agent in the tissue: a higher concentration or higher polarization yields a higher signal, which will be observed upon the background noise. This allows the use of low-magnetic-field MR tomographs to generate images with similar SNRs as those obtained on higher-field MRI scanners.

1.1 Hyperpolarized Gases

The use of nuclei other than ^{1}H has extended the range of feasible diagnostic studies; for example, hyperpolarized noble gases (^{129}Xe and ^{3}He) are being employed for monitoring the lungs and to carry out brain perfusion studies (Kauczor et al. 1998; Moller et al. 2002; Altes and Salerno 2004; Oros and Shah 2004; Albert et al. 1994; Middleton et al. 1995). In this case hyperpolarization is achieved by optical pumping: the noble gas is mixed with an alkali-metal vapor (spin-exchange optical pumping) or with a vapour of metastable atoms (metastability optical exchange), and circularly polarized light from lasers at suitable resonance frequencies passes through the cell containing the mixture. The electrons of alkali or metastable atoms adsorb the angular momentum of the laser light and are polarized. Then, polarization is transferred to the noble gas atoms via "spin exchange" when they come into contact with the alkali or metastable atoms (Van der Waals molecules). In spin-exchange optical pumping, Rb is usually used; its vapour is condensed at the end of the process and the noble gas can be cryogenically extracted (Fig. 1). In metastability, optical

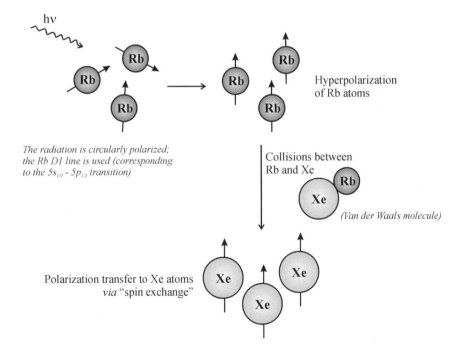

Fig. 1 The process of optical pumping to produce hyperpolarized Xenon

pumping a plasma of ^{3}He atoms is used; in this case the polarization transfer is faster but the technique is limited to hyperpolarized ^{3}He. The hyperpolarized ^{129}Xe and ^{3}He are then packaged into internally coated, iron-free glass cells in order to prevent relaxation and hence to maintain the polarization for as long as possible.

Both ^{129}Xe and ^{3}He have been used in MRI of the lungs, since the lung is a particularly challenging area to study (Cutillo 1996). In fact, even at end expiration, the overall ^{1}H density is only $0.30 \, g/cm^3$; hence, the water content is low and ^{1}H-MRI is not suitable for lung studies. Biomedical hyperpolarized gas MRI has been recently reviewed in many articles (Kauczor et al. 1998; Moller et al. 2002; Altes and Salerno 2004; Oros and Shah 2004; Albert et al. 1994; Middleton et al. 1995). To date, the main clinical application of hyperpolarized noble gases has been the exploitation of ventilation studies with ^{3}He, but other possibilities have been pursued. Utilizing diffusion has already demonstrated applicability in diagnosing emphysema; changes in pO_2 and, hence, abnormal T_1/T^*_2-weighted MRI may provide information about changes in the tissue composition related to the occurrence of a pathological state. Functional MRI may take advantage of the solubility and lipophilic properties of Xe (Mugler et al 1997; Swanson et al. 1997; Wagshul et al. 1996), its binding to haemoglobin has already been utilized to measure blood oxygenation (Wolber et al. 2000). Xe can also be dissolved in some biocompatible carriers to be delivered through intravenous injection (Duhamel et al. 2001; Moller et al. 1999; Wolber et al. 1999; Bifone et al. 1996).

The enormous sensitivity of ^{129}Xe chemical shift to specific interactions may allow to design probe molecules for structural studies of proteins and for the detection of specific biomolecules (Spence et al. 2001). In fact, it has been shown that Xenon biosensors which trap Xe atoms in molecular cages (such as cryptophane-A cage) (Bartik et al. 1998) can be functionalized with suitable vectors in order to target specific analytes. The cage-encapsulated Xe nucleus yields a resonance that is well shifted from that of free Xe and the two chemically different Xe nuclei show exchange on the NMR time scale. Actually, a very interesting development has been recently proposed, aimed at detecting low concentrations of the Xenon biosensor through its effect on the main signal of the free Xe which may eventually be provided by the blood stream in vivo after injection or inhalation (Schroder et al. 2006). The method consists of saturating the adsorption frequency of the Xe resonance in the targeted cage in order to decrease the signal of free Xe which is exchanging with it (Fig. 2). This procedure has been dubbed HYPER-CEST as it recalls the CEST (chemical exchange saturation transfer) protocol, in which a pool of exchangeable protons is selectively irradiated in order to transfer saturated magnetization on the "bulk" water signal (Aime et al. 2005) that, in turn, results in a darkening effect in the corresponding MR images. Analogously to CEST agents, also this Xenon biosensor can allow the detection of multiple targeted epitopes in the same region, provided that the Xe resonances display different chemical shifts for the different targets.

Interestingly, ^{3}He confined in carriers (microbubbles) and targeted to specific isotopes has also been reported. For instance, Tournier and co-workers have been able to visualize endothelial tumor cells by targeting ^{3}He-loaded microbubbles suitably functionalized with a peptide that recognizes over expressed receptors (Callot et al. 2001a, 2001b).

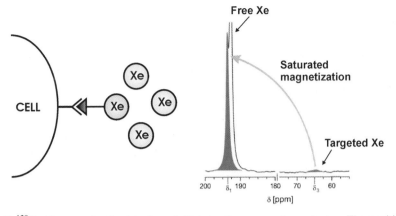

Fig. 2 ^{129}Xe-biosensor for the detection of diluted epitopes on cell membranes. The sensitivity enhancement is obtained by depolarizing the δ_3 resonance (Xe biosensor) and detecting at δ_1 (free Xe)

Table 1 Parameters of interest for the evaluation of the achievable SNR for different nuclei based on the accessible polarization factors P. The estimated SNRs are normalized to yield 100 for ^{1}H

	^{1}H	^{129}Xe	^{3}He	^{13}C
γ [MHz/T]	42.6	11.7	32.5	10.7
P	5×10^{-6}	0.2	0.3	0.15
Conc. [M]	80	0.01	0.002	0.2
Dilution factor	1	60	12	12
Relative SNR	100	2.3	9.5	157

It is of interest to compare the attainable signal to noise ratio for hyperpolarized ^{13}C contrast agents with that from conventional ^{1}H MRI, in order to establish the potential success of hyperpolarized molecules. In Table 1 parameters of interest for the evaluation of the achievable SNR for different nuclei is reported on the basis of accessible polarization factors. The estimated SNRs are normalized to yield 100 for ^{1}H (Svensson 2003).

It is evident that for hyperpolarized natural abundance ^{129}Xe dissolved in bio-carriers and for hyperpolarized ^{3}He encapsulated in microbubbles, the expected SNR is at least one order of magnitude less than for conventional ^{1}H contrast agents, mainly because of the low concentration achievable in blood, and in the case of Xe for a dilution factor due to ventilation of the gas during passage in the pulmonary system. On the contrary, the higher achievable ^{13}C concentrations in blood allow its SNR to be comparable with that from ^{1}H contrast agents, even when a relatively low degree of polarization (15%) is considered. If one takes into account that the polarization could be further increased (up to 30%) by optimization of the used techniques, it is clear that the SNR may increase by one order of magnitude.

1.2 ¹³C *Hyperpolarized Molecules*

Recently much attention has been devoted to ^{13}C hyperpolarized molecules. There is a large degree of expectation on this novel class of MRI reporters as they can distribute all over the body tissues and, with the ^{13}C concentration being low (1.1% natural abundance), no background signal is detected in the image. Furthermore, small molecules may have ^{13}C resonances characterized by relatively long relaxation times (up to 60 s), thus making possible a wide range of studies, from the assessment of flow and perfusion to the detection of abnormalities in the cellular metabolism.

Several methods for achieving ^{13}C hyperpolarization are known, namely the "brute force" approach, dynamic nuclear polarization (DNP) and para-hydrogen induced polarization (PHIP).

1.3 The "Brute Force" Approach

In principle [as stated by (1)], this method is the most straightforward approach to attain hyperpolarized molecules (irrespective of the magnetic nucleus of interest!). The sample must be kept at very low temperatures (mK, Fig. 3) and high magnetic field strength for a sufficiently long period of time that depends upon the relaxation properties of the investigated system. It may be useful to recall that for solid systems at such low temperatures the longitudinal relaxation times are definitively (impossibly!) long. Over the years much work has been done in order to find relaxation switches that allow to shorten this time without compromising the successive maintaining of the hyperpolarization when the sample is brought back to higher temperature for signal detection in a given experimental work-up. A relaxation switch that has received considerable attention is represented by the ^{3}He/^{4}He system: ^{3}He is magnetically active ($I = 1/2$) and it is the only substance that can diffuse (quantum mechanical tunnelling) at temperatures in the mK range. Therefore it may act as a

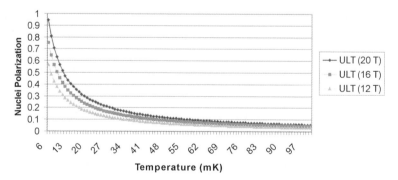

Fig. 3 Nuclear polarization as a function of temperature and magnetic field strength (*ULT*)

relaxation agent, thanks to the dipolar interactions it may have with the substrate molecules to be hyperpolarized. Once the polarization of the nuclei of interest has risen to the expected value, the ^{3}He component is replaced by the magnetically inherent ^{4}He (I $= 0$) (Kalechofsky 2002). The "washing" with ^{4}He should allow the maintaining of the polarization raised thanks to the dipolar interactions with ^{3}He. Although very fashionable, the difficulties of working at such extreme experimental conditions have strongly hampered the development of the "brute force" technique for practical applications.

1.4 DNP

The DNP method takes advantage of the larger polarization of electrons, (due to their higher g value), in respect to the nuclear polarization at the same magnetic field strength. In the solid state, this polarization can be transferred to nuclei by means of the application of a proper radiofrequency, at or near to the electron resonance frequency, promoting flip-flop transitions able to align the nuclear spins by subsequent steps. The slower nuclear relaxation with respect to the electronic one ensures the maintaining of the nuclear spin's alignment during the process. It also makes the entire process possible, even in the presence of a very low concentration of unpaired electrons in the sample (Abragam and Goldman 1978) (Fig. 4).

In practice, the material to be polarized is doped with a stable radical species (usually a nitroxide- or triaryl-based radical) and placed into a suitably strong magnetic field. The solution is frozen (typically at 1.5 K) and the RF irradiation is applied for about 30 min. After the polarization transfer has taken place, the RF is switched off, the sample is raised upon the liquid helium level and is rapidly warmed up (usually by dissolution in hot water) still inside the magnetic field; then it is quickly transferred for observation in the NMR scanner. It has been demonstrated that by using an efficient dissolution method a good level of polarization is maintained (Ardenkjaer-Larsen et al. 2003).

Enhancement of the heteronucleus can be achieved both directly (by direct polarization transfer from electrons to the heteronucleus – single pulse DNP) and indirectly (by ^{1}H DNP and subsequent cross polarization to heteronucleus – DNP-CP).

The method yields ^{13}C polarization of about 10–20% and it has been applied for polarizing also ^{15}N nuclei.

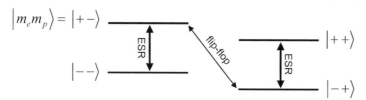

Fig. 4 Schematic representation of the DNP process; m_e and m_p represent, respectively, the spin states of the electron and of the nucleus involved in the dipolar interaction

Selected examples include: ^{15}N single pulse DNP of carbazole, doped with the free stable radical 1,3-bisdiphenylene-2-phenyallyl (BDPA) 1%, with an irradiation frequency of 39.13 GHz (1.4 T), yielding a 930-fold enhancement in the ^{15}N signal of carbazole (Hu et al. 2000); ^{13}C and ^{15}N DNP-CP of amino acids in frozen glycerol-water solutions, doped with 40 mM nitroxide free radical 4-amino-TEMPO (2,2,6,6-tetramethyl-1-piperidinyloxy), yielding 30- and 50-fold enhancements for ^{13}C and ^{15}N, respectively (Hall et al. 1997; Bajaj et al. 2003; Gerfen et al. 1995); high frequency pulsed ^{13}C DNP of fluoranthenyl hexafluorophosphate, showing the usefulness of the application of pulsed rf instead of continuous rf for the polarization transfer (Un et al. 1992); ^{15}N DNP of benzamide doped with BDPA (Hu et al. 1997), ^{13}C and ^{15}N DNP of urea in frozen glycerol solutions, doped with the trityl radical, yielding polarization of 37% for ^{13}C and 7.8% for ^{15}N (Ardenkjaer-Larsen et al. 2003).

Interestingly, a full set-up for the preparation of hyperpolarized molecules by the DNP method is now commercially available (Hyper Sense by Oxford Instruments, UK). The availability of this facility will certainly widen dramatically the studies in the field.

1.5 PHIP

Molecular H_2 occurs into two isomeric spin forms, namely ortho- and para-H_2, corresponding to a triplet spin state (parallel proton spins, 75% at equilibrium) and a singlet state (antiparallel proton spins, 25% at equilibrium), respectively. Enrichment in the para form, which is energetically favoured, is possible by keeping H_2 at low temperature in the presence of a catalyst. A comprehensive study of para-/ortho-hydrogen conversion catalyzed by several dia- and paramagnetic metal complexes has been recently published (Matsumoto and Espenson 2005). An excellent correlation has been observed between the rate of conversion and the paramagnetism of the metal complexes. At liquid N_2 temperature, a 50% enrichment is achieved, while at liquid He temperature, it is possible to obtain a 100% enrichment (Fig. 5). The increase in the population of the para state leads to the hyperpolarization of the H_2 molecule, which can be maintained for days in the absence of the catalyst. Proton spin polarization can then be transferred to the reaction products of para-hydrogen, yielding the characteristic para-H_2 effects in NMR spectra, discovered in 1986 by Weitekamp and Eisenberg (Bowers and Weitekamp 1986; Bowers and Weitekamp 1987; Bowers et al. 1990; Eisenberg 1991). Since then, a number of systems have been investigated, mainly in order to better understand hydrogenation mechanisms (Duckett et al 1994; Bargon and Kandels 1993; Aime et al. 1998, 1999). Typically, when a molecule of para-H_2 is added to an unsaturated substrate, e.g. an alkyne R_1-C $\equiv$ C-R_2 with $R_1 \neq R_2$ (Fig. 6), an AX system is formed, for which four transition frequencies are expected. As the two added hydrogens keep memory of the their spin orientation, only $\alpha\beta$ (ALTADENA experiments) or only $\alpha\beta$ and $\beta\alpha$ states (PASADENA experiments) will be populated and the resulting AX

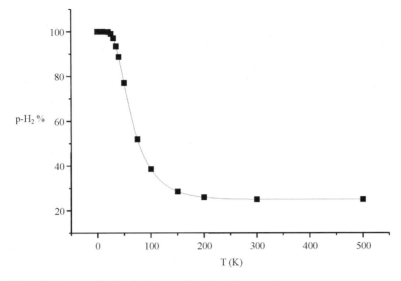

Fig. 5 Equilibrium para-H_2 distribution as a function of temperature

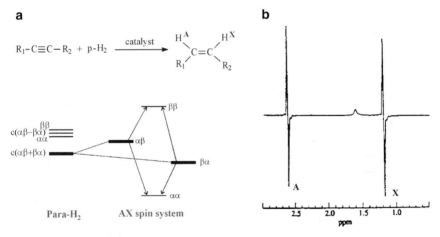

Fig. 6 a Para-hydrogenation of an alkyne yielding the AX spin system; **b** the resulting ^{1}H NMR spectrum under PASADENA conditions

spin system pattern will be strongly affected. In fact, in place of the expected almost equally intense four adsorptions, the AX spin system of a parahydrogenated product yields strong adsorption/emission signals (one adsorption and one emission in the ALTADENA case, two adsorption and two emissions in the PASADENA case, Fig. 6), as the result of the dramatic changes in the populations of the four spin states in respect to the normal Boltzmann distribution. Immediately after the addition (and even when para-H_2 is interacting with the catalytic site), the relaxation process starts to restore the Boltzmann populations and the corresponding intensities in the two doublets of the AX spin-system. The magnetization order transfer from para-H_2 to the hydrogenated product yields extraordinary enhancements in the NMR signal which, in theory, may reach values as high as 10^5-times the signal intensity of the corresponding derivatives produced with normal H_2 (Eisenberg 1991; Bargon et al. 1993; Eisenschmid et al. 1987), allowing the detection of species which are present in solution in very low concentrations. Three conditions need to be satisfied in order to observe para-H_2 enhancements in the NMR spectra; namely, the simultaneous transfer of the two H atoms from the para-H_2 molecule to the same substrate molecule (maintaining of the spin correlation during the reaction), the breakdown of symmetry in the reaction product, and the high hydrogenation rate (necessary to prevent restoration of the equilibrium states populations due to relaxation processes occurring in intermediates or in the reaction products). The PHIP phenomenon has been recently reviewed (Natterer and Bargon 1997; Duckett and Sleigh 1999).

Scalar couplings with heteroatoms or nuclear Overhauser effect (nOe) can cause the polarization to be transferred from H atoms to neighbouring heteronuclei in the hydrogenation products. The heteronucleus hyperpolarization is greater when it is due to scalar couplings; several articles have been published describing the phenomenon not only from a theoretical point of view but also with many examples concerning unsaturated organic molecules (Natterer et al. 1998; Eisenschmid et al. 1989; Stephan et al. 2002; Barkemeyer et al. 1995; Aime et al. 2003). Among them, one may recall the polarization transfer to ^{31}P and ^{13}C in Ir(H_2)Br(CO)(dppe) (Eisenschmid et al. 1989; Duckett et al. 1993), to ^{13}C in various alkenes, obtained by parahydrogenation of alkynes (Stephan et al. 2002), and in particular to the carbonyl ^{13}C atom in para-hydrogenated acetylenedicarboxylate (Barkemeyer et al. 1995), which successively has been the first para-hydrogenated molecule to be used as an MRI contrast agent (Golman et al. 2001) (vide infra); to ^2D in deuterated ethylene obtained by para-hydrogenation of deuterated acetylene (Aime et al. 2003); to ^{13}C in diethylether obtained by para-hydrogenation of ethylvinylether (a substrate that has narcotic properties when inhalated and has been suggested as an alternative to hyperpolarized noble gases) (Bargon et al. 2005).

Basically the pattern of the given heteronucleus resonance appears as an ensemble of strong adsorptions and emissions that, as such, are of limited (if any) utility for MRI applications. Indeed, the non-equilibrium spin order obtained by para-hydrogenation of the substrates can be converted to longitudinal magnetization in order to allow their use in MRI. This can be achieved in two ways: (1) by applying a diabatic field cycling, or (2) by applying suitable pulse sequences.

The diabatic field cycling consists of quickly (diabatically) reducing the magnetic field strength from the earth field value to less than $0.1\,\mu T$, and then slowly (adiabatically) raising it up again to the earth field value. When the field is lowered, the proton-carbon spin system is brought into the strongly coupled regime, enabling intimate coupling between the polarized protons and the coupled carbon atoms. When the field is slowly raised up again, the populations of the spin states are maintained. The result is a ^{13}C NMR spectrum where the allowed transitions are predominantly in phase, corresponding to substantial polarization (Fig. 7). The optimization of the procedure can be achieved by computer simulation of the spin system evolution

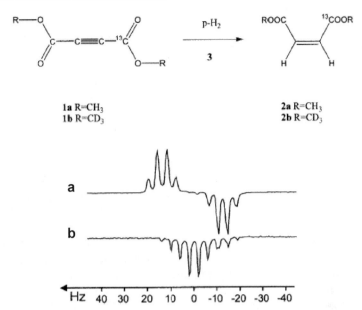

Fig. 7 a ^{13}C NMR spectrum of **2** (carboxylate moiety) after hydrogenation with parahydrogen. **b** Same spectrum after hydrogenation with parahydrogen and subsequent low field cycling (Golman et al. 2001)

and is different for any given molecule. The method was successfully applied (by using a μ-metal shield to lower the field strength to 0.1 μT) for the first time by Golman and co-workers on the product of the para-hydrogenation of acetylenedicarboxylate (Golman et al. 2001) and of hydroxyethylpropionate (Goldman et al. 2005; Johannesson et al. 2004), allowing the attainment of ^{13}C enhancements up to 10^4 with respect to non-polarized molecules, and the substrates have been used as contrast agents for angiographies in rats (vide infra). A theoretical treatment of the polarization transfer process is reported in Goldman et al. (2005).

According to Goldman and Johannesson (2005), the same result can be achieved by using a suitably tailored pulse sequence (Fig. 8). It uses a constant decoupling magnetic field and a continuous rf irradiation of the sample during the hydrogenation reaction, which minimizes the loss of spin order during this stage. Then, a 180x pulse on the proton simply prepares the system for the subsequent series of pulses (90x and 90y on the carbon nucleus), which is effective in the conversion of the spin order into net ^{13}C polarization. Many echoes are introduced in the sequence in order to correct defects due to field inhomogeneity (Goldman and Johannesson 2005). An in-depth description of the pulse method for converting the para spin order into ^{13}C polarization has been reported in Goldman and Johannesson (2005). The final theoretical polarization is close to unity.

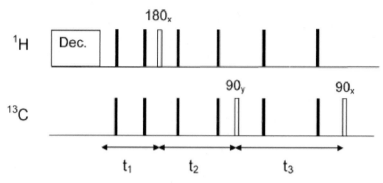

Fig. 8 Pulse sequence for converting para-H_2 spin order to ^{13}C longitudinal magnetization in hydroxyethylpropionate (Goldman and Johannesson 2005)

2 Imaging with Hyperpolarized ^{13}C-containing Molecules: a Survey of the Main Applications

Whereas in conventional MRI the longitudinal magnetization consumed during the image acquisition step can be restored by relaxation processes, this is not possible when using hyperpolarized molecules and the pulse sequences to be used need to take this into account. Two main acquisition protocols have been proposed: (1) to use trains of low flip-angle pulses [fast low angle shot (FLASH)], or (2) to use a single shot sequence. The published MRI works with slowly relaxing ^{13}C hyperpolarized molecules report the use of the RARE (rapid acquisition with relaxation enhancement), EPI (echo planar imaging) and trueFISP (fast imaging with steady-state free precession) sequences. EPI in particular is useful since it converts the initial longitudinal magnetization into transverse magnetization with almost 100% efficiency, thus allowing several images to be acquired and hence to follow the distribution of the contrast agent. The most used pulse sequence is trueFISP, which enables the transverse magnetization from one cycle to be recycled to the next, and it is particularly well suited for slowly relaxing systems because large flip angles can be used (between 160° and 180°), balancing field dishomogeneities well (Svensson 2003; Svensson et al. 2002, 2003).

Several applications of ^{13}C imaging with hyperpolarized (DNP or para-H_2) molecules have been reported, ranging from vascular and perfusion imaging to catheter tracking to highly innovative molecular imaging protocols. Examples of these are described in the following paragraphs.

2.1 Vascular Imaging

^{13}C hyperpolarized angiography is fascinating because the high contrast enhancement (due to the fact that the hyperpolarized agent acts as the direct source of signal, above a very low background) makes it possible to use thick MRI slices to create angiograms, thus obtaining 2D images as good as or even better than the 3D ones obtainable by the classic ^{1}H images in a very short time, and reducing the formation of motion artefacts.

The first example of ^{13}C angiography obtained by using a ^{13}C hyperpolarized molecule as contrast agent was reported by Golman et al. (2001). They were able to acquire a complete angiogram of a rat at 2.4 T, using a 150 mM acetone solution of ^{13}C labelled maleic acid dimethylester, obtained by para-hydrogenation of acetylenedicarboxylic acid dimethyl ester (estimated polarization 0.3%), and the single-shot RARE sequence having a total scan time of 0.9 s (Fig. 9). The para-hydrogenation of the substrate was optimized in order to obtain the higher possible reaction rate. The long ^{13}C relaxation time of the carboxylate group (75 s in

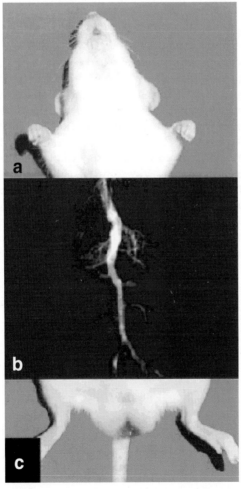

Fig. 9 ^{13}C single-shot RARE image of a rat generated in 0.9 s at 2.4 T (Golman et al. 2001)

acetone-d6 at 7.05 T) in the contrast agent molecule allowed the product to be ma-
nipulated and to be injected into the tail vein of the rat without loosing too much
signal. The net polarization of the ^{13}C resonance was obtained by the field cycling procedure described above. The image clearly showed the vena cava and some
branches, the finest visible structures being <0.5 mm. The work suffered for relatively low ^{13}C polarization (first of all due to the use of only 50% enriched para-H$_2$),
and for the fact that the whole reaction mixture (including the hydrogenation catalyst and the organic solvent) was injected into the rat. Nevertheless, although these
drawbacks, the first image with a ^{13}C-hyperpolarized molecule showed all its huge
potential!

In two patent applications, the same authors reported a method for a quick removal of both the catalyst and the organic solvent from the mixture before the injection. They suggested removing the ionic Rh catalyst used for hydrogenation by ion
exchange and the solvent by spray flash distillation after addition of some amounts
of water to the mixture (Morgensteyerne et al. 2000; Golman et al. 1998). Furthermore, they proposed a number of possible alternative structures as ^{13}C-enriched
substrates for para-hydrogenation.

Clearly, hydrogenation and separation of the catalyst and the organic solvent are
key-steps for a successful application of the para-hydrogen procedure. In our laboratory we have pursued different ways to obtain pure para-hydrogenated water-
soluble compounds. In particular, we have explored the possibility of transferring
a lypophilic compound from the organic to the aqueous solvent by a phase transfer
process (S. Aime, R. Gobetto, D. Santelia, F. Reineri, A. Viale, to be published). The
molecule we tested is bis[(2-methoxyethoxy)ethyl] acetylendicarboxylate, which is
easily para-hydrogenated in acetone by using [Rh(COD)(dppb)][BF$_4$] as catalyst.
The product is not water soluble, but upon adding an equimolar quantity of Li$^+$
a phase transfer process takes place, and the Li$^+$ complex passes from acetone
to water (previously added to the mixture), thus allowing its separation (Fig. 10).

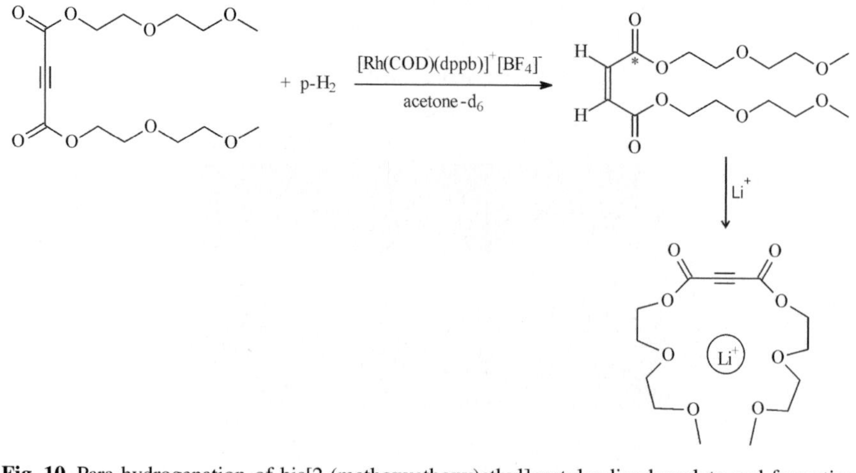

Fig. 10 Para-hydrogenation of bis[2-(methoxyethoxy)ethyl]acetylendicarboxylate and formation
of the water-soluble Li$^+$ complex for phase transfer separation

The ^{13}C polarization detected at the end of the phase transfer process was about 0.1, and allowed the detection of an in-vitro ^{13}C image, by using the single-shot RARE sequence on a spectrometer operating at 75 MHz.

An alternative route to avoid the use of organic solvents in the para-hydrogenation step is the use of water-soluble substrates and catalysts, and high para-H$_2$ pressure. This procedure was used to produce hydroxyethylacrylate by para-hydrogenation of hydroxyethylpropionate, in water, using a water-soluble Rh catalyst (Fig. 11). In this case 95% para-H$_2$ was used at a pressure of 10 bar in a properly designed reaction chamber, which is one part of an automatic apparatus including the magnetic field cycling device and valves to quickly move the reaction mixture. The ^{13}C polarization was estimated to be 21%, more than sufficient to acquire a well-resolved angiogram of the head of a guinea pig by using the trueFISP sequence (Goldman et al. 2005; Johannesson et al. 2004). In Goldman et al. (2005), a series of five successive images is reported, showing the dynamics of the progression of the injected solution through the blood vessels (Fig. 12).

When the polarization is achieved by the DNP method, the problem of removing the hydrogenation catalyst is replaced by the problem of separating the ^{13}C substrate from the organic radical.

The first in-vivo angiographic ^{13}C image of a rat obtained by using a DNP hyperpolarized contrast agent, namely water-soluble bis-1,1-(hydroxymethyl)-1-^{13}C-cyclopropane-d$_8$ (T$_1$ of the ^{13}C nucleus = 82 s at 2.35 T), is reported in Goldman et al. (2005). The DNP procedure was in this case carried out by using the triaryl radical tris(8-carboxy-2,2,6,6-tetra-(hydroxyethyl)benzo[1,2-d:4,5-d']bis(1,3)dithiole-4-yl)methyl sodium salt, which is soluble in the contrast agent, as the doping radical,

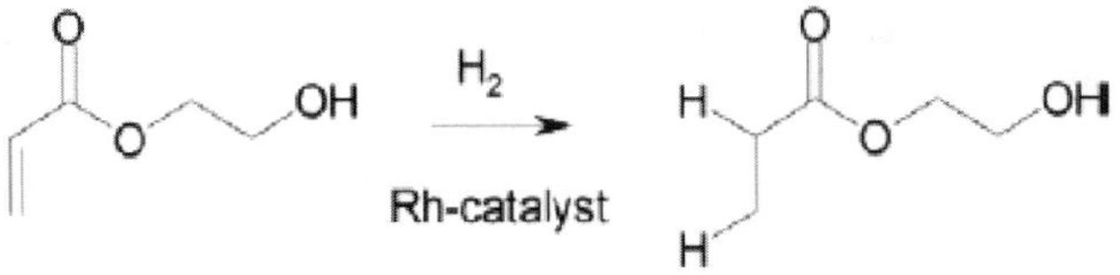

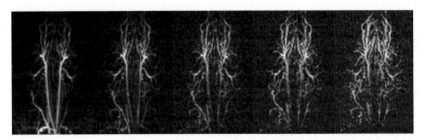

Fig. 11 Para-hydrogenation of hydroxyethylpropionate yielding hyperpolarized hydroxyethylacrylate

Fig. 12 Angiography of a guinea pig head with hyperpolarized hydroxyethylpropionate. Successive ^{13}C images at 480-ms intervals following the injection of the contrast agent (Goldman et al. 2005)

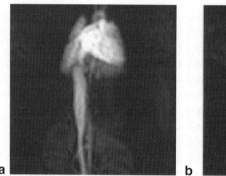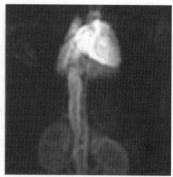

a   b

Fig. 13 a, b Series of angiograms covering the thoracic and abdominal area, acquired immediately after intravenous injections of 3 ml hyperpolarized bis-1,1-(hydroxymethyl)-1-^{13}C-cyclopropane-d$_8$. **a** The first image in the series visualizes several of the main vessels in the area. **b** The fourth image from the same image series (Svensson et al. 2003)

and irradiating the frozen sample at 93.9 GHz. After dissolution in hot water, a 200 mM solution was obtained with a ^{13}C polarization of about 15%. A normal gradient spoiled, gradient echo pulse sequence was used, thus allowing to record only one image, which showed the vena cava, the heart ventricle and several minor vessels with a good SNR. Only blood was visible because the image was obtained during the first pass of the contrast agent in the vascular system.

One year later, a series of in-vivo angiography experiments on rats with the same DNP polarized molecule, by using the trueFISP sequence, has been reported (Svensson et al. 2003). The series of 15 images of the thoracic and abdominal area of the rats (in Fig. 13 two of these are reported) clearly showed the vena cava, aortic arc, carotid arteries and renal arteries, while in those of the head and neck area the carotid arteries, jugular veins and several minor vessels were visible. The loss in signal intensity from one image to the next was mainly determined by the T$_2$ value of the ^{13}C nucleus in blood, and was only slightly influenced by the flow/motion effect.

An angiographic image of a live rabbit was also obtained by using an endogenous substance as contrast agent, namely ^{13}C enriched DNP - hyperpolarized (see above) urea (Kolman et al. 2003): immediately after the injection it was possible to visualize the vena cava, the heart and the pulmonary vascular system; 2 s after completing the injection, the renal vascular system was also clearly detected (Fig. 14).

2.2 Perfusion Studies

Commonly, perfusion parameters such as cerebral blood flow (CBF), cerebral blood volume (CBV) and mean transit time (MTT) can be evaluated by dynamic suscep-tivity contrast MRI, where signal variations following the injection of paramagnetic

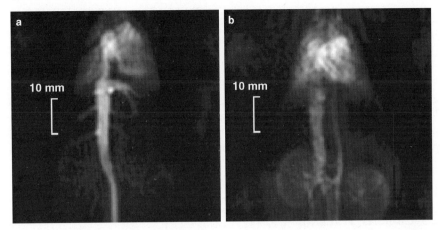

Fig. 14 a, b ^{13}C coronal projection images of a rat. The image acquisitions were started **a** imme-diately and **b** 2 s after completing the injection of the contrast agent. The scan time of each image was 0.24 s (Morgensteyerne et al. 2000)

Gd chelates are analysed on the basis of the bolus tracking theory to yield the perfu-sion parameter values. Nevertheless, problems related to the tissue's vascular com-position, which affects the signal intensity, and the different relaxation mechanisms experienced by the protons in intra- and extravascular spaces make the quantifica-tion of perfusion by this method quite difficult.

These problems are overcome when using hyperpolarized ^{13}C molecules, which act as direct sources of signal (providing therefore a direct relationship between the tracer concentration and the signal intensity over all concentrations), as tracers for flow and perfusion studies. Of course, the depolarization of the tracer must be taken into account since it would produce an apparently faster decrease of the signal, but suitable modifications can be introduced in the bolus tracking theory to take it into account (Johansson et al. 2004a, 2004b), allowing a quite accurate estimation of the perfusion parameters. This has been done, for example, on a rat model, by using ^{13}C DNP hyperpolarized bis-1,1-(hydroxymethyl)-1-^{13}C-cyclopropane-d_8 as the tracer.

The same hyperpolarized tracer has been used to obtain perfusion maps of the myocardium of a pig (Johansson et al. 2005). The tracer was injected both by arterial catheter and by intravenous injection in the femoral vein. In the second case, lower SNR and spatial resolution was achieved.

The properties of a non-equilibrium spin population may also be employed to perform tissue blood flow quantification in a different way. The proposed technique is called bolus differentiation and is based on the fact that the polarization of the hyperpolarized tracer can be destroyed by applying a radiofrequency excitation. An important advantage of this method is that the estimation is independent from the arterial delay and dispersion, and that it can be applied to any tissue in principle.

A study of rabbits' kidneys has been performed by this approach, using ^{13}C-enriched 2-hydroxyethylacrylate polarized by PHIP (20–30% polarization) (Johans-son et al. 2004b). In the reported perfusion maps the aorta and other arteries were apparent, while no blood flow was detected in the inner part of the kidneys maybe because the polarization was destroyed before the tracer arrived in that region (Fig. 15).

Finally, it has been possible to obtain images of the pulmonary arterial circulation of a pig by injection of a ^{13}C hyperpolarized molecule (Fig. 16) (Mansson et al. 2005; Golman et al. 2003). Pulmonary perfusion imaging with hyperpolarized ^{13}C contrast agents may be used in the future to obtain high-resolution perfusion pulmonary maps. Furthermore, it might be possible to also study ventilation and perfusion in real time by injecting simultaneously a ^{13}C and a ^{3}He hyperpolarized contrast agent.

2.3 Catheter Tracking

The absence of ^{13}C background signal when a ^{13}C hyperpolarized contrast agent is used may find an interesting application in interventional endovascular MRI procedures. In this case, ^{1}H images must be acquired simultaneously to the ^{13}C image by using a multinuclei MR scanner, in order to have an anatomical map of the region of interest to be used as an interventional guidance. In addition, 3D maps giving the exact geometrical correspondence between the catheter position and the anatomical images can be constructed.

Examples of 3D reconstruction and fusion with a proton map image are reported by Mansson et al. (2004, 2006) and Golman et al. (2005), where the visualization of a catheter travelling through the aortic arch of a pig is reported. The work reported in Mansson et al. (2006) also shows the visualization of a catheter travelling through the aorta and renal artery of a pig (Fig. 17): in this case, the authors demonstrate the possibility of visualizing both the catheter and the injection of substances during therapy. In the latter case it is sufficient to inject some ^{13}C hyperpolarized contrast agent (2-hydroxyethyl acrylate obtained by PHIP in this particular case) via a separate channel of the catheter into the artery and flushing it into the kidney. This may help in the evaluation of the excretory status of the kidney.

2.4 Molecular Imaging

MR images of live animals injected with a ^{13}C hyperpolarized contrast agents (namely 2-hydroxyethylacrylate obtained by PHIP, polarization 30%) are reported in Golman et al. (2003), to show the distribution pattern of the contrast agent in various rabbits' organs. In particular, the authors followed the ^{13}C molecule distribution at different time points, by recording one image for each rabbit at different times after injection, finding that after 2 s the ^{13}C reporter was mainly located at the heart and the lungs; after 4 s the kidneys and the stomach walls were perfectly visible, while the signal from the heart was diminished, and after 6 s the intestine

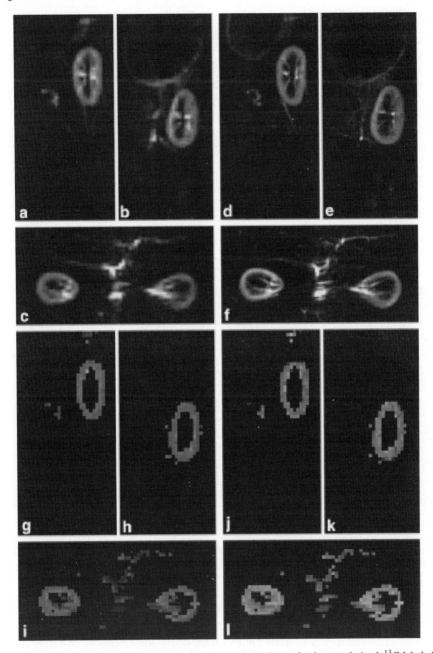

Fig. 15 a–l Parametric maps obtained after venous injections of a hyperpolarized ^{13}C-labeled compound in a rabbit. **a,b,d,e** Renal cortical blood flow assessed in sagittal orientation; **c,f** renal cortical blood flow assessed in transversal orientation. Two in-plane resolutions were used: $2 \times 2\,mm^2$ **a–c** and $1 \times 2\,mm^2$ **d–f**. **g–i** Mean transit time. **j–l** Dispersion. The slice thickness was 10 mm. A TrueFISP sequence with a 90° preparation pulse and a 180° flip angle was employed (Johansson et al. 2004b)

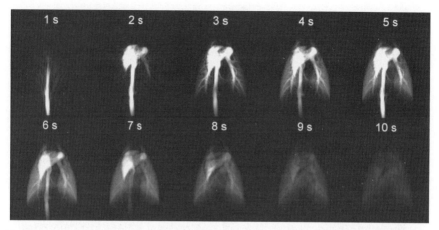

Fig. 16 A series of trueFISP ^{13}C images, showing the lungs of a pig after injection of a hyperpolarized ^{13}C imaging agent. The imaging sequence was repeated with 1-s intervals (Golman et al. 2003)

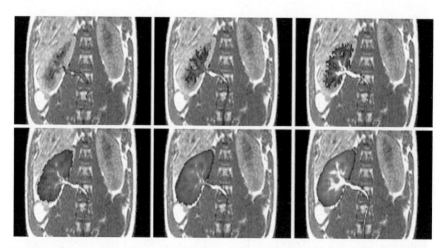

Fig. 17 Catheter tracking of the renal arteries in a pig. A bolus of 2-hydroxyethylacrylate was injected into the kidney via a separate channel of the catheter. The ^{13}C image series was acquired using a true fast imaging with steady state free precision (trueFISP) sequence with in-plane resolution $2 \times 2\,mm^2$ and acquisition time 329 ms/image (Mansson et al. 2006)

also appeared in the images (Fig. 18). Note that the ^{1}H images obtained by usual gadolinium contrast agents did not show either the stomach or the intestine. The authors state that it may be possible to obtain distribution maps by injecting and imaging several hyperpolarized ^{13}C molecules simultaneously, with the possibility of gaining information about membrane structure and permeability.

The information gained from this study is relevant to demonstrate that the crossing of biological barriers does not cause a dramatic loss of the hyperpolarization characteristics of the imaging reporter. This insight has been further substantiated

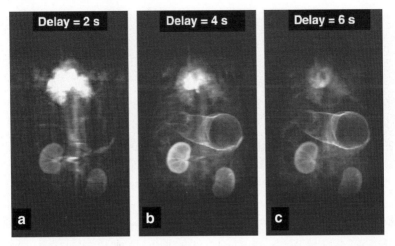

Fig. 18 a–c Images depicting the distribution of the injected hyperpolarized ^{13}C imaging agent at different times after the injection. The delay between injection and imaging is indicated at the top of each image (Golman et al. 2003)

when it has been found that hyperpolarization can be found in the products of a catalyzed transformation of ^{13}C-labelled hyperpolarized pyruvate (from the DNP process). In fact, Golman and coworkers at the Malmo laboratories of GE Health found that the ^{13}C polarization of pyruvate is still found in several products of its metabolic transformation, i.e. alanine, bicarbonate and lactate (Golman et al. 2006b). Two major considerations can be drawn by these findings: (1) the lifetime of the adduct formed by pyruvate and the enzyme responsible for the undergoing transformation is much shorter than the relaxation time of the ^{13}C carboxylate resonance; (2) the rate of tranformation of pyruvate is very high, thus allowing the detection of sufficiently large amounts of polarized product molecules in the short lap of few seconds. These observations represent a real breakthrough in the field of molecular imaging for several reasons. First of all, there is the possibility of visualizing the distribution of molecules that represent key steps of the cellular metabolism (metabolic imaging), therefore providing direct access to physio/pathological changes at the cellular level. Then, by exploiting chemical shift imaging (CSI) procedures it becomes possible to visualize more than one molecule in the same anatomical region. This is clearly not possible for nuclear probes as well as for gadolinium- or iron oxide-based systems in MRI. Possibly, for the latter imaging modality, only the recently introduced class of CEST agents may pursue the same task.

On the basis of the results obtained, the GE Health team has developed a test for assessing prostate tumours based on the relative amounts of alanine and lactate. In fact, it is well established that tumor cell metabolism responds to anoxy conditions by tranforming more pyruvate in lactate rather than in alanine (Fig. 19) (Golman et al. 2006a; Golman and Petersson 2006).

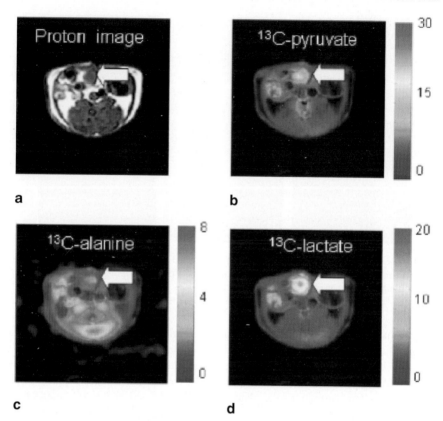

Fig. 19 a–d The metabolic pattern in a tumor model. Maps of the metabolites alanine **c** and lactate **d** obtained in a rat tumor model after injection of hyperpolarized ^{13}C-pyruvate **b**. The first image **a** shows the corresponding proton slice. The ^{13}C maps have all been superimposed on the proton map. In all images, the position of the implanted tumour is indicated by a *white arrow* (Golman et al. 2006a)

3 Final Remarks

The currently used contrast agents based on gadolinium or on iron oxide particles have played an important role in the development of clinical applications of MRI techniques by adding relevant physiological information to the superb anatomical resolution attainable with this imaging modality. Nowadays, the major challenges are in the emerging field of molecular imaging, where the MRI probes are suffering from their limited sensitivity in respect to the reporters available for other imaging modalities. Whereas there is a lot of work currently ongoing that tackles this drawback by designing efficient amplification protocols with the available MRI contrast agents, huge expectation relies on the involvement of hyperpolarized molecules.

Hyperpolarization procedures can have a central role in this context because (1) hyperpolarized imaging reporters allow the sensitivity issue to be overcome and support MRI to compete with nuclear and optical imaging modalities, and (2) the use of hyperpolarized systems make possible the detection of more molecules in the same anatomical region thanks to the acquisition of chemical shift images. Currently this is possible only in optical imaging by using fluorescent dyes, but the problems associated with light penetration and scattering strongly limit this application in the biomedical field. The possibility of comparing high-resolution images reporting on the presence of different metabolites represents a powerful tool to directly access basic information on the function of the cellular machinery and then to assess early diagnoses and efficient monitoring of therapeutic treatments.

References

Abragam A, Goldman M (1978) Principles of dynamic nuclear polarisation. Rep Prog Phys 41:395–467

Aime S, Gobetto R, Canet D (1998) Longitudinal nuclear relaxation in an A_2 spin system initially polarized through para-hydrogen. J Am Chem Soc 120:6770–6773

Aime S, Dastrù W, Gobetto R, Russo A, Viale A, Canet D (1999) A novel application of para H_2: the reversible addition/elimination of H_2 at a Ru_3 cluster revealed by the enhanced nmr emission resonance from molecular hydrogen. J Phys Chem A 103:9702–9705

Aime S, Gobetto R, Reineri F (2003) Hyperpolarization transfer from parahydrogen to deuterium via carbon-13. J Chem Phys 119:8890–8896

Aime S, Carrera C, Delli Caselli D, Geninatti S, Terreno E (2005) Tunable imaging of cells labeled with MRI-PARACEST agents. Angew Chem Int Ed 44:1813–1815

Albert MS, Cates GD, Driehuys B, Happer W, Saam B, Springer CS Jr et al (1994) Biological magnetic resonance imaging using laser-polarized ^{129}Xe. Nature 370:199–201

Altes TA, Salerno M (2004) Hyperpolarized gas MR imaging of the lung. J Thoracic Imag 19:250–258

Ardenkjaer-Larsen JH, Fridlund B, Gram A, Hansson G, Hansson L, Lerche MH, Servin R, Thaning M, Golman K (2003) Increase in signal-to-noise ratio of > 10,000 times in liquid-state NMR. Proc Natl Acad Sci USA 100:10158–10163

Bajaj VS, Farrar CT, Hornstein MK, Mastovsky I, Vieregg J, Bryant J, Elèna B, Kreischer KE, Temkin RJ, Griffin RG (2003) Dynamic nuclear polarization at 9 T using a novel 250 GHz gyrotron microwave source. J Magn Res 160:85–90

Bargon J, Kandels J (1993) Nuclear magnetic resonance studies of homogeneous catalysis using parahydrogen: analysis of nuclear singlet triplet mixing as a diagnostic tool to characterize intermediates. J Chem Phys 98:6150–6153

Bargon J, Kandels J, Woelk KZ (1993) Orthohydrogen and parahydrogen induced nuclear spin polarization. Phys Chem 180:65–93

Bargon J, Bommerich U, Kadlecek S, Ishii M, Fischer MC, Rizi RR (2005) Homogeneous hydrogenation yielding a hyperpolarized form of the inhalation narcotic diethyl ether. Proc Intl Soc Magn Reson Med, 13th Scientific Meeting, Abstracts, p 2572

Barkemeyer J, Haake M, Bargon J (1995) Hetero-NMR enhancement via parahydrogen labelling. J Am Chem Soc 117:2927–2928

Bartik K, Luhmer M, Dutasta P, Collet A, Reisse J (1998) ^{129}Xe and ^1H NMR study of the reversible trapping of xenon by cryptophane-A in organic solution. J Am Chem Soc 120:784–791

Bifone A, Song YQ, Seydoux R, Taylor RE, Goodson BM, Pietrass T, Budinger TF, Navon G, Pines A (1996) NMR of laser-polarized xenon in human blood. Proc Natl Acad Sci USA 93: 12932–12936

Bowers CR, Weitekamp DP (1986) Transformation of symmetrization order to nuclear-spin magnetization by chemical reaction and nuclear magnetic resonance. Phys Rev Lett 57:2645–2648

Bowers CR, Weitekamp DP (1987) Parahydrogen and synthesis allow dramatically enhanced nuclear alignment. J Am Chem Soc 109:5541–5542

Bowers CR, Jones DH, Kurur ND, Labinger JA, Pravica MG, Weitekamp DP (1990) Symmetrization postulate and nuclear magnetic resonance of reacting systems. Adv Magn Res 14:269

Brown TR (2000) Chemical shift imaging. In: Methods in biomedical magnetic resonance imaging and spectroscopy, vol 2. Wiley, Chichester, pp 751–763

Callot V, Canet E, Brochot J, Berthezene Y, Viallon M, Humblot H, Briguet A, Tournier H, Cremillieux Y (2001a) Vascular and perfusion imaging using encapsulated laser-polarized Helium. Magma 12:16–22

Callot V, Canet E, Brochot J, Viallon M, Humblot H, Briguet A, Tournier H, Cremillieux Y (2001b) MR perfusion imaging using encapsulated laser-polarized ^{3}He. Magn Reson Med 46:535–540

Cutillo AG (ed) (1996) Application of magnetic resonance to the study of lung. Futura, Armonk

Duckett SB, Sleigh CJ (1999) Applications of the parahydrogen phenomenon: a chemical perspective. Progr Nucl Magn Reson Spectrosc 34:71–92

Duckett SB, Newell, CL Eisenberg R (1993) More than INEPT: parahydrogen and INEPT + give unprecedented resonance enhancement to carbon-13 by direct proton polarization transfer. J Am Chem Soc 115:1156–1157

Duckett SB, Newell CL, Eisenberg R (1994) Observation of new intermediates in hydrogenation catalyzed by Wilkinson's Catalyst, RhCl(PPh3)3, using parahydrogen-induced polarization. J Am Chem Soc 169:10548–10556

Duhamel G, Choquet P, Grillon E, Lamalle L, Leviel JL, Ziegler A, Constantinesco A (2001) Xenon-129 MR imaging and spectroscopy of rat brain using arterial delivery of hyperpolarized xenon in a lipid emulsion. Magn Reson Med 46:208–212

Eisenberg R (1991) Parahydrogen-induced polarization: a new spin on reactions with molecular hydrogen, Acc Chem Res 24:110–116; and references therein

Eisenschmid TC, Kirss RU, Deusch PP, Hommeltoft SI, Eisenberg R (1987) Para hydrogen induced polarization in hydrogenation reactions. J Am Chem Soc 109:8089–8091

Eisenschmid TC, McDonald J, Eisenberg R (1989) INEPT in a chemical way Polarization transfer from para hydrogen to phosphorus-31 by oxidative addition and dipolar relaxation. J Am Chem Soc 111:7267–7269

Gerfen GJ, Becerra LR, Hall DA, Griffin RG, Temkin RJ, Singel DJ (1995) High-frequency (140 GHz) dynamic nuclear polarization: polarization transfer to a solute in frozen aqueous solution. J Chem Phys 102:9494–9497

Goldman M, Johannesson H (2005) Conversion of a proton pair para order into ^{13}C polarization by RF irradiation, for use in MRI. CR Phisique 6:575–581

Goldman M, Johannesson H, Axelsson O, Karlsson M (2005) Hyperpolarization of ^{13}C through order transfer from parahydrogen: a new contrast agent for MRI. Magn Reson Imag 23:153–157

Golman K, Petersson JS (2006) Metabolic imaging and other applications of hyperpolarized ^{13}C. Acad Radiol 13:932–942

Golman K, Axelsson O, Johanneson H, Olofsson C, Mansson S, Petersson S (1998) Nycomed Innovation AB, patent no. WO9924080

Golman K, Axelsson O, Johannesson H, Mansson S, Olofsson, C, Petersson JS (2001) Parahydrogen-induced polarization in imaging: subsecond ^{13}C angiography. Magn Res Med 46:1–5

Golman K, Ardenkjaer-Larsen JH, Svensson J, Axelsson O, Hansson G, Hansson L, Johannesson H, Leunbach I, Mansson S, Petersson JS, Pettersson G, Servin R, Wistrand LG (2002) ^{13}C-Angiography. Acad Radiol 9(Suppl 2):S507–S510

Golman K, Olsson, LE, Axelsson, O, Mansson S, Karlsson M, Petersson JS (2003) Molecular imaging using hyperpolarized ^{13}C. Br J Radiol 76:S118–S127

Golman K, Olsson LE, Petersson JS (2005) Dynamic interventional MR imaging using hyperpolarized C-13. Acad Radiol 12(Suppl 1):S70–S71

Golman K, in 't Zandt R, Lerche M, Perhson R, Ardenkjaer-Larsen H (2006a) Metabolic imaging by hyperpolarized ^{13}C magnetic resonance imaging for in vivo tumor diagnosis. Cancer Res 66:10855–10860

Golman K, in 't Zandt R, Thaning M (2006b) Real-time metabolic imaging. Proc Natl Acad Sci USA 103:11270–11275

Hall DA, Maus DC, Gerfen GJ, Inati SJ, Becerra LR, Dahlquist FW, Griffin RG (1997) Polarization-enhanced NMR spectroscopy of biomolecules in frozen solution. Science 276:930–932

Hu JZ, Zhou JW, Yang BL, Li LY, Qiu JQ, Ye CH, Solum MS, Wind RA, Pugmire RJ, Grant DM (1997) Dynamic nuclear polarization of nitrogen-15 in benzamide. Solid State Nucl Magn Res 8:129–137

Hu JZ, Solum MS, Wind RA, Nilsson BL, Peterson MA, Pugmire RJ,Grant DM (2000) ^{1}H and ^{15}N dynamic nuclear polarization studies of carbazole. J Phys Chem A 104:4413–4420

Johannesson H, Axelsson O, Karlsson M (2004) Transfer of para-hydrogen spin order into polarization by diabatic field cycling. CR Physique 5:315–324

Johansson E, Mansson, S, Wirestam R, Svensson J, Petersson JS, Golman K, Stahlberg F (2004a) Cerebral perfusion assessment by bolus tracking using hyperpolarized ^{13}C. Magn Reson Med 51:464–472

Johansson E, Olsson LE, Mansson S, Petersson JS, Golman K, Stahlberg F, Wirestam R (2004b) Perfusion assessment with bolus differentiation: a technique applicable to hyperpolarized tracers. Magn Reson Med 52:1043–1051

Johansson E, Magnusson P, Chai CM, Petersson JS, Golman K, Wirestam R, Stahlberg F (2005) Assessing myocardial perfusion using hyperpolarized ^{13}C. In: Proc 21st Annual Meeting ESM-RMB, p 117

Kalechofsky NF (2002) Oxford Instruments Superconductivity Ltd, patent no. WO0155656

Kauczor HU, Surkau, R, Roberts T (1998) MRI using hyperpolarized noble gases. Eur Radiol 8:820–827

Kolman K, Ardenkjaer-Larsen JH, Petersson JS, Mansson S, Leunbach I (2003) Molecular imaging with endogenous substances. Proc Natl Acad Sci USA 100:10435–10439

Lamerichs RM, Luyten PR (2000) Proton decoupling during in vivo whole body phosphorus MRS. In: Methods in biomedical magnetic resonance imaging and spectroscopy, vol 2. Wiley, Chichester, pp 774–777

Mansson, S, Petersson JS, Chai CM, Hansson G, Johansson E (2005) Passive catheter tracking using MRI and hyperpolarized ^{13}C. In: Proc 21st Annual Meeting ESMRMB, p 143

Mansson S, Johansson E, Magnusson, P, Chai CM, Hansson G, Petersson JS, Stahlberg F, Golman K (2006) C-13 imaging – a new diagnostic platform. Eur Radiol 16:56–67

Matsumoto M, Espenson JH (2005) Kinetics of the interconversion of parahydrogen and orthohydrogen catalyzed by paramagnetic complex ions. J Am Chem Soc 127:11447–11453

Middleton H, Balck RD, Saam B, Cates GD, Cofer GP, Guenther R, Happer W, Hedlund LW, Johnson GA, Juvan K, Swartz J (1995) MR-imaging with hyperpolarized He-3 gas. Magn Reson Med 33:271–275

Moller HE, Chawla MS, Chen XJ, Driehuys B, Hedlund LW, Wheeler CT, Johnson GA (1999) Magnetic resonance angiography with hyperpolarized ^{129}Xe dissolved in a lipid emulsion. Magn Reson Med 41:1058–1064

Moller HE, Chen XJ, Saam B, Hagspiel KD, Johnson GA Altes TA, de Lange EE, Kauczor HU (2002) MRI of the lungs using hyperpolarized noble gases. Magn Res Med 47:1029–1051

Morgensteyerne A, Hansson G, Axelsson O, Ardenkjaer-Larsen JH, Johannesson H, Olofsson C (2000) patent no. WO0071166

Mugler JP 3rd, Driehuys B, Brookeman JR, Cates GD, Berr SS, Bryant RG, Daniel TM, de Lange EE, Downs 3rd JH, Erickson CJ, Happer W, Hinton DP, Kassel NF, Maier T, Phillips CD, Saam BT, Sauer KL, Wagshul ME (1997) MR imaging and spectroscopy using hyperpolarized 129Xe gas: preliminary human results. Magn Reson Med 37:809–815

Natterer J, Bargon J (1997) Parahydrogen induced polarization. Progr Nucl Magn Reson Spectrosc 31:293–315

Natterer J, Schedletzky O, Barkemeyer J Bargon J (1998) Investigating catalytic processes with parahydrogen: evolution of zero-quantum coherence in AA'X spin systems. J Magn Res 133:92–97

Oros AM, Shah NJ (2004) Hyperpolarized xenon in NMR and MRI, Phys Med Biol 49: R105–R153

Ortidge RJ, Helpern JA, Hugg JW, Matson GB (2000) Single voxel whole body phosphorus MRS. In Methods in biomedical magnetic resonance imaging and spectroscopy, vol 1. Wiley, Chichester, pp 729–735

Schroder L, Lowery TJ, Hilty C, Wemmer DE, Pines A (2006) molecular imaging using a targeted magnetic resonance hyperpolarized biosensor. Science 314:446–449

Spence MM, Rubin SM, Dimitrov IE, Ruiz EJ, Wemmer DE, Pines A, Yao SQ, Tian F, Schultz PG (2001) Functionalized xenon as a biosensor. Proc Natl Acad Sci USA 98:10654–10657

Stephan M, Kohlman O, Niessen HG, Eichhorn A, Bargon J (2002) ^{13}C PHIP NMR spectra and polarization transfer during the homogeneous hydrogenation of alkynes with parahydrogen. Magn Res Chem 40:157–160

Svensson J (2003) Contrast-enhanced magnetic resonance angiography: development and optimization of techniques for paramagnetic and hyperpolarized contrast media. Acta Radiol 44 Suppl 429:1–30

Svensson J, Mansson S, Petersson JS, Olsson LE (2002) Hyperpolarized 13 MR angiography using trueFISP. Proc Intl Soc Magn Res Med, 10th scientific meeting, Abstracts, p 2010

Svensson J, Mansson S, Johansson E, Petersson JS, Olsson LE (2003) Hyperpolarized ^{13}C MR angiography using trueFISP. Magn Reson Med 50:256–262

Swanson SD, Rosen MS, Agranoff BW, Coulter KP, Welsh RC, Chupp TE (1997) Brain MRI with laser-polarized 129xe. Magn Reson Med 38:695–698

Un S, Prisner T, Weber RT, Seaman MJ, Fishbein KW, McDermott AE, Singel DJ, Griffin RG (1992) Pulsed dynamic nuclear polarization at 5 T. Chem Phys Lett 189:54–59

Wagshul ME, Button TM, Li HF, Liang Z, Springer CS, Zhong K, Wishnia A (1996) In vivo MR imaging and spectroscopy using hyperpolarized 129Xe. Magn Reson Med 36:183–191

Wolber J, Rowland IJ, Leach MO, Bifone A (1999) Perfluorocarbon emulsions as intravenous delivery media for hyperpolarized xenon. Magn Reson Med 41:442–449

Wolber J, Cherubini A, Leach MO, Bifone A (2000) Hyperpolarized ^{129}Xe NMR as a probe for blood oxygenation. Magn Reson Med 43:491–496

Index

Printing: Krips bv, Meppel, The Netherlands
Binding: Stürtz, Würzburg, Germany